Physics
in Anaesthesia

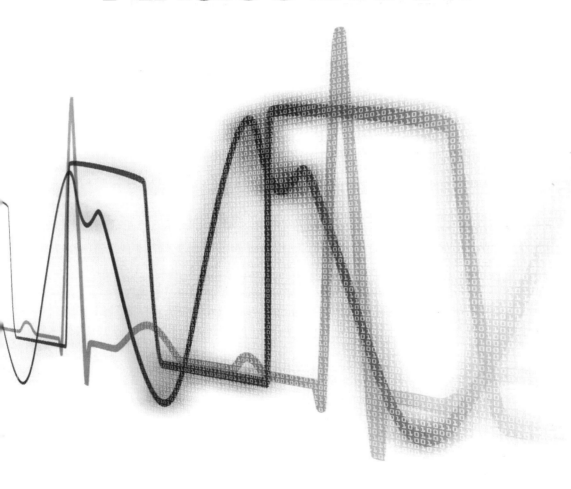

Ben Middleton

Justin Phillips

Rik Thomas

Simon Stacey

Scion

© Scion Publishing Ltd, 2012

ISBN 978 1 904842 98 9

First published in 2012

A CIP catalogue record for this book is available from the British Library.

Scion Publishing Limited

The Old Hayloft, Vantage Business Park, Bloxham Road, Banbury, Oxfordshire OX16 9UX, UK

www.scionpublishing.com

Important Note from the Publisher

The information contained within this book was obtained by Scion Publishing Limited from sources believed by us to be reliable. However, while every effort has been made to ensure its accuracy, no responsibility for loss or injury whatsoever occasioned to any person acting or refraining from action as a result of information contained herein can be accepted by the authors or publishers.

Although every effort has been made to ensure that all owners of copyright material have been acknowledged in this publication, we would be pleased to acknowledge in subsequent reprints or editions any omissions brought to our attention.

Readers should remember that medicine is a constantly evolving science and while the authors and publishers have ensured that all dosages, applications and practices are based on current indications, there may be specific practices which differ between communities. You should always follow the guidelines laid down by the manufacturers of specific products and the relevant authorities in the country in which you are practising.

Cover design by amdesign, Banbury, Oxfordshire, UK

Cover image supplied by Dr. Mark Salmon

Typeset by Manila Typesetting Company, The Philippines

Printed by the MPG Books Group, UK

Contents

Foreword

It has not been long since I sat the 'exam' and like many others, I bought a veritable library! Of all those books, only a handful became indispensable; these were the ones which were not only readable enough from which to learn a topic, but also compact enough to make good revision aids closer to the day.

This book is intended for a broad audience. It does not make the assumption that readers will have studied A-level physics and introduces each topic in a very clear and logical manner, carefully explaining the underlying principles. From this, the text develops to cover the syllabus, explaining how the physics relates to anaesthesia, using examples and analogies that make it easy to understand and reflect the effort the authors have made to produce a book that is easy to comprehend.

Each chapter concludes with a series of MCQs that highlight key points and make a useful revision aid. Even more useful, perhaps, is a brief summary section that is ideal as a rapid refresher, highlighting any problem areas.

Having struggled through the trials of the exam, I wish that this book had been available at the time. The work still has to be done, but having a simple, well-written text is a huge help and I am sure that this book will end up as one of those 'indispensable' volumes.

Dr Mike Cunningham, MBBS FRCA
Specialist Trainee
Barts and the London School of Anaesthesia

Preface

Idle theatre chat during a nocturnal aortic dissection led to a foolhardy commitment to write a book on physics in anaesthesia. We vowed to make it accessible and informative to the many who consider themselves 'non-physicists'. Nothing would be pulled out of thin air, we would start from first principles and then apply it to clinical reality as simply as possible.

The topics have been carefully selected to ensure that they are all relevant for those tackling the FRCA – if you go to www.scionpublishing.com/physicsinanaesthesia and click on "Resources" you will find:

- the latest FRCA syllabus indexed against sections in the book
- a copy of the contents list annotated to let you know which topics it is essential that you learn and which are only for those looking to excel.

This makes for a comprehensive text suitable not only for doctors but also for nurses, operating department practitioners and students. Short, snappy chapters include worked examples to help understanding of tricky areas along with clinical examples to highlight the relevance to anaesthetic practice. All the key terms are highlighted in bold at their first mention and definition. Self-assessment questions can be found at the end of each chapter (MCQs and SBAs in an FRCA style).

The result, we hope, is a book that brings an understanding of physics to those who have long since given up on it, with the minimum of pain and frustration.

Ben, Justin, Rik and Simon
London, December 2011

Acknowledgements

This book was forged with significant help from a number of people: Mike Cunningham transformed the electricity section, Sean Gallagher revascularised the cardiac related passages and Mark Lewis brought the imaging section into focus. Proof-reading by Henry Bishop and Sophie Ata vented much excess gas. Peter Green was generous in his feedback. We received welcome support from our colleagues including Philip Gamston and the perfusion team at Barts and the London. We are thankful to Jonathan Ray, our publisher, who has patiently helped us deliver the book we wanted.

Our families have had to endure the peaks and troughs during this project and we would like to dedicate this book to them: Elwira, Oliver & Jeremy; Deborah; Anandi; Ese, Luke, Harry & Hannah.

About the authors

Simon Stacey (MBBS FRCA) is a Consultant Cardiothoracic Anaesthetist based at the London Chest Hospital. He is co-author of *"Essentials of Anaesthetic Equipment"*, now in its fourth edition.

Rik Thomas (MBBS FRCA) is a Specialist Trainee at Barts and the London School of Anaesthesia. He presents a podcast for trainee anaesthetists at www.gascast.co.uk.

Justin Phillips (BSc PhD MIPEM) is a Senior Lecturer in Biomedical Engineering at City University London. He studied physics at Durham University.

Ben Middleton (BSc SOPGBI RN) is a Lead Perfusionist based at St Bartholomew's Hospital and a Visiting Lecturer at City University London. He studied physics at Bristol University.

Abbreviations

AC	alternating current	LMA	laryngeal mask airway
APL	adjustable pressure limiting	MAC	minimum alveolar concentration
BIS	bispectral analysis	MAP	mean arterial pressure
BMR	basal metabolic rate	MRI	magnetic resonance imaging
BP	blood pressure	NIBP	non-invasive blood pressure
CAT	computer-assisted tomography	NIRS	near-infrared spectroscopy
CO	cardiac output	NNT	number needed to treat
CPAP	continuous positive airway pressure	NPV	negative predictive value
CT	computed tomography	NTC	negative thermal conductivity
CVP	central venous pressure	PET	positron emission tomography
DC	direct current	PMGV	piped medical gas and vacuum
EBM	evidence-based medicine	PPV	positive predictive value
ECG	electrocardiogram	RF	radio frequency
EEG	electroencephalogram	RMS	root mean square
EMF	electromotive force	SMR	standardized mortality ratio
EMG	electromyogram	SPECT	single photon emission computed tomography
EPO	erythropoietin		
ETT	endotracheal tube	STP	standard temperature and pressure
HAFOE	high airflow oxygen enrichment	SVP	saturated vapour pressure
HMEF	heat and moisture exchange filter	TGC	time gain compensation
HSMR	hospital standardized mortality ratio	TOE	trans-oesophageal echocardiogram
		TTE	trans-thoracic echocardiogram
ICD	implantable cardioverter defibrillator	VF	ventricular fibrillation
IV	intravenous	VIC	vaporizer in-circle
LAN	local area network	VIE	vacuum-insulated evaporator
LCD	liquid crystal display	VOC	vaporizer out-of-circle
LED	light emitting diode	VT	ventricular tachycardia

Chapter 1
Atoms and matter

Having read this chapter you will be able to:
- Appreciate the planetary and Bohr models of the atom.
- Define an element's atomic number and atomic mass.
- Recall the key differences between solids, liquids and gases.
- Understand the role of energy in changing states.
- Recognize the value of phase diagrams for showing state, triple point and critical point.

1.1 The atom

The word 'atom' originates from the Greek *atomos* meaning indivisible. In 1912, however, a New Zealand physicist, Ernest Rutherford, caused a sensation by revealing the atom *is* divisible. He had shown that the mass of the atom is concentrated in a tiny positively charged nucleus, surrounded by a tenuous cloud of negatively charged electrons. The new science of atomic physics was born which, for better or worse, heralded the beginning of the atomic age.

> **Definitions**
>
> **Atomic mass:** the atomic mass is the total number of protons and neutrons in the nucleus of an atom.
> **Atomic number:** the atomic number is the number of protons in the nucleus of the atom.

Rutherford's model of the atom

Rutherford created what is now the classic model of the atom, that of an 'atomic planetary model' with the electrons (planets) orbiting the nucleus (the sun). Planets are drawn to the sun due to gravitational force, but the attraction for the atom is due to the particles' electrical charges; the positively charged nucleus attracts the negatively charged electrons.

The nucleus of the atom contains nucleons, and is where virtually all of the atom's mass is held. There are two types of nucleons: protons and neutrons, and both have approximately the same mass, which is about 1840 times the mass of an electron. Protons are positively charged while neutrons have no charge. The number of protons defines the **atomic number** and may be thought of as the 'fingerprint' of an element because it is fixed for a specific element, e.g. hydrogen has atomic number = 1 and carbon has atomic number = 6. The atomic number determines the element's place in the periodic table.

The total number of nucleons is almost exactly equal to the **atomic mass**. Atomic mass is expressed in units of **atomic mass units** (not in units of actual mass). There are small differences between the atomic mass and the nucleon number depending on the element in question.

Atoms of the same element can have different numbers of neutrons in their nucleus, and these are known as **isotopes** of the element. For example, helium (atomic number = 2) has two isotopes: helium-3, and helium-4. Helium-4 is by far the most common isotope and has two protons and two neutrons in its nucleus (see *Figure 1.1*), so has an atomic mass of approximately 4. Helium-3, which is highly sought after for fusion research, has only one neutron so has an atomic mass of approximately 3. On earth, there are less than two atoms of helium-3 for every 10 000 of helium-4.

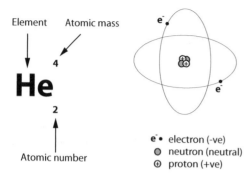

Element   Atomic mass

4

He

2

Atomic number

e•   electron (-ve)
O   neutron (neutral)
⊕   proton (+ve)

Figure 1.1. *The helium-4 atom and Rutherford's model of the atom.*

Some isotopes are stable while some are highly unstable and emit particles or radiation as they disintegrate. These isotopes are described as radioactive and are discussed in more detail in *Chapter 26.*

Units. Atomic mass number was originally standardized so that one atomic mass unit was equal to the mass of a proton (a hydrogen nucleus). This convention has now been changed so that an atomic mass unit is equal to 1/12th of the mass of a carbon-12 nucleus.

The Bohr model and energy levels

Just two years after publication of Rutherford's model of the atom, the Danish physicist Niels Bohr incorporated the idea of energy levels into a new atomic model. Bohr's model had strict rules for electrons: they could only exist in defined energy levels, so they could jump from one level to another but their energy levels were fixed. These energy levels are organized into 'shells' around the atom, an idea which forms a cornerstone of quantum physics and led to the development of the laser (see *Chapter 24*). Sometimes Bohr's model is called the Rutherford–Bohr model as Bohr essentially improved Rutherford's original model.

Chemical bonding

The attraction between atoms is known as a chemical bond, which allows the formation of chemical substances containing two or more atoms. Chemical bonds can be strong interatomic bonds such as **covalent bonds** or **ionic bonds**, or (usually) weaker intermolecular bonds such as **dipole–dipole interactions** or **hydrogen bonding** (see *Section 2.4*).

In covalent bonds, two atoms share one or more of their outer shell electrons. The negatively charged electrons occupy the space between the positively charged nuclei and are attracted to both nuclei simultaneously. The electrons can be thought to exist in a 'cloud' between the nuclei, because they are moving rapidly around an equilibrium position between the atoms. This attraction overcomes the repulsion which would otherwise exist between the two nuclei, so a strong bond is formed. Covalent bonds usually form between non-metallic atoms, for example, in organic compounds, as well as in diatomic gases and water molecules.

In an ionic bond, an outer electron is transferred from one atom to another. The electron is more tightly bound in the new atom so is able to exist at a lower energy level than in the donor atom. The result of the transfer is that the electron-accepting atom becomes a negatively charged ion (an **anion**), while the other becomes a positive ion (a **cation**), resulting in an electrostatic attraction between them. Ionic bonds usually occur between metallic atoms (forming cations) and nonmetals

Table 1.1. *The microscopic properties of substances in different states of matter.*

State	Spacing of molecules	Movement
Gas	• Far apart • Minimal intermolecular forces • No defined position	Random independent collisions
Liquid	• Near enough for weak intermolecular forces • Absence of structure	No independent movement Molecules able to slide past one another
Solid	• Closely packed • Large forces • Distinct patterns	Vibrate around an equilibrium position

(forming anions). The cation and anion bond to form a metal salt, a well known example being sodium chloride, (Na^+Cl^-).

1.2 States of matter

Solids, liquids and gases

The way atoms interact with one another determines the properties of matter. Interatomic and intermolecular bonds both determine the bulk properties of a compound, including whether it exists as a solid, a liquid or a gas at a given temperature. Solids have rigid bonds between their molecules; liquids have looser bonds; gases have minimal bonds. *Table 1.1* summarizes the microscopic properties of solids, liquids and gases. A fourth state of matter: plasma, discussed at the end of this section, can also exist in certain extreme conditions. *Figure 1.2* shows the different states of matter and how matter can change from one state to another.

Definitions

Latent heat: latent heat is the energy required to transform matter from one state to another.
Latent heat of fusion: the latent heat of fusion is the energy required to change one unit of mass from solid to liquid (e.g. when ice melts).
Latent heat of vaporization: the latent heat of vaporization is the energy required to change one unit of mass from liquid to gas (e.g. when water boils).

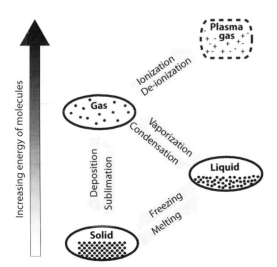

Figure 1.2. *The changes in states of matter, including plasma gas.*

Heat capacity

For an object to increase in temperature, energy in the form of heat must be added and this is covered in more detail in *Chapter 4*. The **specific heat capacity** (*c*) of a substance determines the energy needed to raise 1 kg of the substance by a temperature of 1°C:

$$Q = c \cdot m \cdot \Delta T$$

1.1

where Q is the energy required
         c is the specific heat capacity
         m is the mass
         ΔT is the temperature change

Water has a specific heat capacity of $4.18\,\mathrm{J\,g^{-1}\,°C^{-1}}$, in other words 4.18 joules are needed to raise 1 g of water by 1°C. Liquid water has a constant heat capacity, regardless of its temperature. The heat capacity of ice is different to that of liquid water, however, which is in turn different to the value for steam.

Latent heat

Suppose you are heating a substance in an oven, say a solid block of wax initially at room temperature. The temperature of the wax will rise steadily as the block absorbs thermal energy (*Figure 1.3*). When the melting point is reached (around 59°C for paraffin wax), the temperature stops rising even though the wax continues to absorb thermal energy. This energy is used to break the intermolecular bonds, causing the wax to liquefy. Once all the wax has melted, the temperature of the liquid wax will rise once more. If the oven is hot enough the wax will become a vapour and again the temperature will remain constant during the change of phase. For the same reason, water boiling in a kettle remains at 100°C until the water boils away, no matter how high the heat is turned up.

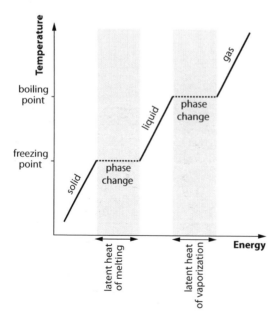

Figure 1.3. *Graph showing the energy needed to produce a change in state.*

Cooling a hypothermic patient is much more effective if melting ice is used, compared to the same mass of freezing water, even if both are at 0°C. With ice, heat is absorbed from the patient to melt the ice, even though the temperature of the ice does not rise until it has thawed.

For matter to change state, energy must either be added or removed and this energy is referred to as **latent heat**. When a solid becomes a liquid or when a liquid becomes a gas, energy must be added to break bonds; similarly when bonds are formed, energy is liberated. Latent heat is quantified by the energy required to change the state of one kilogram of matter. The **latent heat of vaporization** is the energy required to boil one kilogram of liquid. This is the same amount of energy liberated when a kilogram of gas condenses to a liquid (so is also referred to as the latent heat of condensation). Similarly, the **latent heat of fusion** is the amount of energy liberated when one kilogram of liquid freezes.

$$Q = m \cdot L$$

1.2

where Q is the energy required
m is the mass
L is the latent heat

Symbols and units. Latent heat usually has the symbol L along with a subscript: L_f for latent heat of fusion and L_v for latent heat of vaporization. Caution is needed because different terms are used such as latent heat of melting. Latent heat is measured in $J \cdot kg^{-1}$ or, more commonly, $kJ \cdot kg^{-1} = 1 \times 10^3 J \cdot kg^{-1}$. Specific heat capacity takes the symbol, c, and has the units of $J \cdot kg^{-1} \cdot °C^{-1}$.

The fourth state of matter: plasma

Plasma is a gas-like mixture of equal numbers of positive and negative ions making it electrically neutral. It is created at very high temperatures when molecules are ripped apart and electrons are stripped from their atoms; the resulting high-energy ions form plasma. Plasma is not encountered under normal conditions, though it should be noted that the sun is composed mainly of matter in the plasma phase. With the aid of electricity, plasma can be used to generate light such as in the fluorescent strip light or a plasma television; a plasma screen consists of thousands of pockets of gases each located between two tiny electrodes.

1.3 Phase diagrams

Temperature has an effect on whether an object is a solid, liquid or gas. Water turns from a liquid to a gas as it boils at 100°C and from liquid to solid as it freezes at 0°C. These temperatures only apply to substances at one particular pressure: atmospheric pressure at sea level. A pan of water on a camping stove near the summit of Mount Everest will boil at less than 80°C as a result of the lower atmospheric pressure at altitude. A pressure cooker maintains higher-than-atmospheric pressure within the cooker, typically allowing water to boil at around 125°C, significantly reducing cooking times.

Definition
Phase diagram: a phase diagram is a graph that displays the relationship between the solid, liquid, and gaseous states of a substance as a function of temperature, volume and pressure.

If the temperature and pressure are known, then a phase diagram can be used to predict what state a substance will be in. *Figure 1.4* shows the phase diagram for water, but all substances have a different phase diagram. The point where all three states, solid, liquid and gas, intersect is referred to as the **triple point**. For water, the triple point is at a temperature of 0.001°C and a pressure of only

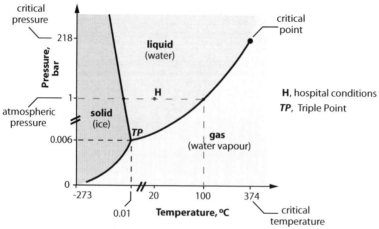

Figure 1.4. *Phase diagram for water (not to scale).*

0.006 atmospheres. For carbon dioxide, however, the triple point temperature is lower at –56.4°C while the pressure is five times higher than atmospheric pressure.

Above a certain temperature and pressure, known as the **critical point**, a substance can exist only as a gas, no matter how high the pressure. For water the critical point is 374°C at a pressure of 218 bar. *Table 1.2* shows some example elements and compounds with their critical temperatures and pressures.

For water the solid–liquid equilibrium line (the melting point line) slopes backwards rather than forwards. The solid phase, ice, is less dense than the liquid phase, which explains why ice floats in water. It has been postulated that life could not have evolved in the sea if water did not have this highly unusual property.

Is steam a gas?

When water boils it changes state from a liquid to a gas or vapour. 'White steam' consists of tiny droplets of condensed vapour, so is in fact a liquid! True steam is a vapour, invisible to the human eye and is present close to the spout of the kettle.

> **Definitions**
>
> **Triple point:** the triple point is a combination of pressure and temperature where all three states, solid, liquid and gas, can coexist.
> **Critical temperature:** the critical temperature of a gas is the temperature at or above which no amount of pressure, however great, will cause the gas to liquefy.
> **Critical pressure:** the critical pressure is the minimum pressure required to liquefy the gas at the critical temperature.

Table 1.2. *Critical temperatures and pressures.*

Substance		Critical pressure (bar)	Critical temperature (°C)
Water	H_2O	218	374
Nitrous oxide	N_2O	71.7	36.5
Carbon dioxide	CO_2	73	31.1
Oxygen	O_2	50	–119
Xenon	Xe	0.8	–112

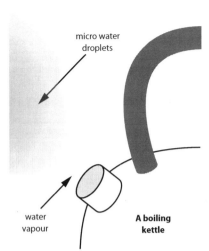

micro water
droplets

water
vapour

**A boiling
kettle**

Figure 1.5. *A boiling kettle showing white steam, a collection of micro water droplets and water vapour, an invisible gas.*

What is the difference between a gas and a vapour?

The language surrounding gases is confusing, as scientific terms have been mixed in with day-to-day bywords. A vapour is a type of gas, and is any substance in the gas phase at a temperature lower than its critical temperature. This means that the vapour can be condensed to a liquid or to a solid by increasing the pressure without reducing the temperature. Carbon dioxide, for example, has a critical temperature of 31.03°C, so may be described as a vapour below this temperature.

Summary

- Elements are characterized by their atomic number which is equal to the number of protons in the nucleus.
- Isotopes of an element have the same atomic number but different atomic mass. The atomic mass is approximately equal to the number of nucleons.
- The Rutherford–Bohr model describes the atom as a positively charged nucleus surrounded by a cloud of negative electrons in different energy states or 'shells'.
- When a substance changes state, latent heat is transferred to or from the substance.
- Energy is required to break bonds, while energy is liberated when bonds are made.
- The heat capacity describes how much the temperature of a substance increases if it absorbs a known amount of energy.
- The phase diagram allows us to predict the state of matter of a substance at a given pressure and temperature.
- The triple point is the temperature and pressure where solid, liquid and gas states of a substance can coexist.

Single best answer questions

For each of these questions, only one option is correct.

1. What do carbon-14 and nitrogen-14 have in common?
   (a) they have exactly the same atomic mass
   (b) they have exactly the same atomic number
   (c) they have approximately the same atomic number
   (d) they have approximately the same atomic mass
   (e) they are isotopes of carbon-14

2. A molecular liquid differs from a molecular gas because
   (a) it has a higher density
   (b) it has stronger intermolecular forces
   (c) it has stronger interatomic forces
   (d) it has a lower temperature
   (e) its molecules have less thermal motion

3. Regarding plasma, which one of the following is true?
   (a) A plasma can exist in a liquid or gaseous state.
   (b) Plasma forms at very low pressures.
   (c) Plasma forms at very high temperatures.
   (d) An electric field is needed to form a plasma.
   (e) Plasma is highly stable.

4. 20.9 kJ of energy would raise the temperature of 1 kilogram of water at atmospheric pressure by:
   (a) 0.2°C
   (b) 0.5°C
   (c) 2°C
   (d) 5°C
   (e) 20°C

5. Which one of the following statements is true?
   (a) The freezing point temperature is lower than the melting point temperature.
   (b) The latent heat of vaporization is the same as the latent heat of fusion.
   (c) The boiling temperature is the same as the condensation temperature.
   (d) The triple point pressure of water is below 1 atmosphere.
   (e) The heat capacity of water is the same as that of steam.

Multiple choice questions

For each of these questions, more than one option may be correct.

1. The latent heat of fusion:
   (a) is the amount of heat required to raise the temperature of water by 1°C
   (b) is the amount of heat required to boil 1 kg of water
   (c) is the amount of heat liberated when 1 kg of water freezes
   (d) is the amount of heat liberated when 1 kg of steam condenses
   (e) is the amount of heat required to melt 1 kg of ice

2. Which of the following are vapours?
   (a) Fog at 12°C.
   (b) Nitrogen at 375°C.
   (c) Nitrous oxide at 25°C.
   (d) Isoflurane at 50°C.
   (e) 'Invisible steam' at the spout of a kettle at 100°C.

3. Which of the following are true of water?
   (a) It is a vapour at 100°C on Mount Everest.
   (b) Increasing the pressure of liquid water can cause it to freeze.
   (c) Increasing the pressure of steam can cause it to condense.
   (d) Has a triple point temperature greater than 0°C.
   (e) Can exist only as a gas or a solid in a vacuum.

4. Which of the following processes liberate energy?
   (a) Ionization.
   (b) Condensation.
   (c) Freezing.
   (d) Melting.
   (e) Deposition.

5. Which of the following are true for any substance?
   (a) The gaseous state cannot exist at temperatures below the triple point.
   (b) The liquid state cannot exist at pressures below the triple point.
   (c) The liquid state cannot exist at pressures above the critical pressure.
   (d) At 1 atmosphere of pressure, all gases become liquids if cooled sufficiently.
   (e) All liquids expand when they solidify.

Chapter 2
Simple mechanics

Having read this chapter you will be able to:
- Distinguish between force, velocity, speed and acceleration.
- Be familiar with Newton's laws of motion.
- Understand the vector nature of velocity.
- Distinguish between Newtonian and non-Newtonian viscosity.
- List the properties that affect the viscosity of blood.
- Define surface tension and wall tension.
- Apply Laplace's law to alveoli.
- Explain the role played by surfactant.
- Appreciate the critical point in vessel collapse.

2.1 Force, velocity and acceleration

The English philosopher and mathematician Isaac Newton is famous for observing an apple falling to the ground and concluding that all objects with mass are attracted to all others, explaining, among other things, how the moon orbits the earth. This work is embodied in the more general three Laws of Motion, which describe the relationship between velocity, force and acceleration.

> **Definition**
>
> **Force:** a force is an influence capable of producing a change in the velocity of a mass.

Newton's first law: constant velocity

Newton's first law outlines that any change in motion is the result of the application of a force. A ball bearing rolling across a glass surface has almost no friction acting on it so it rolls with almost constant velocity. The Voyager 1 spacecraft left the outer solar system at a speed of 63 000 km·h^{-1} and will continue to move at this speed forever unless it comes close to a star or other object.

> **Definitions**
>
> **Velocity:** the velocity of an object refers to the speed and direction in which it moves.
> **Newton's first law:** objects move in a straight line at constant speed, or remain stationary, unless a force acts upon the object.

Physics makes a distinction between speed and velocity though they both refer to the rate of travel. **Speed** is scalar and does not have a direction linked to it whereas velocity is a vector and does include direction. **Velocity** can be thought of as speed with direction. So if a car drives around a roundabout at a constant 20 km·h^{-1} then, despite this constant speed, the velocity has changed because the direction of travel has altered. Newton's laws apply to liquids and gases flowing through a tube; every time a change in direction is required, such as at the junction in a T-piece, forces are needed to produce this change. Fluid flow is examined in more detail in *Chapter 8*.

Newton's second law: force and acceleration

Definitions
Acceleration: this is the rate of change of velocity with respect to time. **Newton's second law:** a force acting on a body produces an acceleration proportional to the force.

Newton's second law states that acceleration of a body is proportional to the force applied, and inversely proportional to the mass of the object. Massive objects require more force to generate the same acceleration than small objects. This is why you have to push a loaded shopping trolley much harder than an empty one.

Acceleration is a change in velocity, either speed or direction (or both speed and direction). A tennis ball attached to a string and whirled around your head is accelerating, because the force in the string acts inwards on the ball, causing a change in velocity, despite its speed remaining constant. The earth orbits the sun in exactly the same way, except that gravity replaces the string. Similarly, every twist and turn in the breathing circuit causes the flow of air to change direction, so acceleration of the gas takes place.

$$F = m \cdot a$$

2.1 **Learn**

where F is the force applied (N)
m is the mass of the object (kg)
a is the acceleration of the object (m·s^{-2})

Newton's third law: action and reaction

Definition
Newton's third law: every action of a force produces an equal and opposite reaction.

Newton's third law can be thought of as the 'bookkeeper's law': that is, the forces must add up. If an apple is hanging on a tree, the force of gravity acting downwards on the apple is balanced by an equal upwards force, which is the tension in the apple's stalk, holding it to the tree. If the force in the opposite direction is greater than gravity the apple moves upwards, but if it is less than the force of gravity the apple will move downwards. Another example of Newton's third law is the kick (or 'recoil') felt by someone firing a shotgun. The force to the shot propelled in one direction is equalled in the opposite direction by the recoil of the shotgun.

Units. The symbol for force is usually F and the unit for force is the newton (N). The newton is defined as the force that provides a mass of one kilogram with an acceleration of 1 m·s^{-2}. In SI base units a newton can be written as kg·m·s^{-2}. The units are summarized in *Table 2.1*.

Table 2.1. *Units of force, mass, velocity and acceleration.*

	Symbol	Unit		SI base units
Force	F	Newton	N	kg·m·s^{-2}
Mass	m	Kilogram	kg	kg
Velocity	v	Metres per second	m·s^{-1}	m·s^{-1}
Acceleration	a	Metres per second-squared	m·s^{-2}	m·s^{-2}

2.2 Force, weight and pressure

Weight

The weight of a body is a measurement of the gravitational force exerted upon it, and so is measured in newtons (N), although in everyday life we incorrectly quote weights in units of mass (kg or pounds). A person who 'weighs' 70 kg has in actual fact a mass of 70 kg. The actual weight of the person is dependent on the size of the planet and the distance you are from the planet. The earth has a **gravitational acceleration** (g) of 9.81 m·s⁻² whereas the moon's is only 1.62 m·s⁻². Weight (w) is given by:

$$w = m \cdot g$$

2.2

where w is the weight (N)
m is the mass of the object (kg)
g is the acceleration due to gravity (m·s⁻²)

If your mass was 70 kg, your weight on the earth would be almost 700 N, but on the moon it would be just 177 N, although your mass would still be 70 kg. In deep space you would be weightless although, since you have mass, a force would be required to accelerate you.

Pressure and force

When a drawing pin is pushed into a board, there must be a force exerted on the back of the pin with the thumb. According to Newton's third law, the same force is applied to the board surface by the sharp end of the pin. The pin deforms the board surface because it exerts a very high pressure on the board, due to

> **Definition**
>
> **Pressure:** this is the force applied to an object per unit surface area.

the pin having a small cross-sectional area. This also illustrates why it is much harder to cut a slice of bread with a blunt knife than with one that is sharp; to exert the same effect (pressure), more force is required because the blunt knife has a relatively large surface area. The pressure exerted by a force is calculated using the following equation:

$$P = \frac{F}{A}$$

2.3 **Learn**

where P is the pressure (pascal or N·m⁻²)
F is the force (N)
A is the area (m²)

Hooke's law

When a spring or a piece of elastic is extended, it will exert a force and will try to regain its initial equilibrium length. The force exerted by the spring is directly proportional to the extension (see *Figure 2.1*). This is Hooke's law:

$$F = -k \cdot x$$

2.4

> **Definition**
>
> **Hooke's law** (applied to a spring): there is a linear relationship between the force applied and the extension of a spring, within the elastic limits for that spring.

where F is the force applied
x is the extension
k is the **spring constant**

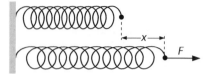

Figure 2.1. *A force F causes a displacement of the end of the spring from its equilibrium position. The displacement x is directly proportional to the force.*

The **spring constant** is the degree of stiffness or 'springiness'. The higher the spring constant, the more difficult the spring is to extend. The amount of displacement from the equilibrium position can be positive (extension) or negative (compression). The minus sign before the spring constant indicates that the spring exerts a force in the opposite direction to the displacement. Spring-loaded diaphragm pressure valves utilize Hooke's law, as outlined in *Section 6.4*.

2.3 Viscosity

Definitions
Viscosity: a measure of a fluid's resistance to flow. **Newtonian fluid:** a Newtonian fluid has a constant viscosity regardless of flow rate. **Non-Newtonian fluid:** a non-Newtonian fluid has a viscosity that changes with flow rate.

Newtonian and non-Newtonian fluids

Milk pours from a jug with ease, but pouring maple syrup from a jug is tiresome. The property of the two liquids that differs is viscosity, with the maple syrup being far more viscous than milk. A moving fluid can be considered as a series of layers with one layer moving over another and the viscosity is a result of the fluid's internal friction between these layers; in engineering terms it is a result of shear stress. Gases also have viscosity.

A fluid such as water, a collection of the small and uniform H_2O molecules, has a viscosity that is constant no matter how fast it is flowing and so it is described as a Newtonian fluid. Although blood has a high water content it differs from pure water because approximately two-fifths of its volume is made up of red blood cells. The red cells thicken the blood because they have a tendency to aggregate (clump together) as they try to move over one another, as shown in *Figure 2.2*. These cells change shape the faster they travel, becoming more elongated, and they also tend to fall into a line. This results in a lower resistance between layers of fluid travelling quickly and as a result there is a drop in viscosity as the rate of flow increases. This change in viscosity at differing flow rates makes blood a non-Newtonian fluid. It should be noted that not all non-Newtonian fluids become less viscous with increased flow rate; some become more viscous.

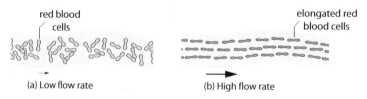

(a) Low flow rate   (b) High flow rate

Figure 2.2. *(a) Red blood cells aggregate at low flow rates. (b) At high flow rates, blood cells elongate and fall into line, leading to lower viscosity.*

Factors affecting viscosity

Pouring maple syrup from a jug when it is cold takes longer than at room temperature: when the temperature drops the syrup becomes even more viscous. Although not so obvious, water and blood both become more viscous at lower temperatures. Haematocrit is a reflection of cellular content in blood, and a rise in the proportion of cells in the blood changes the flow dynamics of blood; the higher the haematocrit, the greater the viscosity of blood and therefore impedance to flow. This makes the blood more likely to clot due to venous stasis, which is why athletes who abuse erythropoietin (EPO) are at increased risk of thromboembolic events.

Units. The SI unit of viscosity is the pascal second (Pa·s), also known as the poiseuille; however, the poise (dyne·sec·cm^{-2}) is more commonly used. One poise is equal to 0.1 Pa·s.

Clinical examples

Frostbite
In extreme cold the extremities of the body dramatically cool down, as does the temperature of the blood in these zones, and this leads to an increase in viscosity which hampers circulation. Victims of frostbite are usually dehydrated, adding to the viscous nature of their blood. As a result, the blood becomes sludge-like and circulation in the affected parts is compromised.

Polycythaemia
An increase in haematocrit (the proportion of red blood cells in blood) raises viscosity, though moderate variations in haematocrit are well tolerated. However, polycythaemia results in a significant increase in haematocrit, which in turn leads to increased viscosity of blood, and the result may be potential blockages in the arterioles and capillaries.

2.4 Surface tension and wall tension

In the absence of gravity, a drop of water will always tend to form a sphere (see *Figure 2.3b*). The reason for this lies in the attraction between water molecules. Molecules close to the surface have fewer attracting partners than those deep within the droplet, so form stronger bonds with the available molecules. The attractive forces pull the molecules as close together as possible and the droplet forms the shape that has the lowest possible surface area for a given volume, i.e. a sphere. The downward force of gravity stretches a suspended droplet vertically, making for a more ellipsoidal shape. The effect known as **surface tension** explains many observations, including the apparent ability of certain small objects to 'float', despite them being denser than water. Pond skaters and other aquatic insects exploit this property of water.

Definitions

Surface tension: this is a result of the attraction between molecules across the surface of a liquid (see *Figure 2.3a*).
Wall tension: this is similar to surface tension, but refers to a vessel wall that is an elasticated solid, as opposed to a liquid.
Laplace's law: the larger the radius of a vessel, the greater the wall tension required to withstand a given internal fluid pressure.

Intermolecular forces arise from irregularities in charge within each molecule, forming what are known as **dipoles**. In water molecules, the oxygen atom attracts the electrons more strongly than the two hydrogen atoms, forming a negative dipole and two positive dipoles. The hydrogen atoms can be visualized by imagining a partially 'bare' hydrogen nucleus (in actual fact a proton) because the single electron that normally accompanies each atom has migrated towards the oxygen. The hydrogen atoms thus develop a positive dipole, which is attracted to the negative dipole on an oxygen atom within an adjacent molecule. These **hydrogen bonds** are strong electrostatic intermolecular bonds, but are much weaker than the covalent bonds within the molecules.

The surface tension of a water drop is a product of these hydrogen bonds and acts parallel to the surface. The surface tension of water provides the necessary wall tension for the formation of

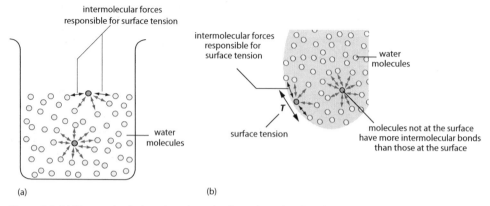

Figure 2.3. *(a) Water molecules in a glass: the molecules at the surface form fewer intermolecular bonds than those not at the surface. (b) Cross-section of a falling rain drop showing intermolecular forces.*

gas bubbles within liquids. As with droplets, this wall tension causes bubbles to form spherical shapes. The pressure difference between the inside and outside of a bubble depends upon the surface tension and the radius of the bubble and was first described by the French mathematician Pierre-Simon Laplace. The surface tension compresses the gas slightly, so that the pressure inside the bubble is always larger than the liquid pressure. **Laplace's equation for a spherical bubble** is:

$$\Delta P = \frac{2 \cdot T_{sph}}{R}$$

2.5 **Learn**

where   *T* is the surface tension
   R is the bubble radius
   ΔP is the pressure difference between the inside and the outside of the bubble

Laplace's equation has been adapted for different shapes. **Laplace's equation for a cylinder** can be applied to the pressure within a blood vessel. The tension is the combination of the surface tension and the elastic wall tension.

$$\Delta P = \frac{T_{cyl}}{R}$$

2.6 **Learn**

where   *T* is the total of the surface tension and the elastic wall tension
   R is the vessel radius
   ΔP is the pressure difference between the inside and the outside of the vessel

Units. Wall and surface tension, *T*, are measured as the force per unit length. The SI unit for surface tension is N·m⁻¹.

Clinical examples

Critical closing pressure
The blood pressure at which a blood vessel suffers complete collapse and a halting of all blood flow is known as the critical closing pressure. For this to happen, the pressure outside a blood vessel must exceed the intravascular pressure. Surface tension plays a decisive role in this, but other factors including blood viscosity and vascular smooth muscle tone also play a part. A low surface tension reduces the critical closing pressure.

Dilated cardiomyopathy
An abnormally enlarged heart struggles to pump blood. The distended radius (*r*) of the left ventricle has increased but the same pressure (*P*) during ejection is needed. From Laplace's equation for a sphere (Equation 2.5) the wall tension T must be greater than for a heart of normal (smaller) dimensions. As a consequence, the dilated heart strains to generate the necessary tension in the ventricular walls. One option for treatment is the surgical remodelling of the ventricle to reduce the effective radius.

Aortic aneurysm
If a weak spot in an arterial wall gives way and starts to bulge then the effective radius of that artery starts to increase. If the blood pressure remains constant and the radius has increased then Laplace's Law dictates that the wall tension of the artery rises. This becomes a vicious circle as the artery becomes further strained, dilating more and more. The only way of decreasing wall tension is for the cylindrical shaped bulge to move towards a sphere-like form. The wall tension of a sphere is half that of a cylinder with the same radius (as is shown by Equations 2.5 and 2.6). This explains why aneurysms often form a spherical bulge, as shown in *Figure 2.4*.

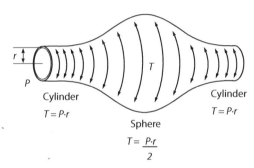

Cylinder
$T = P \cdot r$

Cylinder
$T = P \cdot r$

Sphere
$T = \dfrac{P \cdot r}{2}$

Figure 2.4. *An aneurysm's spherical shape requires less wall tension than a cylinder of equal radius for a given pressure.*

2.5 Surfactant and surface tension

The alveoli in the lungs are lined with fluid which, comprising mainly water, has a significant surface tension. This surface tension, like that in a bubble, tends to collapse the lung. Laplace's law shows us that this effect is greater when the alveoli are small; a balloon is more difficult to blow up when it is empty compared to when it is half full. As a consequence, a large effort would be needed to overcome the initial inflation phase. In health, **surfactant** is excreted by the alveolar cells and mixes with the alveolar fluid, significantly reducing surface tension. The compliance of the lung is greatly increased, despite the fact

Definitions

Surfactant: surfactants are compounds that lower the surface tension of a liquid.
Pulmonary surfactant: this reduces surface tension in the fluid lining the alveoli, reducing pulmonary compliance and thus reducing the work of breathing.

that the surface tension (even with surfactant present) exceeds the elastic forces produced by the connective tissue of the lung. The effect of surfactant is illustrated in *Table 2.2* which shows the comparative pressures required to inflate different sized alveoli with and without surfactant.

The bubble analogy is helpful, because we can apply Laplace's law for a sphere (Equation 2.5) to the alveoli. The equation states that a high pressure is needed to oppose a given surface tension if the radius is small. Because alveoli are very small and very numerous, it is easy to see how their combined surface tension can potentially cause a formidable restriction to breathing. This is illustrated in cases of infant respiratory distress syndrome, where premature neonates with underdeveloped lungs lack surfactant so cannot overcome the surface tension forces in the lung.

Table 2.2. *Effect of surfactant on surface tension of large and small alveoli.*

| Alveoli radius | Pressure required to inflate alveoli sac (approximate) | |
	Without surfactant	With surfactant
0.005 mm	15 mmHg	1 mmHg
0.01 mm	7.5 mmHg	1 mmHg

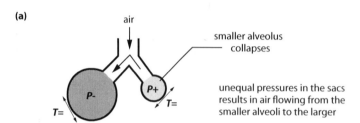

(a)

Surfactant absent from alveoli: surface tensions (T) are equal but pressures (P) are unequal.

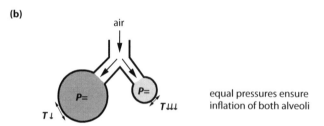

(b)

Surfactant present: surface tensions (T) unequal but pressures (P) equal.

Figure 2.5. *A pair of connected alveoli. (a) When surfactant is not present the surface tensions are equal, while the pressures are unequal. (b) When surfactant is present, surface tensions are unequal, but pressures are equal.*

Surfactant allows alveoli of differing sizes to exist and function. As shown by Laplace's law, the smaller the radius of the alveoli, the higher the pressure needed to inflate the sac. The air in smaller alveoli would simply flow into neighbouring larger alveoli, as there would be a pressure gradient between them (see *Figure 2.5*). This is avoided by surfactant being excreted in greater proportions in the smaller sacs, balancing out the pressure needed for inflation.

Worked example

Question
The surface tension of an alveolar sac of radius 0.10 mm is 0.02 N·m⁻¹ and its neighbour has radius 0.05 mm with an unknown surface tension. What would its surface tension have to be for the pressures in both alveoli to be equal?

Key points
- Alveoli can be treated as sphere-like shapes.
- To help the with the algebra the two alveoli will be called large (lg) and small (sm).
- The radii are in millimetres and for clarity are converted to metres.

Step 1
- Expressing the pressure for each alveolus in terms of surface tension and radius, using Laplace's equation for a sphere (Equation 2.5):

$$\text{pressure for large alveolus} = \frac{2 \cdot T_{lg}}{r_{lg}}$$

$$\text{pressure for small alveolus} = \frac{2 \cdot T_{sm}}{r_{sm}}$$

Step 2
- The pressure in both alveoli are the same, so combining the equations in Step 1:

$$\frac{2 \cdot T_{sm}}{r_{sm}} = \frac{2 \cdot T_{lg}}{r_{lg}}$$

isolating T_{sm} the equation becomes

$$T_{sm} = \frac{T_{lg} \cdot r_{sm}}{r_{lg}}$$

Step 3
- Substituting the numbers into the equation from Step 2:

$$r_{sm} = 0.05\,\text{mm} = 5 \times 10^{-5}\,\text{m}$$

$$r_{lg} = 0.10 = 1 \times 10^{-4}\,\text{m}$$

$$T_{lg} = 0.02\,\text{N·m}^{-1}$$

$$T_{sm} = \frac{T_{lg} \cdot r_{sm}}{r_{lg}} = \frac{0.02 \times 5 \times 10^{-5}}{1 \times 10^{-4}}\,\text{N·m}^{-1}$$

$$T_{sm} = 0.01\,\text{N·m}^{-1}$$

Answer
The surface tension would have to be 0.01 N·m^{-2}, half that of the larger neighbouring alveoli, for the pressure to be equal. This is achieved by the increased presence of surfactant in the smaller alveolus.

Menisci

The free surface of a liquid is called the meniscus and this can assume a flat, convex or concave shape; the shape is dependent on the liquid and its attraction to the material of the container holding it. With a concave shape, such as water held in a glass container, the water molecules have a high attraction (or **affinity**) to the glass relative to the affinity the water molecules have to each other,

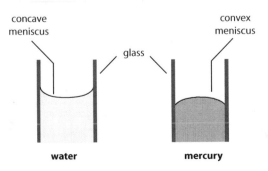

concave
meniscus

convex
meniscus

glass

water

mercury

Figure 2.6. *The shape of the meniscus is determined by the relative attractions between liquid molecules and the container surface and between the liquid molecules themselves.*

such that the water appears to hug the glass (as shown in *Figure 2.6*). Conversely, the meniscus for mercury in a glass exhibits a convex shape – a result of a high affinity between the atoms in the liquid, and a comparatively low affinity between mercury atoms and the glass.

Summary

- Newton's laws of motion explain the relationship between force, acceleration and velocity.
- The acceleration of an object is equal to the force acting on the object divided by its mass.
- An object following a curved path is accelerating, even if its speed is constant, because it is changing direction.
- Weight is expressed in newtons, while mass is expressed in kilograms.
- Pressure is the force acting per unit of area.
- A Newtonian fluid is one whose viscosity does not change with flow rate. Blood is an example of a non-Newtonian fluid.
- Surface tension arises from the strong intermolecular forces between molecules (of water and also other liquids). The molecules at the surface do not have other molecules on all sides of them, so are pulled inwards. Surface tension explains why water droplets and bubbles tend to form spherical shapes.
- Surfactant is a compound which reduces surface tension.
- Laplace's law describes surface and wall tension in a sphere or a cylinder.
- Pulmonary surfactant increases lung compliance, reducing the work of breathing.

Single best answer questions

For each of these questions, only one option is correct.

1. Weight depends on:
    (a) velocity and mass
    (b) acceleration and mass
    (c) acceleration due to gravity and velocity
    (d) mass and acceleration due to gravity
    (e) mass and momentum

2. A person whose mass is 100 kg weighs how much on the earth?
    (a) 98.1 N
    (b) 981 N
    (c) 9810 N
    (d) 9.81 N
    (e) 100 N

3. Acceleration can be defined as:
    (a) force per unit velocity
    (b) mass per unit time
    (c) rate of change of velocity
    (d) rate of change of force
    (e) velocity in a scalar format

4. Newton's second law states that force is the:
    (a) product of mass and velocity
    (b) mass divided by acceleration
    (c) product of mass and acceleration
    (d) product of mass and acceleration
    (e) product of velocity and weight

5. The pressure exerted onto the ice by the blade of an ice skater standing on one leg depends on:
    (a) their mass, the acceleration due to gravity and their velocity
    (b) their mass, the surface area of the blade and the acceleration due to gravity
    (c) the surface area of the blade, their mass and their velocity
    (d) the acceleration due to gravity and their velocity
    (e) their mass and the surface area of the blade

6. The units of surface tension are:
   (a) $N \cdot m^{-1}$
   (b) N
   (c) $N \cdot m$
   (d) $J \cdot m^{-1}$
   (e) $J \cdot m$

7. Surfactant works so as to:
   (a) prevent gas moving from larger alveoli into smaller alveoli due to differences in surface tension
   (b) decrease surface tension in pulmonary capillaries
   (c) prevent gas moving from smaller alveoli into larger alveoli due to differences in surface tension
   (d) increase surface tension in larger alveoli
   (e) increase surface tension in smaller alveoli

8. Which is true of a water meniscus in a glass vessel?
   (a) It curves upwards because the water molecules attract the glass molecules more than each other.
   (b) It curves upwards because the water molecules repel the glass.
   (c) It curves downwards because the water molecules attract the glass molecules more than each other.
   (d) It curves downwards because the water molecules repel the glass.
   (e) It curves downwards because the water molecules attract each other more than the glass molecules.

Multiple choice questions

For each of these questions, more than one option may be correct.

1. Which of the following are true?
   (a) The moon orbits the earth with constant velocity.
   (b) The earth exerts constant gravitational force on the moon.
   (c) The moon orbits the earth with variable speed.
   (d) The moon orbits the earth with constant speed.
   (e) The moon exerts a gravitational pull on the earth.

2. The viscosity of blood increases with:
   (a) an increase in temperature
   (b) an increase in haematocrit
   (c) an increase in blood flow rate
   (d) a decrease in temperature
   (e) a decrease in haematocrit

3. For a fluid that travels around a bend in a circuit at a constant flow rate, which of the flowing is false?
   (a) The fluid has exhibited constant velocity.
   (b) The fluid has accelerated.
   (c) A force was needed to change the direction of travel.
   (d) The speed could have been constant.
   (e) Newton's Second Law is not applicable.

4. Regarding an aortic aneurysm, which are true?
   (a) Wall tension decreases as the aneurysm gets larger.
   (b) Wall tension of a spherical aneurysm is greater than for a cylindrical vessel of the same radius.
   (c) Wall tension of a spherical aneurysm is smaller than for a cylindrical vessel of the same radius.
   (d) Wall tension is inversely proportional to radius in a spherical aneurysm.
   (e) Wall tension is proportional to pressure in a cylindrical vessel.

5. Connected alveoli of differing radius in the lung:
   (a) have the same pressure when surfactant is present
   (b) have the same tension when surfactant is present
   (c) have the same tension when surfactant is not present
   (d) have different pressure and different tension when surfactant is not present
   (e) have different pressure and the same tension when surfactant is not present

6. The menisci formed by water and mercury curve upwards and downwards, respectively, because:
   (a) mercury has a higher density than water
   (b) mercury has weaker intermolecular forces than water
   (c) mercury has stronger intermolecular forces than water
   (d) mercury has a higher viscosity than water
   (e) water has a higher affinity for glass than between its own atoms

Chapter 3
Energy and power

Having read this chapter you will be able to:
- Distinguish between work done and energy.
- Understand the concept of energy efficiency.
- Appreciate the significance of the pressure–volume loop and the phenomenon of hysteresis.
- Recognize the work done by the heart.
- Analyse the work done by the lungs without assistance and during ventilation.

3.1 Work and energy

Definitions

Work done: the work done by a force acting on an object is a product of the force applied and the distance the object has moved.
Energy: the capacity for doing work.

What constitutes work? A simple example is pushing a box along the floor: this involves work and the work done is by the person who is pushing the box. Though work is a widely used day-to-day term, for physicists work is a carefully defined term: it refers to the amount of energy applied by (or applied to) a system and is given the title *work done*.

Continuing the example from before, work done is the product of the distance the box has moved and the force needed to push it. This force will be enough to overcome the friction between box and floor: so the force to push the box over a highly polished floor is less than the force needed to push the box over a thick carpet that offers considerable resistance. More work was done pushing on the carpet and this is the same as saying more energy was needed to complete the task.

What does not constitute work? Lifting a shopping bag up from the floor is considered work because a force has been applied over a distance: this is the force applied by the person to overcome gravity and the distance being the height the bag has been lifted. However, standing still whilst holding a heavy shopping bag does not constitute physical work, even if it feels like hard work, because the shopping bag is not being moved. The equation for work done is:

$$\text{work done} = F \cdot d$$

3.1 Learn

where F is force
         d is distance the force has acted over

While work is restricted to acts (or processes) where energy has been utilized, the term **energy** is more general. Energy can be thought of as the capacity to do work. Work done by a system can have a positive or a negative value, depending on whether energy is transferred *from* or *to* the system, respectively. When work is done, energy is usually converted from one form into another. *Table 3.1* summarizes some of the different forms of energy encountered in everyday life.

Table 3.1. *Different forms of energy.*

Energy form	Description
Kinetic energy	Energy possessed by an object by virtue of its motion
Potential energy	A general term for stored energy; usually refers to energy stored by an object with mass in a gravitational field
Electrical energy	Energy related to the storage of electric charge
Thermal energy	Energy of vibrating molecules; differences in temperature cause heat to flow from one place to another
Radiant energy	Energy transferred by emission or absorption of light or other electromagnetic radiation
Sound energy	Energy transferred by mechanical vibration of air molecules in a wave-like manner
Chemical energy	The potential energy stored in chemical bonds
Elastic energy	The potential energy stored in a deformed (or stretched) elastic material

Conservation of energy

A solar-powered radio gains energy by light waves hitting the solar panels, that is then converted into electrical energy by a solar cell. This electrical energy is then used to power a radio to produce sound to listen to and it also produces some heat from the electrical components. The energy balance sheet for the energy coming in (from the rays of the sun) minus the energy going out (heat, sound and others) must tally up to zero. This principle is known as the **conservation of energy**.

> **Definition**
>
> **Conservation of energy:** energy can neither be created nor destroyed, only changed from one form to another.

The principle that energy cannot be created nor can it be destroyed is fundamental to physics. Energy is only converted from one form to another, different form and this means that energy gained by one system must equal the amount lost by another.

3.2 Efficiency and power

Energy efficiency

When the solar-powered radio uses the energy gained from the sun's rays, some of that energy is loosely described as 'lost'. Of course, the principle of conservation of energy dictates that the energy is not really lost, but is converted into another form; in this case the radio generates heat as a by-product. Similarly, when chemical energy in the form of petrol is converted by a car engine into kinetic energy, the engine gets hot. Tungsten filament light bulbs convert only around 2% of the electrical energy supplied to them into visible light, with the remaining 98% being radiated as heat. No physical process is 100% efficient; an unshakeable consequence of the laws of thermodynamics:

$$\text{Efficiency} = \frac{\text{Energy output}}{\text{Energy input}} \times 100\% \qquad \textbf{3.2}$$

Units. Energy efficiency is quoted as a percentage (or a ratio) and therefore has no units.

Power

What is the power being delivered by the person pushing the box along the carpet? Power is simply the rate at which work is done (or energy is transferred):

> **Definition**
>
> **Power:** the rate at which work is done or the rate of transfer of energy.

$$\text{power} = \frac{\text{work done}}{\text{time taken}}$$

So for the person pushing the box it would be the work done in pushing the box divided by the time taken to push it.

Units.

- The unit of energy is the joule (J) and one joule is the amount of energy required to exert a force of one newton through a distance of one metre.
- The unit for power is the watt, which is equivalent to $1\ \text{J}\cdot\text{s}^{-1}$.

The non-SI unit, the **calorie** is another unit for energy and is equal to approximately 4.2 J (there are five different values for a calorie!).

3.3 Work of respiration

Work done by a ventilator during inspiration

The key condition for a fluid or gas to flow is that there must be a difference in pressure between where the fluid or gas is and where it is going. To generate a pressure, work has to be done on the fluid or gas by either a **fan** or a **pump**. Fans are used to generate gas flow while pumps generate flow in liquids. In the clinical setting, **ventilator** is a term used for a system that assists the flow of air in and out of the lungs.

To calculate how much work is done by a ventilator, consider a ventilator supplying air to a patient's lungs at constant pressure, as shown in *Figure 3.1*. The ventilator bellows produce a force F and move a distance d. Because pressure P is defined as force per unit area, for bellows of area A we can write:

$$P = \frac{F}{A} \quad \text{or} \quad F = P \cdot A \qquad \qquad \text{3.4}$$

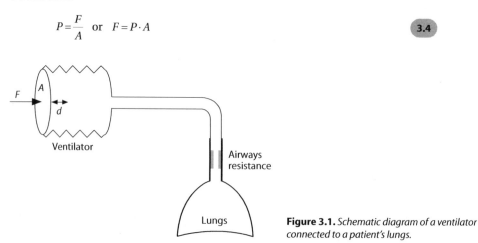

Figure 3.1. *Schematic diagram of a ventilator connected to a patient's lungs.*

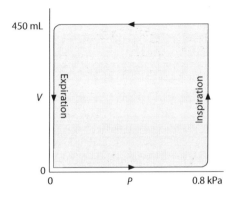

$$W = F \times D.$$

$$W = (P \times A) \times D.$$

Figure 3.2. *Graph of volume against pressure for a constant pressure ventilator.*

Substituting (Equation 3.1) into Equation 3.4 we get:

work done = $P \cdot A \cdot d$ **3.5**

But volume V is equal to area multiplied by length, i.e.

$A \cdot d = V$, so that Equation 3.5 becomes:

work done = $P \cdot V$ **3.6 Learn**

Figure 3.2 shows a graph of volume against pressure for one inspiration and expiration produced by a constant pressure ventilator. The shaded area enclosed by the graph represents the work done by the ventilator. Note that the pressure on the *x*-axis refers to the pressure within the ventilator bellows; the lung pressure builds up more gradually as the lung inflates, due to the resistance of the airways of the lung.

Worked example

Question
How much work is done by a ventilator each time a breath of 450 mL is given at a constant pressure of 0.8 kPa?

Key points
- lungs inflated with a volume (V) of 450 mL ($= 0.45$ L $= 4.5 \times 10^{-4}$ m³)
- pressure of inflation (P) a constant 0.8 kPa ($= 0.8 \times 10^{3}$ Pa)

Calculation
The work done by a ventilator (from Equation 3.6):
$P_{vent} = P \cdot V = (0.8 \times 10^{3}) \times (4.5 \times 10^{-4}) = 0.36$ J

Answer
The work done by the ventilator is 0.36 J.

Work done in the lung

So far we have only considered the pressure in the bellows of the ventilator. Because of airway resistance, the pressure within the lung is not equal to the ventilator pressure, except at the points of maximal and minimal inspiration (where there is no airflow). The volume–pressure response of the lung itself is shown by a dotted line in *Figure 3.3*. The lighter shaded area enclosed by the dotted

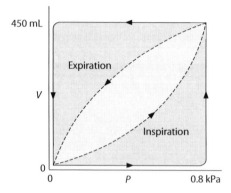

Figure 3.3. *Graph of volume against pressure for a model ventilator.*

line represents the energy required to inflate and deflate the lung. The elastic forces of the lungs' connective tissue, the chest wall, in addition to the surface tension forces in the alveoli, must be overcome each time the lung expands. The remaining (darker) shaded area is energy lost through friction, caused by the resistance of the airway.

Hysteresis

The lungs, like many elastic materials, do not return to their original size in an identical fashion to the manner in which they expanded: they retain a 'memory' after having been stretched. So for the lungs, whilst at identical pressures during inhalation and exhalation, the volumes are actually different, with the volume being less during exhalation. This phenomenon is known as **elastic hysteresis**. The dotted line in *Figure 3.3* takes the form of a **hysteresis loop**, and the area within the loop represents the energy lost in the lung and chest wall during one respiratory cycle.

3.4 Compliance

Definition

Compliance: this is the change of volume with respect to pressure and is a measure of the ease of expansion.

Imagine two yet to be inflated balloons, one is thin- and the other thick-walled. When blowing up the two balloons the thinner walled balloon expands with considerably less effort than the thicker one. The thinner walled balloon is said to be more compliant.

Compliance can be thought of as the ease of expansion and it is expressed as a change in volume divided by a change in pressure:

$$C = \frac{\Delta V}{\Delta P}$$

3.7 **Learn**

where C is compliance
             ΔV is change in volume
             ΔP is the change in pressure

The gradient on the volume (*y*-axis)–pressure (*x*-axis) graph (*Figure 3.4*) is the compliance. Note how the compliance is greater during the expiratory phase due to hysteresis of the lung tissue.

Units. The units of compliance are metres per newton, $m \cdot N^{-1}$. **Elastance** is the opposite of compliance, and its value is the reciprocal of the compliance value.

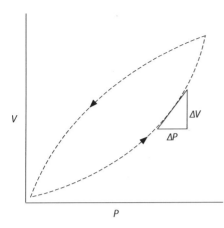

Figure 3.4. *The compliance of the lung is equal to the gradient of the volume–pressure curve.*

Compliance and the lungs

The compliance of the lungs is a balancing act. If the pulmonary compliance is too high then the elastic recoil is diminished, passive exhalation is undermined and the respiratory muscles associated with exhalation have to do more work. On the other hand if the compliance is too low then the lungs might be described as 'stiff' and the work done by the respiratory muscles during inhalation increases. Pulmonary compliance has two contributing variables: the compliance of the lungs themselves and the compliance of the chest wall.

High compliance in the lungs. Like a well-used rubber band, compliance in the lungs also increases with age, and the elasticity decreases. This increase is accelerated in diseases such as emphysema. Extra work is required to breathe during exhalation when the elastic recoil is diminished and muscles associated with exhalation have to work harder.

Low compliance in the lungs. Diseases that cause a decrease in the compliance of the lungs mean that extra work is required to expand the lungs and chest wall during inhalation. The decreased compliance in the lungs results in higher pressures being needed for inspiration of the same volume of air. Examples of conditions associated with low compliance are atelectasis, pulmonary fibrosis, pneumonia, a deficit of surfactant, oedema and pneumonia.

3.5 Work done during spontaneous breathing

The lungs are elastic structures prevented from collapsing by adhesion to the pleural membrane lining the interior of the chest wall. During a spontaneous inspiration the diaphragm moves down by 1–1.5 cm and the intercostal muscles cause the ribcage to move outwards, increasing the volume of the chest cavity. The intrapleural pressure becomes sub-atmospheric, so the pressure in the lungs falls slightly and air rushes in through the mouth and nose to equalize the pressure difference. Expiration occurs by relaxation of the respiratory muscles and the combined passive contraction of the elastic lung tissues and alveolar surface tension.

The respiratory muscles are inefficient; 90% of the energy supplied to them is lost as heat. The remaining 10% is mechanical energy used to do work to expand the lungs and some of that energy is stored in the lungs as elastic potential energy. This stored energy is released on exhalation and is often referred to as the recoil energy. The remainder is lost through hysteresis and airways resistance.

When the body is functioning normally the work done whilst breathing feels inconsequential. When there is a severe increase in resistance in the airway then breathing can become laboured, and the effort required to breathe can become exhausting.

Power of breathing

It was shown in the example above that the work of one inspiration is typically around 0.36 J. For a respiratory rate of 15 breaths per minute, the power of breathing can easily be calculated:

$$\text{Power of breathing} = 0.36\,\text{J} \times \frac{15}{60} = 0.09\,\text{J}\cdot\text{s}^{-1} = 90\,\text{mW}$$

Because the respiratory muscles are only approximately 10% efficient, the power required for resting breathing is actually closer to 900 mW. The total metabolic rate of a subject at rest is 80–90 W, so the respiratory power represents approximately 1% of the energy consumed by the body. The power of breathing during exercise is greatly increased due to a much greater tidal volume in addition to increased airway resistance (see *Section 3.6* below) and respiratory rate. During strenuous exercise the power of breathing can rise to 25% of the total metabolism.

3.6 Flow characteristics during breathing

Power of fluid flowing through a tube

During normal respiration the lungs exhibit a mixture of laminar and turbulent flow (see *Chapter 8*). In the large airways, turbulent flow dominates but in the smaller airways, where the velocities are lower, laminar flow dominates. Consider a fluid flowing through a tube driven by a pressure difference *P*. The amount of energy required to move a volume *V* through the tube is the product of the volume and the pressure difference (Equation 3.6):

$$E = P \cdot V$$

If the pressure difference remains constant, it follows that the power is equal to the pressure times the rate of change of volume (or flow rate *Q*).

$$\dot{E} = P \cdot \dot{V} = P \cdot Q \qquad \text{3.8}$$

Note that the small dot above the symbol indicates a rate of change of the quantity.

Power in laminar flow

From Equation 8.3 the relationship between pressure and laminar flow is linear:

$$P \propto Q$$

Substituting Equation 3.8 into the above equation gives:

$$\text{Power} \propto Q^2 \qquad \text{for laminar flow.} \qquad \text{3.9 Learn}$$

Power in turbulent flow. From Equation 3.9, the relationship between turbulent flow rate is proportional to pressure squared:

$$P \propto Q^2$$

Substituting Equation 3.8 into the above equation gives:

$$\text{Power} \propto Q^3 \quad \text{for turbulent flow.}$$

 3.10 Learn

Clearly laminar flow is more energy efficient, requiring less power to maintain a given flow rate than turbulent flow.

Hyperventilation

Rapid breathing generates air flow at higher rates than normal and as a result considerably more turbulence occurs. Turbulent flow requires more power than laminar flow for a given flow rate, which means a higher energy consumption by the respiratory muscles. The oxygen demands of the muscles associated with respiration can outstrip the extra oxygen supply gained by faster breathing. This outstripping of demand over the supply of oxygen can lead to hypoxia; in patients with respiratory diseases the over-stimulation of respiration by medical interventions can cause a danger of hypoxia as a result.

3.7 Work done by the heart

The heart does mechanical work as it pumps a mass of blood through the vasculature, overcoming the resistance of the network. Metabolic energy is converted into the kinetic energy of the flowing blood. The heart acts as a dual pump, the right side pump supplying the pulmonary system and the left side supplying the systemic circulation. The right ventricle only does about a fifth of the work of the left ventricle. *Figure 3.5* shows how the pressure and volume in the left ventricle vary over one cardiac cycle (the pressure–volume 'loop').

Power of the heart

At rest, the mechanical output power of the human heart is approximately 1.3 W. During exercise both heart rate and blood pressure rise, both of which increase the power, or work rate, of the heart.

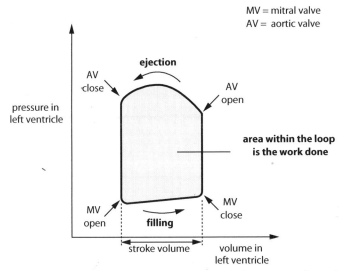

Figure 3.5. *The pressure–volume loop for the left ventricle over one cardiac cycle.*

Efficiency of the heart

Only 10% of the energy supplied to the heart is converted into mechanical energy, with the other 90% being converted into heat, and so like most engines the energy efficiency is low. The heart therefore requires approximately 13 W of power input to function at rest.

Worked example

Question
A heart is beating at a rate of 80 beats min⁻¹, average ventricular pressures in the left and right ventricles are 100 mmHg and 20 mmHg, respectively, and the heart is ejecting 75 mL per cycle. What is the work done in one cardiac cycle and what is the power?

Key points
- The heart ejects a volume (V) estimated at 75 mL per cardiac cycle
- Average pressure in the left ventricle, P_{LV}, is 100 mmHg or 13.3 kPa
- Average pressure in the right ventricle, P_{RV}, is 20 mmHg or 2.7 kPa

Step 1
Using Equation 3.8, the work done by the left ventricle, W_{LV}:

$W_{LV} = P_{LV} \cdot \Delta V = (13.3 \times 10^3) \times (7.5 \times 10^{-5}) = 0.9975$ J

$W_{LV} \simeq 1$ J

The work done by the right ventricle, W_{RV}:

$W_{RV} = P_{RV} \cdot \Delta V = (2.7 \times 10^3) \times (7.5 \times 10^{-5}) = 0.2025$ J

$W_{RV} \simeq 0.2$ J

Step 2
Total work done per cardiac cycle is:

$W = W_{LV} + W_{RV} = 1 + 0.2 = 1.2$ J

Step 3
Work done in one minute: = work done in one cardiac cycle × heart rate
= 1.2 × 80 = 96 J

Power is work done per second so:

$\text{Power} = \dfrac{\text{work done in one minute}}{60} = \dfrac{96}{60} = 1.6$ W

Answer
In one cardiac cycle the work done is 1.2 joule and at a heart rate of 80 the power is 1.6 watt.

Summary

- Work done is the amount of energy transferred from one system to another.
- Energy is the capacity to do work.
- Power is the rate of energy transfer per unit time, or work done per unit time.
- Energy cannot be created or destroyed, merely converted from one form to another.
- Energy is required during respiration to overcome elastic forces in the lung and chest wall as well as airways resistance.
- Turbulent airflow in the lungs is considerably less efficient than laminar flow.
- The mechanical efficiency of the respiratory muscles and the heart are both approximately 10%.

Single best answer questions

For each of these questions, only one option is correct.

1. Which forms of energy are involved when a wind generator powers an electric hairdryer?
   (a) Kinetic, chemical, potential, electrical.
   (b) Kinetic, potential, electrical, heat.
   (c) Kinetic, electrical, heat.
   (d) Kinetic, potential, heat.
   (e) Potential, electrical, heat.

2. Which is true of laminar flow?
   (a) Pressure proportional to square of flow, power proportional to square root of flow.
   (b) Pressure proportional to square of flow, power proportional to square of flow.
   (c) Pressure proportional to square of flow, power proportional to flow.
   (d) Pressure proportional to flow, power proportional to square of flow.
   (e) Pressure proportional to square of flow, power proportional to cube of flow.

3. Which of the following have no effect on the work of breathing?
   (a) The compliance of the lungs.
   (b) Airway resistance.
   (c) Respiratory rate.
   (d) Viscosity of inhaled gas.
   (e) Pulmonary blood flow.

Multiple choice questions

For each of these questions, more than one option may be correct.

1. Which of the following constitute work done?
   (a) Lifting a 1 kg weight above your head.
   (b) Holding a 1 kg weight above your head.
   (c) Blowing up a balloon.
   (d) A car colliding with a wall.
   (e) A ball bearing rolling across a glass surface.

2. Which of the following conditions decrease lung compliance?
   (a) Fibrosing alveolitis.
   (b) Deficiency of pulmonary surfactant.
   (c) Emphysema.
   (d) Allergic asthma.
   (e) Atelectasis.

3. Which of the processes associated with respiration store recoverable energy?
   (a) Hysteresis.
   (b) Recoil of alveolar surface tension.
   (c) Large airways resistance.
   (d) Recoil of lung tissue.
   (e) Small airways resistance.

Chapter 4
Temperature and heat

Having read this chapter you will be able to:
- Understand the concept of heat and thermal energy.
- Explain temperature and understand temperature scales.
- Understand heat transfer through conduction, convection and radiation.
- Appreciate the significance of the laws of thermodynamics.
- Appreciate the adiabatic model relevant to a discharging cylinder of gas and associated cooling.

4.1 Heat

Definition

Heat: the quantity of thermal energy contained in a substance.

A lit match reaches a temperature fierce enough to burn skin, but the heat it generates could not warm a cup of water. In contrast, the water in a radiator can warm a room even though it is at a significantly lower temperature – the radiator can transfer far more heat than the hotter match. Temperature is a measure of how hot or cold an object is. Above absolute zero, a body's atoms or molecules are in constant motion and the amplitude of their vibrations determines the temperature of the body. Adding heat to a body raises its temperature. Heat is the thermal energy that flows from one body in contact with another when they are at differing temperatures.

Heat capacity

Definition

Specific heat capacity: the specific heat capacity of a solid or liquid is defined as the heat required to raise unit mass of the substance by one degree of temperature.

Although not immediately obvious, a bucket of water at room temperature contains more thermal energy than a red-hot nail. This is because the water has a much larger mass, and thus a larger **heat capacity** than the nail so it can store more energy without raising its temperature considerably.

If the nail is quenched in the water in the bucket there will be a small rise in temperature, but this will be much smaller than the drop in temperature of the nail. The material of the nail (iron) and the water can also be defined in terms of a quantity called the **specific heat capacity**, which is the heat capacity per unit mass. Iron has a value of 0.450 $J \cdot g^{-1} \cdot K^{-1}$, compared to a much greater 4.18 $J \cdot g^{-1} \cdot K^{-1}$ for water, meaning that the nail could be quenched effectively by a fairly small amount of water. The amount of heat (Q) needed to raise the temperature of a body is given by the following equation:

$$Q = m \cdot c \cdot \Delta T$$

4.1

where ΔT is the temperature change
         c is the specific heat capacity
         m is the mass of the body

Units. Thermal energy is another form of energy so is expressed in joules, J (or kg·m²·s⁻²). In some countries, the calorie is used as a unit of thermal energy, where 1 calorie = 4.18 J. One calorie is defined as the energy required to raise the temperature of 1 gram of water from 15°C to 16°C. Specific heat capacity is normally expressed in units of J·g⁻¹·K⁻¹.

Clinical examples

Respiratory heat loss
The heat lost by the body through respiration may be categorized as roughly 25% through warming of surrounding air, and 75% through humidification of air.

Shivering generates heat
Shivering raises the metabolic rate from a resting power of 80 W to around 320 W, a fourfold increase. The majority of this power is converted into heat (through the inefficiency of the muscles), warming the body.

4.2 Temperature

The more a substance is heated, the more kinetic energy the molecules gain. Temperature quantifies the average kinetic energy of the atoms or molecules, i.e. how fast they are moving around. As a substance is heated, its atoms or molecules move faster. In solids, the atoms vibrate more vigorously; for example, atoms in a crystal lattice vibrate around their average position dictated by their lattice bonds. In a gas or liquid, the atoms or molecules move faster and bump into each other more energetically. At any temperature, these tiny particles have a wide range of kinetic energies and the temperature represents the average kinetic energy. Even at low temperatures, a small proportion are moving or vibrating very fast.

Definition

Temperature: when a body is at any temperature the individual molecules are at a range of energy levels; the temperature is related to the mean energy of the molecules.

Temperature scales

Temperature scales are based on known, repeatable temperature points of reference. The Celsius scale uses the boiling and freezing points of pure water at atmospheric pressure. Zero on the Fahrenheit scale was set at the lowest freezing point obtainable with an ice–water–salt mixture. The freezing point of water is 32°F and the boiling point is 212°F, being 180 degrees apart. *Figure 4.1* shows the kelvin, Celsius and Fahrenheit temperature scales.

Temperature sensors don't measure temperature directly, but instead measure a change in a physical property sensitive to temperature. For example, a simple thermometer relies on expansion of a liquid, such as mercury, inside a glass tube. Modern thermometers use an electrical device such as a thermocouple and display the temperature on a digital read-out.

Absolute zero

The theoretical temperature of absolute zero is the starting point of the kelvin scale. At 0 K, absolute zero, molecules contain no kinetic energy. Though attempts to reach absolute zero have come very, very close, true absolute zero can never be reached.

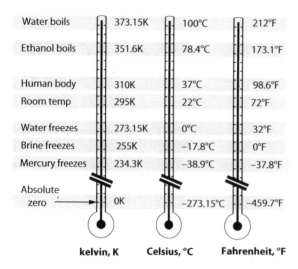

Figure 4.1. *Temperature scales: kelvin, Celsius and Fahrenheit.*

Worked example

Question
Does a temperature rise from 50°C to 100°C represent a doubling of the absolute temperature?

Answer
No. Temperature starts at −273°C (0 kelvin) where the body holds no thermal energy. Zero on the Celsius scale is simply the freezing point of water at sea level (1 atmosphere). So an increase of 50°C is actually only an 18% increase in absolute temperature.

Body temperature

Humans, like all mammals and birds, are **homeothermic**; that is, they control their core body temperature within a narrow range. For humans this is 36.8 ± 0.4°C, although this depends on the level of activity. Temperature also varies by around 0.4°C during normal circadian rhythm, being lowest in the early hours of the morning and highest in the evening. The mean temperature of the body's central core is steady, while the forehead skin temperature ranges from 29 to 33°C.

4.3 Transfer of heat

Consider a hot cup of coffee left on a table overnight. The next morning the coffee is at room temperature because heat flows from the hot coffee to the surroundings. In the presence of a temperature gradient, heat flows from hot to cold until thermal equilibrium is reached. The coffee, the table and the room air all settle at the same temperature. Heat transfer from one body to another can occur by three main methods: conduction, convection and radiation.

Conduction

Holding metal or wooden objects on a winter's day are very different sensations. Metal feels notably colder, yet both objects are in the same environment so are at the same temperature. The hand is at a higher temperature (than the metal or wood), so heat is conducted from the skin due to the temperature difference. The heat is conducted at a much faster rate to the metal because metal is a far better conductor of heat than wood.

Conduction is the process of kinetic energy in the form of heat being transferred from one body to another. In other words, it is the direct transfer of heat energy from molecule to molecule. Some materials, such as metals, are very good at conducting heat, whereas plastics are generally not and are therefore described as good **insulators**. Conduction cannot occur in a vacuum, as it is an exchange of thermal energy between bodies. Gases are poor conductors; for example, copper is an incredible 16 000 times better at conducting heat than air; this means that the heat loss during breathing is low.

Units. The units of conductivity are $W \cdot K^{-1} \cdot m^{-1}$.

> **Definition**
>
> **Conduction:** the flow of heat by conduction occurs via direct collisions between the atoms and molecules of warmer and cooler regions and the resultant transfer of kinetic energy. Conduction can occur in solids, liquid and gases.

> **Worked example**
>
> **Question**
> Why does a string vest still offer a degree of warmth to the wearer?
>
> **Answer**
> Static air is held amongst the holes in the vest. Gases in general are poor conductors of heat and air is typical of this. Similarly, hospital blankets are often of a knitted design with many holes to take advantage of this principle.

Convection

Once on the operating table, if not appropriately covered, patients cool down very quickly due to convection. Heat is transferred due to the temperature gradient between the patient and the cooler air immediately surrounding the patient. This warmed air is then moved by the operating theatre's laminar flow system and is replaced by colder air, once again establishing a temperature gradient through which heat is lost.

The heat loss from breathing involves convection. For ventilated patients or patients with supplemental oxygen the dry air/oxygen from cylinders means that energy is lost in humidifying inhaled air. Like conduction, convection cannot exist in a vacuum, as it needs a medium through which the thermal energy can be transported. Convection can be a passive or an active process:

> **Definition**
>
> **Convection:** the transfer of heat from a body by the liquid or gas which surrounds it. The fluid has a tendency to rise if it is hotter because it is less dense; colder, denser material sinks under the influence of gravity.

- **passive convection** can be seen in a hot object cooling in still air (note that some heat loss also occurs by radiation and conduction)
- **active convection** can be achieved by blowing cool air over the object with a fan.

Clinical example

Warming and cooling blankets
Controlling patient temperature is most commonly achieved with the aid of a warming blanket where a fan drives hot air through an inflatable blanket. This method of convection has also been adapted to cool patients following a cerebral insult, with the hope that a reduced metabolic rate will reduce oxygen demand and minimize ischaemic insult. Instead of air, hyper-hypothermia water therapy systems can be employed. The water is pumped through a collection of garments such as a head wrap, patient vest and lower body blanket.

Radiation of heat

Definition

Radiation: hot bodies emit thermal energy in the form of electromagnetic radiation; this radiation is absorbed by the surroundings, resulting in heat transfer.

When the sun emerges from behind a cloud its warmth is immediately apparent, despite the fact that the heat has travelled from over 93 million miles away! Neither convection nor conduction can adequately explain how this heat is transferred, because both rely on a medium to carry the heat and yet space is virtually a vacuum with very few molecules present. The answer lies in radiant heat: the sun's heat is carried by electromagnetic waves (see *Chapter 5*), most of which are invisible to the naked eye. When electromagnetic waves are being discussed in terms of the energy they are carrying they are often referred to as **electromagnetic radiation**.

The phenomenon of thermal radiation is not limited to the sun: imagine two objects, one hot and one cold, placed in a vacuum with no physical contact between them. Heat transfer via either conduction or convection is impossible because in the vacuum there is no transporting medium, yet the two objects will eventually reach a common temperature. The heat transfer occurs because both objects continually release and absorb energy in the form of electromagnetic radiation: the emitted energy is commonly called **thermal radiation**: it can also be referred to as **radiant heat**.

4.4 Black-body radiation

Definition

Stefan–Boltzmann law: the radiation energy per unit time from a black body is proportional to the fourth power of the temperature.

A black body is a body that absorbs all radiation that falls upon it. It follows that dark-coloured objects are the best absorbers, as shown in *Figure 4.2*. Black bodies are also the best emitters. Painting a radiator matt black increases its efficiency at heating a room.

The amount of radiation emitted by a black body depends on its temperature, and is described by the **Stefan–Boltzmann law**. This law states that the emitted power is equal to the fourth power of the absolute temperature (the temperature relative to absolute zero).

$$P = e \cdot \sigma \cdot A \cdot T^4$$

(4.2)

where P is the radiated power
T is the temperature
A is the surface area
σ is the Stefan constant ($= 5.67 \times 10^{-8}$ J·m^{-2}·s^{-1}·K^{-4})
e is the **emissivity**

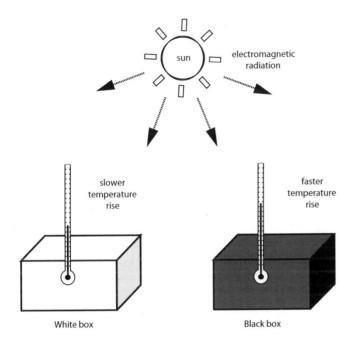

Figure 4.2. *Absorption of thermal radiation by black and white bodies.*

The radiant power is also proportional to the emissivity, a dimensionless quantity (i.e. it has no units), which quantifies the ability of a body to radiate heat; this is established by a comparison to a perfect black body surface at the same temperature. The emissivity of a black body is 1, while true bodies have a value of less than 1.

The wavelength of the emitted radiation also depends on the temperature. At room temperature, or body temperature, a body will emit electromagnetic radiation over a range of wavelengths within the infrared region of the electromagnetic spectrum. At higher temperatures, the body will emit a shorter wavelength radiation, as shown in *Figure 4.3*, until at very high temperatures (greater than 800 K), the object begins to glow red-hot as electromagnetic radiation in the visible region is emitted (the visible region spans the wavelength range from approximately 380 to 700 nanometres). At higher temperatures still, the object glows orange, yellow and eventually white as shorter and shorter wavelengths of radiation are emitted. The sun's surface is at a temperature of approximately 5000 K, so although a wide range of wavelengths are emitted, it appears bright white to the eye. Astronomers observe the black-body radiation spectrum of distant stars and from this it is possible to calculate the stars' surface temperature and energy output.

Clinical example

Thermogram scans
A thermogram records the temperatures of a subject. Breast thermography is a non-invasive screening procedure that detects and records temperatures from predominantly infrared heat emissions. Metabolic and vascular activity in pre-cancerous tissue, and also the area surrounding developing breast cancer, is often high. Different colours are used to represent the temperature zones.

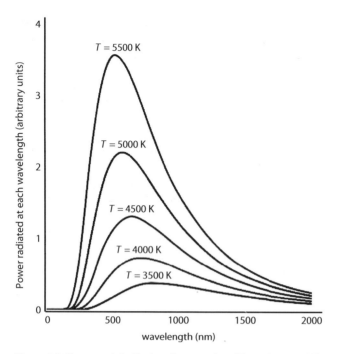

Figure 4.3. *The spectral distribution of power radiated from objects at different temperatures.*

4.5 Regulation of body temperature

Mammals and other warm–blooded animals continuously produce heat and this is evident by the rapid cooling that follows death. An average healthy male at rest emits approximately 50 watts per square metre of body surface, or approximately 80 watts. The rate of thermal emission is affected by the basal metabolic rate (BMR), which increases after eating and during exercise, leading to an increase in the core temperature of the body. In cold ambient conditions, increased heat production can also be achieved by shivering and through voluntary muscular activity. There is no direct mechanism for a reduction in heat production to compensate for overheating; instead the body relies on cooling mechanisms such as sweating.

There are several routes of heat loss from the body, summarized in *Table 4.1*. Clearly the statement that 90% of body heat is lost through the head is nonsense; the actual figure is probably somewhere between 20 and 40%.

Table 4.1. *Routes of heat loss from the body.*

Heat loss	Fraction
Radiation	40%
Convection	30%
Evaporation of skin moisture (sweating)	20%
Respiration	10%

When the body temperature rises as cutaneous blood flow increases and heat loss is increased via radiation, the temperature differential between the body and the environment increases the rate of heat loss. Clothing decreases loss through radiation as well as via convection. In neonates, heat loss through radiation accounts for a higher rate of heat loss than in adults, due to a much higher relative body surface area.

Sweating is an efficient means of cooling the body, because moisture excreted onto the skin surface will evaporate readily in dry air. Since energy is needed to turn water into vapour, thermal energy is removed from the skin. In humid conditions, evaporation is much slower, so people tend to become much more hot and uncomfortable than in dry conditions at comparable temperatures. In certain conditions, evaporation of sweat can be a critical means of cooling the body. For example, it is highly inadvisable to undertake vigorous exercise in a wetsuit out of water: evaporation is prevented by the wetsuit and, coupled with the thermal insulation given by the wetsuit itself, rapid overheating of the body would occur.

Clinical example

Reflective blankets
Human bodies are no different to any other objects in that they both absorb and also emit thermal radiation. When the peripheral circulation is dilated there an increased emission of thermal radiation so that after strenuous exercise, such as a triathlon, competitors are often given reflective blankets that reflect back emitted thermal radiation, greatly reducing one source of thermal heat loss. Similarly patients who are hypothermic might have a reflective blanket wrapped around them.

Fluid warmers
Infusing fluids that are below the core temperature of the body will lower the temperature of a patient. When the volume of fluid infused is low and the patient is warm, this drop in thermal energy is compensated for easily. Anaesthetized patients who are already cooling down and receiving significant infusion volumes, require fluids that are warmed to approximately their core temperature. A fluid warmer will also warm any gases present and Charles's law (see *Chapter 9*) tells us that these gas bubbles will expand on warming, which is why a bubble trap is often present downstream of the warming device.

4.6 Measuring temperature

Thermometric properties

All thermometers work by exploiting a particular physical, or **thermometric** property that changes with temperature in a predictable fashion. A simple relationship between temperature and the variable allows for easy measurement. *Table 4.2* lists the most commonly used thermometric properties. Ideally the property that changes with temperature should be linearly

Definition

Thermometric property: this is a physical property that changes in a known, consistent way with temperature.

proportional to temperature; for example, the length of a liquid column in a liquid-in-glass thermometer. Many thermometers, however, utilize non-linear thermometric properties; for example, a thermistor.

The liquid-in-glass thermometer

The liquid-in-glass thermometer (*Figure 4.4*) is used to measure temperatures in the oral, axillary and rectal regions. The liquid expands linearly as the temperature rises, but the expansion is only 1–2% of the total volume so the glass casing of the column is designed to magnify the narrow liquid column. Originally filled with mercury, thermometers are now filled with an alcohol-based liquid. There is a constriction between the bulb and the column and this allows the thermometer to be

Table 4.2. *Thermometric properties utilized in thermometers.*

Thermometer	Thermometric property
Liquid-in-glass	Expansion of a liquid
Bimetallic strip	Expansion of solid
Bourdon	Pressure change of gas
Resistance	Resistance of coil of wire
Thermistor	Resistance of metal oxides
Thermocouple	Seebeck effect
Infrared	Thermal radiation

removed from the patient and read at leisure; the thermometer has to be shaken to return the liquid to the bulb. Though not particularly sensitive, liquid-in-glass thermometers have the advantage of simplicity and low cost. They are limited by their fragility and slow response time.

Bourdon thermometer

The Bourdon thermometer is popular in industry because it is capable of measuring high temperatures accurately. It is based on the principle described in Charles's law: as the temperature of a gas increases, the pressure proportionately increases with it (see *Chapter 9*). The gas is held in a reservoir or bulb and is linked by a capillary tube to a hollow Bourdon tube. As the temperature increases the gas expands, the pressure increases and the Bourdon tube uncoils – this is linked to a pointer behind which is a temperature on a calibrated dial. The Bourdon thermometer is similar to the Bourdon pressure gauge (see *Chapter 6*) because they both measure the expansion of a fluid. The filling for the bulb of the Bourdon thermometer can be either liquid or gas, because they both expand as temperature increases.

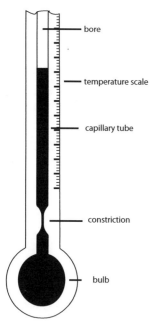

Figure 4.4. *A liquid-in-glass thermometer.*

Electronic thermometers

Modern medical thermometers are usually electronic, and are either of the handheld type, or are part of an integrated patient monitoring system. Electronic thermometers normally utilize either a temperature-dependent resistor or a simple temperature sensing device called a thermocouple. Electronic thermometers are now relatively cheap, have highly sensitive sensors and can be calibrated accurately. They also have the advantage that they are easy to read and can be logged automatically, a useful feature for long-term patient monitoring.

Platinum resistance thermometers

This is the simplest type of electronic thermometer. The resistance of a thin platinum wire has a linear relationship with temperature, as shown in *Figure 4.5*. The device measures resistance and this is then converted to temperature using a simple calibration equation. This type of thermometer has the disadvantage that it is not sensitive compared to a thermistor (see below).

Thermistors

A thermistor is a temperature-sensitive resistor whose resistance changes with temperature. Most temperature-sensitive resistors are constructed from a semiconductor material (carefully chosen metal oxides) and the resistance increases with a fall in temperature (they have a negative temperature coefficient) and they are known as **negative thermal conductivity** (NTC) thermistors. A Wheatstone bridge circuit (see *Chapter 18*) is used to measure the resistance accurately.

The main disadvantage of thermistors is the non-linear resistance versus temperature characteristic, although this can be compensated for using an appropriate calibration equation programmed into an electronic measurement system. Thermistors remain highly popular due to their cost, miniature size and convenience. Thermistor probes are commonly placed in the naso-pharynx, oesophagus, rectum or bladder (integrated with a urinary catheter). They have excellent accuracy and their small mass means that there is a quick response to variations in temperature.

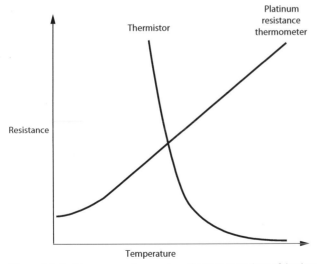

Figure 4.5. *Resistance versus temperature: the steeper gradient of the thermistor as opposed to platinum wire means it is more sensitive to variations in temperature.*

Thermocouples

Definition
Seebeck effect: this is the conversion of a temperature difference directly to an electric current; for small changes in temperature, the Seebeck voltage is linearly proportional to temperature.

Thermocouples rely on the Seebeck effect: when a junction is formed between two dissimilar metals a small voltage is produced across the junction and this voltage varies with temperature.

Temperature-measuring thermocouples are traditionally constructed with two junctions, as shown in *Figure 4.6*. One junction is used as the measurement probe while the other (the 'reference' junction) is held at a fixed, known temperature, for example, melting ice at 0°C. The most common thermocouples are made from copper and constantan (an alloy of copper with 40% nickel). The voltage across the thermocouple is known as Seebeck voltage, given by:

$$V = \alpha \cdot (T_1 - T_2)$$

4.3

where α is the Seebeck coefficient ($V \cdot K^{-1}$)
   T_1 and T_2 are the temperatures at the two end junctions
   V is the voltage generated

The **Seebeck coefficient** is a constant that depends on the two metals used. Modern thermocouple-based thermometers use a single junction, making the reference junction redundant, instead using a special circuit called a cold-junction compensator. This circuit contains a thermistor, which senses the ambient temperature, and thus compensates the output of the thermocouple for any temperature. Thermocouples can be made extremely small and as a result have very low heat capacity. They therefore respond rapidly and can be used to measure the temperature of very small volumes of matter. Thermocouples can also produce very accurate readings if correctly calibrated.

Infrared tympanic thermometers

A tympanic thermometer measures the temperature in the middle ear by detecting the radiation emitted by the eardrum. The sensor in this type of thermometer is a **thermopile**, an electronic device which converts thermal energy into electrical energy. Infrared radiation emitted from the eardrum causes a temperature rise in the thermopile and, as explained in *Section 4.4*, the radiated power of the infrared energy provides an indication of the emitter temperature. The tympanic membrane is a

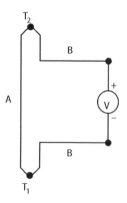

Figure 4.6. *A thermocouple, where A and B are different metals.*

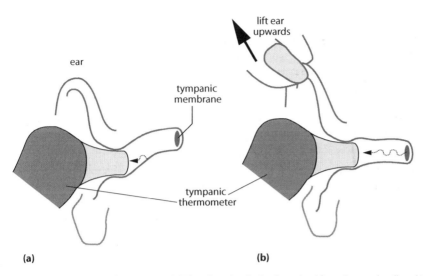

Figure 4.7. *A tympanic thermometer. (a) The infrared radiation is received from the canal wall, making it inaccurate. (b) The ear is lifted and the infrared radiation received is from the tympanic membrane, giving an accurate reading.*

suitable site because its blood supply is similar in temperature and location to the blood supplying the hypothalamus, the site of the body's thermoregulatory centre and, therefore, an ideal location for core temperature estimation.

Tympanic thermometers can give falsely low temperature readings depending on the anatomy of the ear, the build-up of earwax or other debris, or poor user technique. The most accurate readings are obtained if the user lifts the ear upwards, giving the instrument a clear line of sight to the tympanic membrane, as shown in *Figure 4.7*. Otherwise it responds to infrared rays from the ear canal that are approximately 2°C lower than the tympanic membrane, giving a falsely low reading. This type of thermometer is obviously limited by the fact it can only be used in one area of the body to sample temperature.

4.7 Laws of thermodynamics

Thermodynamics deals with the transfer of heat energy to other forms of energy, most notably mechanical work. The temperature, pressure and volume of a gas are all related to their thermal energy. Study of the laws of thermodynamics allows an understanding of these relationships and from this, predictions about a wide range of physical processes can be made.

> **Definition**
>
> **Thermodynamics:** the branch of physics that deals with the interaction between heat (thermal energy) and other forms of energy.

First law of thermodynamics

Imagine an enclosed chamber that has absolutely no communication with the outside world: it is perfectly insulated. Can the total energy inside that chamber ever change? The first law of thermodynamics categorically says no: the only change of energy can come about by energy being added or subtracted externally.

> **Definition**
>
> **First law of thermodynamics:** the change in internal energy of a system is equal to the heat added minus the work done by the system.

In essence it is a law about the conservation of energy: although energy assumes many forms, the total quantity of energy is constant, and when energy disappears in one form it appears simultaneously in other forms. Put simply, energy can neither be created nor destroyed. An equation accompanies this law that can be considered the bookkeeping of energy states:

$$\Delta U = Q \pm W \qquad \text{4.4}$$

where: ΔU is the change in the total energy of the system
Q is heat added to the system
W is work done by the system

By convention if energy leaves the system the change in energy is classed as positive, but negative if energy is gained by the system.

Clinical example

The human body
The first law of thermodynamics can be considered as another way of writing the conservation of energy.

$$\Delta U \text{ (stored energy)} = Q \text{ (heat loss/gain)} - W \text{ (work done)} \qquad \text{4.5}$$

where: ΔU is the stored energy in the form of food, fat and heat
Q is the heat loss from or gain to the body (e.g. heat lost swimming in cold sea (-ve) or heat gained in a hot sauna (+ve))
W is the work done, such as when climbing a flight of stairs

Second law of thermodynamics

Heat cannot pass naturally from a colder body to a hotter one; work is required, which is why a fridge requires energy. Work is done to pump heat from the fridge's interior to the external environment.

$$\Delta S = \frac{\Delta Q}{T} \qquad \text{4.6}$$

Definition

Second law of thermodynamics: heat generally cannot flow spontaneously from a material at lower temperature to a material at higher temperature.

where: ΔS is the change in entropy
ΔQ is the heat entering the system
T is the temperature

Units. Entropy does not have units – it is a measure of disorder. The most probable state of a system is the state with the largest entropy.

Third law of thermodynamics

Definition

Third law of thermodynamics: the temperature absolute zero is unattainable.

As a system approaches absolute zero, all processes cease and the entropy (a measure of disorder) of the system approaches a minimum value. It is impossible by any procedure, no matter how idealized, to reduce any system to the absolute zero of temperature (0 K) in a finite number of operations.

Units. The Kelvin scale has absolute zero as the lowest temperature theoretically possible. However, the third law states that it can never be quite reached!

> In other words..., scientist, politician and author C.P. Snow put the three laws in a more memorable way:
> 1. You cannot win (that is, you cannot get something for nothing, because matter and energy are conserved).
> 2. You cannot break even (you cannot return to the same energy state, because there is always an increase in disorder; entropy always increases).
> 3. You cannot get out of the game (because absolute zero is unattainable).

Heat lost by gas expansion

When a gas expands it does work. **Adiabatic expansion** simply refers to a process that involves no external heat transfer, so any work done by an adiabatic system is at the expense of the system's existing internal energy. In other words, an adiabatic system can be considered entirely insulated.

For a process of gas expansion that is adiabatic, there is no change in the system's total energy, so $\Delta U = 0$ and Equation 4.4 becomes:

$$0 = Q \pm W \qquad \text{for an adiabatic process} \qquad \boxed{4.7}$$

Joule–Thomson effect

After enthusiastically pumping up a bike tyre, the valve of the pump feels hot to the touch. Work is done to compress the gas into the tyre so the temperature of the gas rises. If the tyre is pumped more slowly the valve would not heat up, as the heat would have dissipated to the surroundings. The enthusiastic cyclist temporarily creates an adiabatic process because minimal heat had time to enter or leave the system (the system being the enclosed pump, valve and tyre).

Definition
Joule–Thomson effect: a gas changes temperature when it moves from a higher pressure to a lower pressure and for most gases they cool.

The temperature rises when a gas is compressed. Conversely, when gas expands its temperature drops. As a medical gas cylinder empties there is a drop in temperature in the gas expelled and there is a danger that the valve will be obstructed by ice as the gas cools on exit from the cylinder – this is why gases are stored as dry gases. This principle is utilized by a **cryoprobe**, which is cooled by rapid expansion of compressed gas.

If gas in the clinical setting rapidly undergoes compression its temperature will rise. So if the gases in the piping of the anaesthetic machine are compressed from atmospheric pressure to cylinder pressure there is a resultant rise in temperature.

Summary
- Heat is the amount of thermal energy contained by an object.
- The specific heat capacity of a substance determines how much heat is required to raise its temperature.
- Heat flows from a region of high temperature to a region of lower temperature by conduction.
- Thermal energy can travel though a vacuum by the process of radiation.

- Thermometers rely on thermometric properties, that is, properties which change with temperature.
- Thermistors and thermocouples are sensitive temperature-sensing devices commonly used in electronic medical thermometers.
- Thermocouples rely on the Seebeck effect, where a voltage is produced across a two-junction thermocouple if each junction is at a different temperature.

Single best answer questions

For each of these questions, only one option is correct.

1. Thermistors are better temperature sensors than platinum wires because they:
   - (a) have a more linear response
   - (b) have a positive temperature coefficient of resistance
   - (c) are more sensitive
   - (d) give better repeatability
   - (e) are cheaper

2. The body loses heat by which processes and by what proportion?
   - (a) Convection 40%; radiation 30%; evaporation and respiration 20%
   - (b) Convection 40%; radiation 40%; evaporation and respiration 20%
   - (c) Convection 30%; radiation 40%; evaporation and respiration 30%
   - (d) Convection 30%; radiation 30%; evaporation and respiration 40%
   - (e) Convection 20%; radiation 40%; evaporation and respiration 40%

3. The total radiated power of an object is proportional to the objects:
   - (a) temperature
   - (b) temperature-squared
   - (c) emittance
   - (d) surface area
   - (e) mass

4. The temperature of the human body on the Kelvin scale is:
   - (a) 37 K
   - (b) 298.15 K
   - (c) 300 K
   - (d) 310 K
   - (e) 335 K

5. An infrared tympanic thermometer:
   - (a) must be in good thermal contact with the ear canal
   - (b) must have a clear line of sight to the tympanic membrane
   - (c) requires several seconds to obtain a reading
   - (d) is insensitive to debris in the ear
   - (e) may be used in other measurement sites

Multiple choice questions

For each of these questions, more than one option may be correct.

1. Which of the following statements are true of thermistors?
   (a) They have a rapid response time.
   (b) They are not suitable for internal use due to harmful metal content.
   (c) They are small.
   (d) Readings can be taken continuously.
   (e) Expense prohibits manufacture as disposable items.

2. If two bodies are in thermal equilibrium:
   (a) they have the same temperature
   (b) they contain the same quantity of heat
   (c) they have the same heat capacity
   (d) no heat flows between them
   (e) they have the same specific heat capacity

3. A body of emissivity 0.8 compared to a body of emissivity 0.4:
   (a) is a better emitter and a less good absorber of thermal radiation
   (b) is a better emitter and a better absorber of thermal radiation
   (c) is a better emitter but the absorptive abilities are not known
   (d) is more likely to be visibly lighter
   (e) is more likely to be visibly darker

4. 1 kg of iron at 25°C contains more heat than 100 mL of water at 50°C because:
   (a) the iron has a higher heat capacity than the water
   (b) iron has a higher specific heat capacity than water
   (c) the iron has a higher mass than the water
   (d) the iron atoms have a higher mean kinetic energy than the water molecules
   (e) iron has a higher density than water

5. On a cold day, metal feels colder to the touch than wood because:
   (a) metal has a higher specific heat capacity than wood
   (b) the metal is at a lower temperature than the wood
   (c) the metal is a better thermal conductor than wood
   (d) the metal has a lower specific heat capacity than the wood
   (e) the metal contains less heat than the wood

Chapter 5
Waves

Having read this chapter you will be able to:
- State the relationship between frequency and wavelength.
- Define wavelength, frequency, period and amplitude.
- Compare and contrast transverse and longitudinal waves.
- Appreciate how a wave can be interrogated using Fourier analysis.
- Understand the concepts of damping and resonance and their clinical significance.
- Understand the principle of the Doppler effect.

5.1 Properties of waves

Definitions

Waves: a wave is a series of repeating disturbances that propagates in space and time.
Longitudinal waves: a longitudinal wave has oscillations occurring in the direction of travel.
Transverse waves: a transverse wave has oscillations perpendicular to the direction of travel.

When listening to a radio it is interesting to think about how the signal from the transmitter gets to the radio's aerial and how the sound travels from the loudspeaker to your ears. Sound waves and radio waves are markedly different in nature, but have some important properties in common. All waves propagate through space carrying energy from one place to another. The medium itself, for example, the air through which a sound wave is travelling, oscillates around its undisturbed (equilibrium) position as the wave passes. The frequency of the wave, which is measured in hertz, is simply the number of oscillations, or cycles, made by the medium each second. Electromagnetic waves are oscillating electric and magnetic fields and are unique in that they can travel through the vacuum of space. There are two fundamental types of waves: longitudinal and transverse.

- **Longitudinal waves**, such as sound waves, oscillate back and forth in the same direction that the wave is travelling. Imagine a queue of people standing in a line. If you were to push the person at the back, they would bump into the person in front of them and so on. The longitudinal 'wave' of disturbance would travel from one person to the next.
- **Transverse waves** oscillate in a direction perpendicular to the direction of propagation. A Mexican wave in a sports arena is an example of a transverse wave: the spectators stand up and sit down, perpendicular to the direction of the wave. Another example is a mechanical wave travelling along a taut string. All electromagnetic waves are also transverse waves. *Figure 5.1* shows the directions of oscillation of longitudinal and transverse waves relative to their propagation direction.

All waves have certain features in common. *Figure 5.2* shows how a wave produces an effect, in this case a disturbance from equilibrium, which changes periodically with time. The **frequency** is simply the number of oscillations occurring in one second, and is expressed in cycles per second or hertz. The **amplitude** of the wave is the maximum disturbance caused by the wave; for a wave travelling

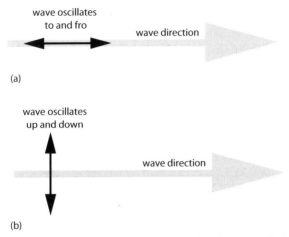

(a)

(b)

Figure 5.1. *Direction of oscillation relative to direction of travel for longitudinal (a) and transverse (b) waves.*

through water, the amplitude is simply the height of the wave, and for sound, the amplitude would be the maximum pressure, above the normal equilibrium value, produced by the wave. The **period** of the wave is defined as the time it takes to complete one oscillation, so:

$$f = \frac{1}{T}$$

5.1 (Learn)

where f is the frequency (the number of cycles per unit time)
    T is the period for one full cycle

Waves can also be described by their **wavelength**, the physical length of one complete cycle. Higher frequency waves have shorter wavelengths than lower frequency waves. The product of a wave's frequency and wavelength gives the velocity of the wave:

$$v = f \cdot \lambda$$

5.2

where λ is the wavelength
    v is the velocity of the wave

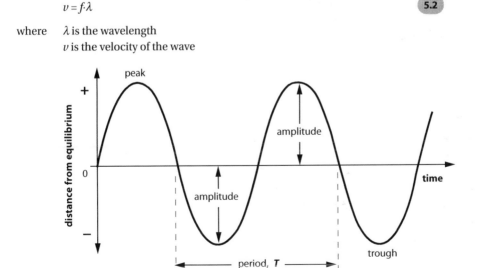

Figure 5.2. *The amplitude and period for a wave.*

5.2 Sound waves

Sound occurs as a series of physical vibrations spreading out from a source. As the wave passes by, the medium experiences changes in pressure. Higher amplitudes are heard as louder sounds and correspond to larger changes from the equilibrium pressure. The molecules are successively bunched together (compressed) and then stretched apart (rarefied), as shown in *Figure 5.3*. Energy is passed on in the form of vibrations that occur in a direction parallel to the direction of propagation. The speed of sound is determined by the density of the medium, and is independent of frequency and amplitude. Generally, the lower the density of the medium, the slower the speed of the sound wave travelling through it. At the extreme, in the near vacuum of outer space, there is silence because there is a lack of a medium to transmit the vibrations of sound. The speed of sound in dry air at sea level is approximately 340 m·s⁻¹, while the speed of sound in water is over four times this value.

Sound can be divided into three sub-categories:
- **ultrasonic** waves with frequencies above the audible range
- **audible** waves that can be detectable by the human ear
- **infrasonic** waves with frequencies below the audible range (as seen in *Figure 5.4*)

Some species of animal can detect a greater range of frequencies, and even within a species the young can generally hear higher frequencies which are inaudible to older subjects. In music, the frequency of a sound wave is referred to as pitch. The A below middle C on the piano keyboard has a frequency of 440 Hz. If the frequency is doubled, the pitch increases by one octave.

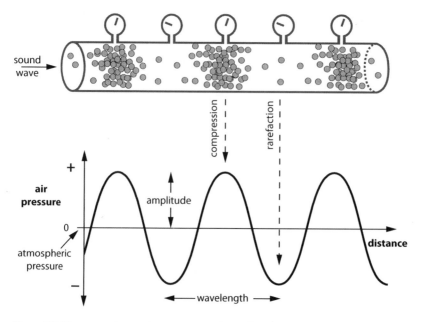

Figure 5.3. *The pressure in sound waves: compression and rarefaction.*

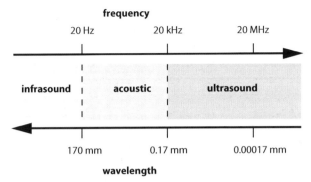

Figure 5.4. *Sound wave spectrum (note that the scale is logarithmic).*

5.3 Electromagnetic waves

Wave behaviour

A light wave is an electromagnetic wave. It manifests as an oscillating electric field and a magnetic field; both perpendicular to the direction of travel and to each other, as shown in *Figure 5.5*. It may be difficult to visualize this, but consider a radio transmitter, essentially an aerial in the form of a vertical wire. The transmitter is operated by applying an alternating current (see *Chapter 18*), so that the electrons in the wire vibrate up and down. Because the electrons have an electric charge, they are surrounded by a tiny electric field that also vibrates up and down. This disturbance spreads

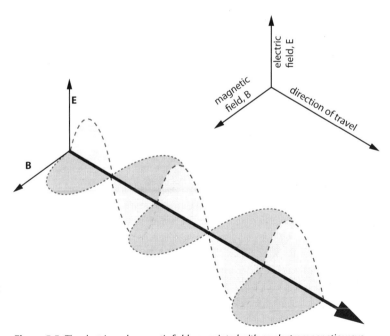

Figure 5.5. *The electric and magnetic fields associated with an electromagnetic wave.*

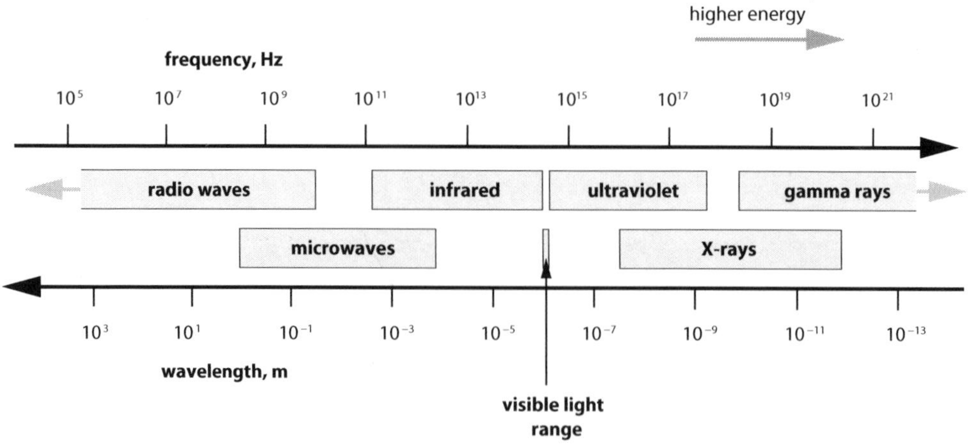

higher energy

frequency, Hz

| 10^5 | 10^7 | 10^9 | 10^{11} | 10^{13} | 10^{15} | 10^{17} | 10^{19} | 10^{21} |

radio waves   infrared   ultraviolet   gamma rays

microwaves   X-rays

| 10^3 | 10^1 | 10^{-1} | 10^{-3} | 10^{-5} | 10^{-7} | 10^{-9} | 10^{-11} | 10^{-13} |

wavelength, m

visible light
range

Figure 5.6. *The electromagnetic spectrum.*

out like ripples on a pond carrying energy away from the source. The magnetic field occurs as a consequence of the principle of induction (*Chapter 19*) which states that a changing electric field induces a magnetic field and vice versa. Unlike sound waves, electromagnetic waves can travel through a vacuum.

The properties and effects of electromagnetic waves vary greatly according to their frequency. *Figure 5.6* shows a diagram of the **electromagnetic spectrum**. At one end of the spectrum waves of the lowest frequency are called radio waves and wavelengths vary from hundreds of metres down to several centimetres. At shorter wavelengths there are microwaves, and then come infrared radiation, visible light and ultraviolet light. At the highest frequencies are X-rays and gamma rays. Different types of electromagnetic radiation have different properties; for example, X-rays can penetrate solid objects much more readily than visible light. There are no definite boundaries between different radiation types and so, for example, short wavelength infrared (near infrared) radiation behaves in a similar way to visible light. Despite their different properties, all electromagnetic waves travel at the same speed, the speed of light, though the speed varies according to the medium's density. However, unlike sound, light travels faster through lower density materials. In glass, for example, the speed of light is roughly two-thirds the value in air.

Photons

Electromagnetic waves behave very much like other types of wave; for example, they can be shown to interfere with each other. In experiments conducted at the beginning of the last century, however, electromagnetic energy was found to behave more like a stream of particles. This behaviour becomes very apparent at high frequencies. Gamma rays are detected as separate bursts of energy, heard as 'clicks' on a Geiger counter. At lower frequencies this particle-like behaviour may be demonstrated using very sensitive detectors and low-intensity sources.

So is electromagnetic radiation really a wave or a particle? When energy is emitted or absorbed by an atom (*Chapter 1*), the interaction is best described in terms of the transfer of a quantum of energy. These quanta or packets of electromagnetic energy are called photons. However, when electromagnetic energy travels through space and interacts with radiation from other sources, it seems to behave more like a wave. So the correct answer is that it is both a wave and a particle.

Electromagnetic waves apparently exist simultaneously as waves and as photons, very small bundles of energy. The energy E carried by a photon is directly proportional to the wave's frequency:

$$E = h \cdot f$$

5.3

where f is the frequency of the wave
       h is Planck's constant (6.6×10^{-34} m²·kg·s⁻¹)

  Visible light photons each carry a tiny amount of energy; around 10^{-20} joules. A huge number of photons are thus emitted from even the dimmest light source. Gamma ray and X-ray photons, however, have such a high energy that when they impact on objects they can knock out electrons from atoms and molecules, which is why this radiation is known as **ionizing** electromagnetic radiation.

Polarization

Imagine trying to throw a frisbee through iron railings: unless it enters exactly parallel to the iron bars the frisbee will simply bounce off the rails. The railings act as a filter, not letting through any frisbees that are not parallel to the rails. Similarly, **plane-polarized** light is light that has its electric field oscillating in one direction only. The associated magnetic field is as always

> **Definition**
>
> **Polarization:** plane-polarized light consists of waves that have associated electric fields all in the same plane.

perpendicular to the electric field and both fields are, of course, perpendicular to the direction of travel. Vertically polarized light, for example, has a vertical electric field and a horizontal magnetic field. Non-polarized light consists of waves whose electric and magnetic fields are in random orientations perpendicular to the direction of travel. Note that sound waves cannot be polarized because they are longitudinal waves and only oscillate in the direction the wave is moving.

  Like the vertical iron railings, a polarizing filter only lets through the component of light that is in one particular plane of polarization. Rotating the filter causes the plane to change; for example, moving the filter through 90° would change the polarization of the emerging light by the same angle. Two polarizing filters will block all light if their planes of polarization are at 90° to each other, as shown in *Figure 5.7* – you may have noticed this if you have ever tried to look at a petrol pump read-out while wearing sunglasses.

Unpolarized light

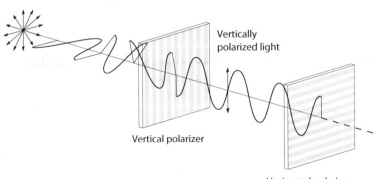

Vertically polarized light

Vertical polarizer

Horizontal polarizer

Figure 5.7. *Unpolarized light is vertically polarized by a vertical polarizing filter. This light is then blocked by a second polarizer orientated at 90° to the first.*

Polarized sunglasses have a polarizing coating, so let through roughly 50% of light. They also have the desirable property of reducing glare from reflected light. This is because light reflecting off a surface such as snow or water will tend to be horizontally polarized, so skiers find polarizing goggles to be very effective. Fishermen also wear sunglasses with a polarizing coating as the water's reflection is blocked, making the water appear more transparent and thus revealing the fish close to the water's surface. Paparazzi use polarizing filters on their camera lenses to snap pictures of celebrities through glass car windscreens.

Constructive and destructive interference

When two waves are superimposed upon one another the waves add together. The wave that emerges is dependent on the relative timing, or **phase**, of the two waves. The phase relates to the point in the cycle one wave is relative to another. If the waves are in phase, i.e. the oscillations are in time with each other, then the resultant wave is bigger. This is known as constructive interference and is shown in *Figure 5.8*. Conversely, if one wave starts its cycle when the other wave is halfway through, then the waves are said to be in **anti-phase**, or are 180° out of phase. The resultant wave becomes smaller; this is destructive interference. This constructive or destructive interference is known as the superposition of waves. For constructive interference the combined wave has the amplitude of the sum of the combining waves. In destructive interference the resultant amplitude of the wave is the difference between the amplitudes of the two waves, so if both waves have equal amplitude they cancel one another out.

Noise-cancelling earphones provide a practical demonstration of destructive interference. A tiny microphone on the outside of each earphone sends the ambient sound signal to an electronic circuit, which 'flips' the signal so it is effectively 180° out of phase with the incoming sound. This signal is

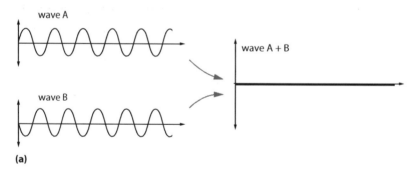

(a)

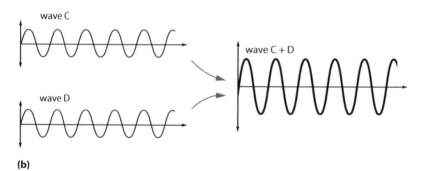

(b)

Figure 5.8. *Destructive interference (a) and constructive interference (b).*

amplified and immediately played back to the listener at just the right amplitude to cause almost complete destructive interference with the unwanted sound. When listening to music, the noise-cancelling signal is added to the musical signal so the listener hears nothing but uninterrupted music.

5.4 Simple harmonic motion

Imagine a child on a swing. Before the first push the swing is as close to the ground as possible, the swing is at equilibrium (or in its natural state) – this is the fixed point. At any point whilst swinging the distance between where the swing is and the equilibrium or fixed point is called the displacement. Simple harmonic motion is characterized by periodic oscillation about the equilibrium position and each oscillation is one cycle.

> **Definition**
>
> **Simple harmonic motion:** occurs when the acceleration of an object is proportional and in opposition to its displacement from the equilibrium position.

Simple harmonic motion describes a motion that repeats over and over again and the time taken to execute one cycle, the period, is constant. The relationship between the mass and time vary in a **sinusoidal** fashion. The graph plotting time against displacement from the equilibrium forms a sine wave, as shown in *Figure 5.9*. Simple harmonic motion may be observed in many everyday phenomena: a swinging pendulum, the vibrating prongs of a tuning fork, a mass bobbing up and down on a spring, or a loudspeaker vibrating.

When a mass oscillates with simple harmonic motion, a force acts on the mass, accelerating the mass back to its original position. For true simple harmonic motion to occur, this force must be proportional to the displacement from equilibrium, so at the equilibrium position there is no force, but the further the mass travels, the greater the force. In the example of the child on the swing the force is provided by gravity, and in the case of the mass on the spring the force is provided by the elasticity of the spring.

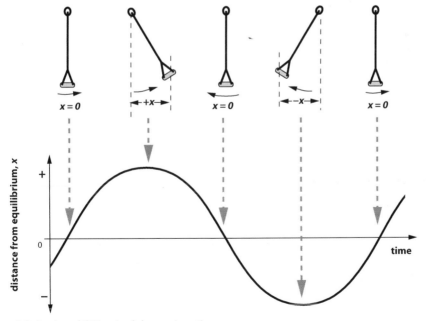

Figure 5.9. *A swing exhibiting simple harmonic motion.*

The frequency of the oscillation is dependent on the amount of acceleration acting for a given displacement. Returning to the mass on the spring, the smaller the mass, the higher the frequency because at any given displacement the force of the spring will accelerate the mass more easily. A higher **spring constant**, i.e. a stiffer spring, will also increase frequency because the accelerating force will be greater throughout the cycle. In the case of the pendulum, mass has no effect since the acceleration due to gravity is the same for all objects. Amplitude also does not affect the frequency; however, the length of the pendulum does affect frequency (a fact proved by Galileo in 1602), with the period being proportional to the square root of the pendulum length.

5.5 Resonance and damping

Resonance

Definitions
Resonance: the natural tendency to oscillate. **Natural/resonant frequency:** a frequency that can exist without any driving source.

When pushing a child on a swing the maximum return for effort is realized if the parent's push is well timed. A series of ill-timed pushes would ensure that the child would still move to and fro but with a much reduced amplitude. If the force applied is in time with the **natural frequency** of the swing then the maximum amplitude is gained for the effort put into each push – this effect is known as **resonance**.

Objects that tend to vibrate or oscillate need less energy to vibrate at their resonant frequencies and conversely more effort is needed to make them oscillate at other frequencies. Many musical instruments rely on resonance to produce sound: a violinist makes a violin string resonate at its natural frequency by creating a vibration in the string using the bow, and wind instruments make use of resonating columns of air to produce sound.

Of course, not all resonance is a good thing. For example, a bridge must not resonate in response to wind-induced oscillatory forces. Failure to prevent this can result in a bridge resonating at low frequency, causing alarming swinging and in severe cases breaking up. London's Millennium footbridge spanning the Thames swayed at a resonant frequency generated by multiple pedestrians' footsteps. Fitting strategically placed dampers to the bridge eventually cured the 'Millennium Wobble'.

Damping

Definition
Damping: the tendency to resist oscillation.

A car has suspension which makes the ride comfortable whilst still allowing the car to be driven safely. The use of springs for the suspension created a problem: what was there to stop the car just bouncing up and down like a child on a trampoline? This solution was shock absorbers: they act to **damp** the oscillation of the springs. Damping is a crucial consideration in equipment design. *Figure 5.10* shows a graph of displacement against time for a general damped oscillator.

Critical damping is an important element in equipment design. In the example of the car, heavy damping would cause the system to very slowly return to equilibrium after a bump in the road, rendering the suspension ineffective, whereas light damping would cause an extremely bouncy ride. Oscillations can occur in some unexpected places, an important medical example being an arterial blood pressure catheter and transducer. The transducer diaphragm has a tendency to oscillate, while friction in the catheter produces damping. Too much or too little damping will produce distortion of the recorded waveform, and errors in blood pressure measurement. This phenomenon is described in more detail in *Section 6.8*.

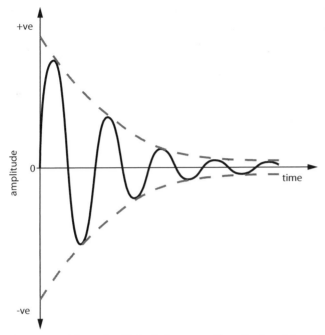

Figure 5.10. *A damped oscillation is characterized by a vibration of decreasing amplitude.*

5.6 Harmonic series and Fourier analysis

Harmonic series

Consider again the violinist. Drawing the bow across the string causes resonance of the string at the natural frequency. Because the string is fixed at each end, this fundamental vibration has two points where there is no vibration, known as nodes. A beginner often creates screeching sounds by unskilfully bowing the string in such a way that only higher harmonic vibrations occur, as shown in *Figure 5.11*; each harmonic has one extra node, with nodes distributed equally along the string. Even when played correctly the string also vibrates at these higher

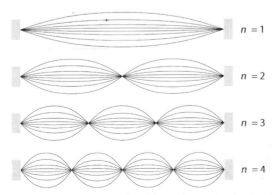

Figure 5.11. *First (n = 1) to fourth (n = 4) harmonics of a vibrating string.*

frequencies. In fact the tone, or *timbre,* of the violin is characterized by the fundamental note overlaid with overtones of decreasing amplitude, known as a harmonic series. The lowest frequency wave in the series is called the fundamental frequency, *f,* and all the other waves in the series have a frequency which is an exact multiple of the fundamental frequency, e.g. 2*f,* 3*f,* ... etc. Most oscillators have a tendency to resonate at several frequencies, the higher frequencies being harmonics (whole number multiples) of the lowest resonant frequency. String instruments tend to have a rich sound due to the presence of many higher harmonic overtones. Wind instruments such as organ pipes are essentially resonating columns of air and their hollow sound is due to the presence of mostly odd-numbered harmonics in their overall sound.

Fourier analysis

Definition
Fourier analysis: a mathematical method for analysing a periodic waveform to find its component frequencies.

Fourier analysis is a commonly used method of analysing a periodic waveform and so is very useful for application to biological signals such as blood pressure or ECG signals. Joseph Fourier, an exceptional mathematician, developed a method of mathematically manipulating periodic waveforms. If a simple fundamental vibration or wave can be represented by a sine wave, then any periodic waveform, regardless of its shape, could be replicated by adding together a series of sine (and cosine) waves of different amplitudes and frequencies. In other words, any periodic wave can be thought of as a harmonic series and separated into a series of sine and cosine waves. The difference in amplitudes of each wave in the series defines the shape of the initial waveform.

Fourier analysis allows complex waves to be analysed, often with surprisingly simple results: very few sine and cosine waves need to be combined to create a reasonably accurate model of most waveforms. Fourier analysis is a useful tool for studying biological signals: arterial blood pressure, ECG and EEG are all periodic waveforms. An aortic pressure wave can normally be represented with 95% accuracy by just four sine waves, and adding higher harmonics increases the accuracy of the Fourier approximation still further. *Figure 5.12* shows an aortic pressure waveform approximated by combining two sine waves of appropriate frequency, amplitude and phase.

Because complex calculations are needed, Fourier analysis is usually performed using a computer. The result of the analysis is a spectrum of frequencies, i.e. a plot of amplitude against frequency, as shown in *Figure 5.13*. The aortic waveform produces a Fourier spectrum with a large peak at the cardiac frequency (75 b.p.m. = 1.25 Hz) with higher harmonics at 2.5 Hz and 3.75 Hz, each

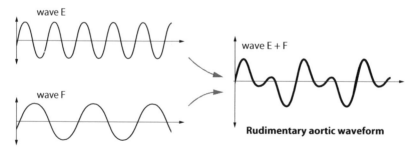

Figure 5.12. *Fourier analysis: two sine waves combining to produce a rudimentary aortic pressure waveform.*

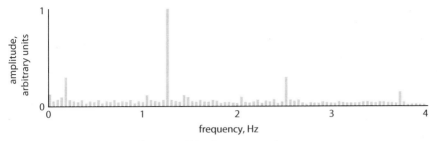

Figure 5.13. *Fourier spectrum of an arterial blood pressure waveform.*

with diminishing amplitude. In ventilated patients a respiratory modulation at 0.15 Hz also appears, revealing that blood pressure is affected by respiration.

5.7 The Doppler effect

The Doppler effect was first described by Christian Doppler in 1842 and is commonly observed in everyday life. For example, when travelling on a train past a stationary sound source, the pitch (frequency) of the sound rises when approaching the source, and falls when moving away. The observer encounters wave fronts more frequently when approaching the source because they are travelling relative to the sound waves.

The Doppler effect may also be observed from a moving source by a stationary observer, such as the siren of a passing ambulance. The velocity of sound does not change relative to the observer; however, the wave fronts are 'bunched up' in front of the source and 'stretched out' behind as shown in *Figure 5.14*.

The Doppler effect may be used for measurement of velocity. Police use radar (radio waves) and measure the Doppler shift (Δf, the difference between the source frequency and the detected radiation reflected from the car) to catch speeding drivers. The moving object reflects the radiation from the source, and acts as a source itself. The radiation is reflected at the frequency 'seen' by the moving object. This is again Doppler-shifted because the source is moving relative to the observer. The observer thus detects a double Doppler shift. The fractional Doppler shift is equal to:

$$\frac{\Delta f}{f} = \frac{2v\cos\theta}{c} \qquad \text{5.4}$$

so

$$v = \frac{\Delta fc}{2f\cos\theta} \qquad \text{5.5}$$

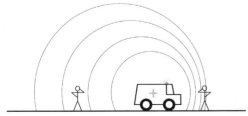

Figure 5.14. *The Doppler effect as a speeding ambulance passes by stationary observers.*

where θ is the angle between the direction of motion and the detector
         v is the velocity
         c is the speed of the waves (i.e. the speed of light)

Astronomers observe the Doppler effect in 'red-shifted' light from distant galaxies which are moving away at very high velocities due to expansion of the Universe. In medicine, the Doppler effect is widely applied to the measurement of blood flow using ultrasound as well as laser light. These techniques are discussed in detail in *Chapters 6* and *23*.

5.8 Flux, intensity and luminance

A cardiac surgeon complaining about inadequate theatre lighting is a well-known phenomenon. What is less well known is how lighting levels are quantified. The humble candle was the first measure of brightness or luminance and the first standardized unit was known as a Candle or candlepower. It was taken from a candle made of a specific kind of wax derived from sperm whales. The modern equivalent is the candela, the unit of luminous intensity, and it is one of the seven SI base units.

A light source, like any other energy source, emits energy. A light bulb emits energy over a wide range of frequencies, so it appears to be approximately white. The energy emitted by a laser, on the other hand, is concentrated over a very narrow frequency range; in fact a laser is usually considered a monochromatic source, i.e. emits only a single wavelength.

The output power (or **radiant flux**) of a light source is simply the number of joules of energy emitted each second and is expressed in watts. The **intensity** (or **irradiance**) describes how much energy falls on a surface and is measured in watts per square metre. Light from a bulb is emitted roughly equally in all directions so the intensity decreases with increasing distance, as shown in *Figure 5.15*. The total power is spread over the surface of a sphere, so the intensity I at a distance r from the source is related to the output power by the following equation:

$$I = \frac{P}{4 \cdot \pi \cdot r^2}$$

5.6

where P is the radiant flux
         r is the distance from the source

The field of science associated with the measurement of visible light as perceived by human eyes is known as photometry. The perception of brightness has a complex relationship with measured levels of intensity, since the eye is more sensitive to certain wavelengths. The bright-

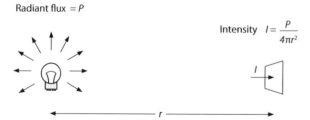

Radiant flux $= P$

Intensity $I = \dfrac{P}{4\pi r^2}$

Figure 5.15. *The intensity is the amount of radiant power passing through unit area and decreases with the square of distance r from the source.*

adapted eye is most sensitive to light of an approximate wavelength of 555 nanometres, i.e. in the yellow–green part of the spectrum. As a result, a blue light looks dimmer than a yellow light of the same radiant flux.

Special units have been devised to account for the eye's sensitivity profile. The **luminance** (or luminous intensity) is equal to the intensity multiplied by a weighting function called the **luminosity function**. The units of luminance are candelas per square metre (cd·m^{-2}). The **luminant flux** is equal to the total radiated power, adjusted for the eye's sensitivity in the same way, and is expressed in candela (cd). As a result of the luminosity function, a yellow light has a greater luminant flux than a blue light of the same power (radiant flux).

Summary

- Sound waves are longitudinal waves comprising periodic compressions and rarefactions of air.
- Electromagnetic waves are transverse waves capable of propagating through a vacuum.
- The frequency of a wave is inversely proportional to its wavelength.
- Waves in phase undergo constructive interference, while waves in anti-phase tend to cancel each other out.
- All electromagnetic waves travel at the speed of light and exhibit wave-like and particle-like behaviour.
- The characteristic sound of musical instruments depends on the frequencies present in their sound; each produces a harmonic series.
- Fourier analysis produces a frequency spectrum of a periodic waveform.
- Sound waves heard from a moving source are detected with a frequency shift by a stationary observer, due to the Doppler effect.
- The intensity of a light source depends on the radiant flux and is proportional to the inverse square of the distance from the source.
- The luminance of a light source depends on the wavelength-dependent sensitivity of the human eye.

Single best answer questions

For each of these questions, only one option is correct.

1. In water, compared to air:
    (a) the speed of sound and the speed of light are both slower
    (b) the speed of sound is slower and the speed of light is the same
    (c) the speed of sound is slower and the speed of light is faster
    (d) the speed of sound is faster and the speed of light is slower
    (e) the speed of sound and the speed of light are both faster

2. The Doppler effect has what effect on the sound waves from a moving source observed by a stationary observer?
    (a) Change in frequency, wavelength and velocity.
    (b) Change in frequency and wavelength.
    (c) Change in velocity and wavelength.
    (d) Change in velocity and frequency.
    (e) Change in frequency only.

3. What is the ratio of the frequency of two
   pendulums if the ratio of their lengths is 1:2?
   (a) 1:2
   (b) 1:1.41
   (c) 1:0.71
   (d) 0.71:1
   (e) 1.41:1

4. How many nodes does a string vibrating at the
   nth harmonic have?
   (a) n
   (b) $n+1$
   (c) $n-1$
   (d) $2n$
   (e) $n/2$

5. Calculate the approximate luminance measured
   at a distance of 2.5 m from a spherical light source
   of total luminant flux of 25 candelas.
   (a) 0.32 cd·m^{-2}
   (b) 0.64 cd·m^{-2}
   (c) 3.2 cd·m^{-2}
   (d) 6.4 cd·m^{-2}
   (e) 8.0 cd·m^{-2}

Multiple choice questions

For each of these questions, more than one option may be correct.

1. Two identical light bulbs of equal power are
   viewed at distances of 1 m and 4 m. Which are
   true?
   (a) The flux is the same but the intensity
       different.
   (b) The flux is the same but the luminance
       different.
   (c) The intensity is the same but the flux
       different.
   (d) The luminant flux is the same but the
       luminance is different.
   (e) The luminance is the same but the luminant
       flux is different.

2. X-ray photons compared to ultra-violet photons:
   (a) have more energetic photons
   (b) have the same properties
   (c) are more ionizing
   (d) have a higher velocity
   (e) have a lower frequency

3. Which of the following statements are true?
   (a) Light reflected from a flat surface is
       polarized.
   (b) Sound waves passing through vertical metal
       bars are vertically polarized.
   (c) Horizontally polarized light passing
       through a vertical polarizer has its plane of
       polarization rotated by 90°.
   (d) All light is either vertically or horizontally
       polarized.
   (e) Vertically polarized light has a horizontally
       polarized magnetic field component.

4. Which of the following groups are in order of
   increasing frequency?
   (a) Gamma rays, visible light, infrared.
   (b) Visible light, X-rays, gamma rays.
   (c) Radio waves, microwaves, infrared.
   (d) Infrared, X-rays, ultraviolet.
   (e) Red light, green light, yellow light.

5. Which is true of simple harmonic motion?
   (a) Acceleration is proportional to
       displacement.
   (b) Velocity is proportional to displacement.
   (c) Velocity is zero at maximum displacement.
   (d) Frequency is affected by the
       force:displacement ratio.
   (e) Frequency is affected by maximum
       displacement.

Chapter 6
Pressure measurement

Having read this chapter you will be able to:

- Define pressure in terms of force and area.
- Understand the concepts of gauge and absolute pressure.
- Explain the origins and significance of Korotkoff's sounds.
- Apply Pascal's principle to comprehend the importance of the levelling of the pressure transducer.
- Appreciate the siphon effect applied to infusions.
- Understand the workings of basic gas valves in clinical use.

6.1 Absolute and relative pressure

A gas in a box contains many millions of molecules zipping around in all directions, bouncing off one another and also bouncing off the walls of the box. The combined effect of the collisions with the walls of the box (see *Figure. 6.1*) creates the effect known as

> **Definition**
>
> **Pressure:** the force acting per unit of area.

pressure. Pressure is simply the force of these collisions acting on a given area and is standardized as force per *unit* area.

The lowest possible pressure is a vacuum, i.e. zero pressure. This would occur if there were no molecules present to bounce off the walls. A true vacuum is extremely difficult to create; the nearest nature comes to a true vacuum is deep space, where there are just one or two gas molecules per cubic metre.

We live and breathe at the bottom of a huge volume of air and we experience a pressure from the weight of the air above us. As a mountaineer climbs higher and higher, the pressure gradually drops because there is less weight of air above to create a pressure. Atmospheric pressure or barometric pressure refers to the pressure of the air, and is dependent on altitude as well as the weather.

> **Clinical example**
>
> *Pressurizing a plane's cabin*
> When a commercial airliner takes off, it quickly climbs to an altitude of approximately 11 000 m. Outside of the aircraft the partial pressure of oxygen in the atmosphere is too low for adequate oxygenation of blood in the pulmonary capillaries. To counter this, the aircraft cabin zone is pressurized, but only to approximately three-quarters of the pressure at sea level, reducing stress on the aircraft body. Air travellers with severe chronic respiratory disease who can only just adequately oxygenate at sea level may require supplemental oxygen to fly.

Pressure can be recorded in two ways, as an **absolute** pressure with a vacuum being the zero point, or as **relative** pressure (also known as **gauge** pressure) where a reference pressure is nominated as the zero point:

$$\text{gauge pressure} = \text{absolute pressure} - \text{reference pressure}$$

6.1

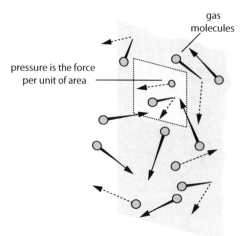

gas
molecules

pressure is the force
per unit of area

Figure 6.1. *Pressure generated by gas molecules on a wall. The pressure is the combined force of the impact of gas molecules repeatedly bouncing off the wall.*

Absolute pressure cannot have a negative value because the zero point has been set at the absolute minimum pressure can be. Gauge pressure can have a negative value if the measured pressure is less than the reference pressure.

Definitions
Absolute pressure: gives a *true* pressure, where zero is the pressure of a vacuum with no molecules being present to generate a pressure. **Gauge pressure:** this is a *relative* pressure taking the zero point of the scale as a convenient reference pressure.

Gauge pressures are almost always used in the clinical setting with the reference point for zero usually set as the atmospheric pressure. Once the reference pressure is chosen, all pressure is stated relative to this pressure level. Blood pressure is therefore measured relative to atmospheric pressure. If the systolic pressure (gauge) is 120 mmHg and the value of atmospheric pressure at sea level is 760 mmHg, the absolute systolic blood pressure at sea level is 120 + 760 = 880 mmHg.

The SI unit for pressure is the pascal (Pa), but kPa is often more convenient to use (1 kPa = 1000 Pa). Atmospheric pressure at sea level has the following values:

101.3 kPa = 760 mmHg = 1033 cmH_2O = 1 atm

There is a dizzying array of units applied to pressure, both in medicine and in other applications (*Table 6.1* lists those used most commonly).

Table 6.1. *Units of pressure.*

Name (abbreviation)	Equivalent value in kPa	Example application
Kilopascal (kPa)	1	Gas partial pressure
Millimetres of mercury (mmHg)	0.1333	Blood pressure
Atmosphere (atm)	101.3	Scuba divers' tank pressure
Bar (Bar)	100	Cylinder pressure
Millibar (mbar)	0.1	Meteorology
Centimetres of water (cmH_2O)	0.09807	Airway pressures
Pounds per square inch (psi)	6.895	Tyre pressures

Worked example

Question
A central venous pressure (CVP) is measured via a pressure transducer and the pressure displayed as 0.4 kPa (kilopascals). What would the pressure be in cmH₂O (centimetres of water)?

Key points
- From *Table 6.1*: 1 kPa = 10.2 cmH$_2$O because 1 cmH$_2$0 = 0.09807 kPa

Step 1
- CVP = 0.4 × 10.2 = 4.08 cmH$_2$O

Answer
A CVP of 4.1 cmH$_2$O is equivalent to 0.4 kPa.
Note that CVP is often measured in centimetres of water because it was originally measured using a manometer filled with normal saline, prior to the emergence of pressure transducers.

6.2 Simple pressure-measuring devices

The manometer

A manometer compares the pressure of two gases, one being a reference pressure and the other being the sample pressure. At its most simple it consists of a U-shaped tube of glass partially filled with a liquid, as shown in *Figure 6.2*. The columns change height in direct proportion to the pressure difference between the sample and the reference pressures. If both the density of the

Definition

Manometer: an instrument to measure the pressure in a gas by the vertical displacement of a liquid in a tube.

liquid and the reference pressure are known then the pressure applied to the sampling tube can be calculated from the difference in heights of the two adjoining columns. In a manometer, the reference tube is usually open to the atmosphere, so the gauge pressure relative to atmospheric pressure is measured.

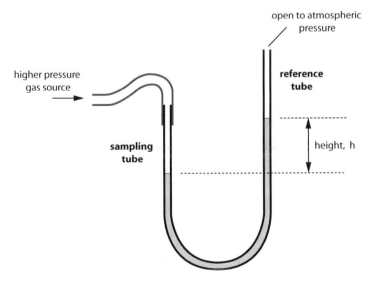

Figure 6.2. *A manometer for measuring gas pressure. The height of elevation of the liquid allows the gas pressure to be measured. The denser the liquid in the tube, the lower the displacement.*

The relationship between height and pressure may be understood by considering the weight (gravitational force) exerted by the column of liquid (*Figure 6.3*). The pressure exerted as a result of a liquid's weight is known as **hydrostatic pressure**.

Pressure is equal to force divided by area (see *Chapter 2*):

$$P = \frac{F}{A}$$

6.2

The force of gravity is mass, *m*, times acceleration due to gravity, *g*:

$$P = \frac{m \cdot g}{A}$$

6.3

The mass of the column is the density times the volume (area × height):

$$P = \frac{(\rho \cdot A \cdot h) \cdot g}{A}$$

6.4

The measured gauge pressure *P* is therefore related to the manometer height, *h*, by the following equation:

$$P = \rho \cdot g \cdot h$$

6.5

where ρ is the liquid density

g is acceleration due to gravity ($9.81 \ \mathrm{m \cdot s^{-1}}$)

The density of the liquid used in the manometer determines the sensitivity of the manometer. A liquid of low density delivers greater accuracy whereas a liquid of higher density allows for a more compact manometer.

Manometer for measuring central venous pressure

A manometer is most commonly used to measure the central venous pressure (CVP) and is configured as shown in *Figure 6.4*.

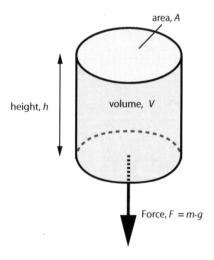

area, *A*

volume, *V*

height, *h*

Force, $F = m \cdot g$

Figure 6.3. *Gravitational force acting on a column of liquid.*

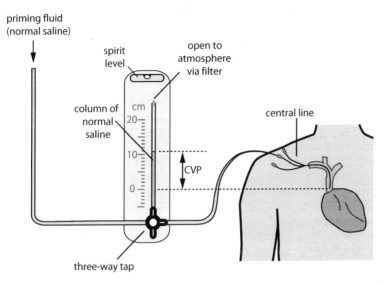

priming fluid
(normal saline)

spirit
level

open to
atmosphere
via filter

column of
normal
saline

cm

20—

10—

0—

CVP

central line

three-way tap

Figure 6.4. *Manometer setup for measuring central venous pressure.*

Bourdon tube gauge

The Bourdon tube measures gauge pressure and it is named after the French industrialist Eugène Bourdon. The 'C'-shaped hollow spring-like tube extends outwards at the sealed end when the pressure within it rises. It gives a comparison of the pressure within the tube to the pressure outside. This is in agreement with Boyle's Law (see *Chapter 9*): as the pressure rises then so does the volume of a gas. When the hollow tube expands or contracts this change is relayed to a pointer that indicates the pressure on a calibrated dial, as shown in *Figure 6.5*.

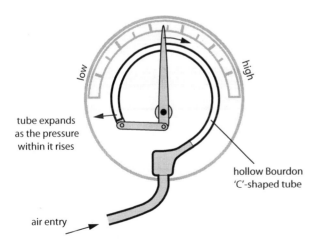

low

high

tube expands
as the pressure
within it rises

hollow Bourdon
'C'-shaped tube

air entry

Figure 6.5. *Bourdon tube gauge.*

The barometer

The traditional barometer (*Figure 6.6*) is a special type of manometer for measurement of atmospheric (or **barometric**) pressure. Unlike a normal manometer, instead of measuring pressure relative to a reference pressure, the barometer measures absolute atmospheric pressure. The reference pressure is a vacuum (zero pressure) formed by a closed tube filled with liquid. Gravity pulls the liquid downward and a gap forms at the top of the closed tube while a reservoir of liquid is exposed directly to atmospheric pressure, which pushes down on the liquid and 'balances' the weight of the liquid in the tube. In other words, atmospheric pressure is equal to the hydrostatic pressure exerted by the mercury, so the height of the liquid is directly proportional to the atmospheric pressure. Mercury is an ideal liquid for this purpose because of its high density.

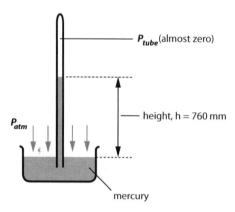

P_{tube} (almost zero)

height, h = 760 mm

P_{atm}

mercury

Figure 6.6. *A mercury barometer. The height of the mercury column is proportional to the atmospheric pressure pushing down on the mercury in the reservoir.*

Worked example

Question
A mercury barometer shows a height of 760 mm at a standard atmospheric pressure. If the liquid in the barometer is changed to water (rather than mercury) how high would the column of fluid be?

Key points
- Density, the mass per unit volume, of water is 1 g·cm⁻³ = 1000 kg·m⁻³
- Atmospheric pressure at sea level is 101.3 kPa = 101 300 Pa.

Step 1
Use Equation 6.5 and convert quantities to SI units:

$$P = \rho \cdot g \cdot h, \text{rewriting}: h = \frac{P}{\rho \cdot g}$$

$$h = \frac{101\,300\,(\text{Pa})}{1000(\text{kg}\cdot\text{m}^{-3}) \cdot 9.81(\text{m}\cdot\text{s}^{-2})} = 10.3\,\text{m}$$

Answer
The height of water that is equivalent to atmospheric pressure is 10.3 m.

Notes
- At a height of 10.3 m for atmospheric pressure the water-filled barometer is too large to be practical.
- Equation 6.5 shows that the pressure is independent of the surface area or the length of the column. Rather than the length of the tube being critical it is the **vertical height** of the column that is directly proportional to pressure.

Worked example

Question
A 2 mL and a 50 mL syringe (see *Figure 6.7*) have the same force applied to depress their plungers: which syringe will deliver the greater pressure?

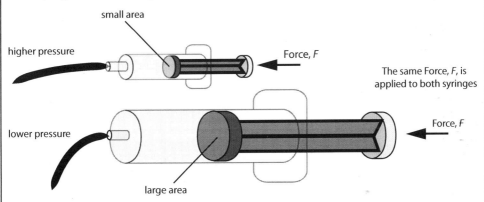

Figure 6.7. *Comparative pressure generated by a 2 mL and 50 mL syringe.*

Key points
- The two syringes (2 mL and 50 mL) have plunger cross-sectional areas of $A_{2\,mL}$ and $A_{50\,mL}$.
- The force, F, is applied equally to both plungers.

Step 1
Pressure is the force per unit area.

$$P_{2\,mL} = \frac{F_{2\,mL}}{A_{2\,mL}} \qquad P_{50\,mL} = \frac{F_{50\,mL}}{A_{50\,mL}}$$

rewritten

$$F_{2\,mL} = P_{2\,mL} \cdot A_{2\,mL} \qquad F_{50\,mL} = P_{50\,mL} \cdot A_{50\,mL}$$

Step 2
The force applied to both plungers is equal so $F_{2\,mL} = F_{50\,mL}$ so from Step 1

$$F = P_{2\,mL} \cdot A_{2\,mL} = P_{50\,mL} \cdot A_{50\,mL}$$

rearranging

$$P_{2\,mL} = P_{50\,mL} \frac{A_{50\,mL}}{A_{2\,mL}}$$

But $A_{2\,mL} < A_{50\,mL}$ dictating that $P_{2\,mL} > P_{50\,mL}$

Answer
The 2 mL syringe generates more pressure than the 50 mL syringe.

6.3 Pressure relief valves

The pressure-relieving valve is sometimes referred to as a safety valve and allows a gas (or a liquid) to be expelled if a certain pressure has been reached. There are several variations on the basic design, but most are based around the simple principle of a spring-loaded diaphragm.

Adjustable pressure limit (APL) relief valve

In this design (*Figure 6.8*) the diaphragm is pushed upwards and reaches a point where gas can escape. The adjustable pressure limit valve allows the 'blow-off' pressure to be altered. This is achieved by turning a screw on top of the valve that either raises or lowers the spring and diaphragm. When the spring is lowered, the spring must be compressed further so greater pressure is needed to raise the diaphragm sufficiently before the gas can escape. It is simple, cheap and adaptable. This type of valve is classed as a 'non-return' valve and has the disadvantage that it does not conserve gas, as the gas is expelled into the surroundings.

From Hooke's law, the spring exerts a force proportional to its compression (see Equation 2.4):

$$F = -k \cdot x$$

Since pressure is force per unit area (Equation 6.2):

$$P \cdot A = -k \cdot -x, \quad \text{rearranging} \quad x = \frac{P \cdot A}{k}$$

6.6

so x is the amount the valve attached to a diaphragm of area A moves under a pressure P.

Note the minus sign on the x which signifies that the pressure acts in the opposite direction to the force of the spring.

(a) Valve closed

(b) Valve open

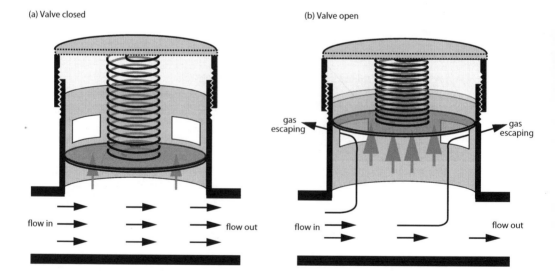

Figure 6.8. *Adjustable pressure limit (APL) relief valve at (a) lower pressure and (b) higher pressure.*

Fixed pressure relief valve

Fixed relief valves are used on equipment such as non-invasive positive pressure support devices. The relief pressure is fixed, so to change this a new valve has to be attached.

6.4 Pressure regulator valves

A pressure-reducing (or regulating) valve, an adaptation of the variable pressure relief valve, is used to supply a flow of gas to an outlet (e.g. a facemask) at a much lower pressure than the supply pressure (e.g. a cylinder). Gas flows out of a chamber below a diaphragm attached to a spring, as shown in *Figure 6.9*. The chamber pressure is maintained by gas from the supply flowing

> **Definition**
>
> **Pressure regulator:** a valve that automatically cuts off the flow of a gas (or liquid) at a certain pressure.

into the chamber through a piston attached to the underside of the diaphragm, but only when the chamber pressure is lower than a preset outlet pressure. Once the chamber pressure reaches the desired pressure, gas pushing upwards on the diaphragm moves the piston upwards, reducing the aperture. The small aperture restricts the flow of gas sufficiently to cause a significant reduction in gas pressure. During use, the piston moves up and down in response to changes in pressure at the patient end to ensure the gas is supplied at a constant pressure. Unlike the pressure-relieving (safety) valve it does not release gas into the surroundings but instead conserves gas.

Pressure regulator of a cylinder (or piped gas)

A pressure regulator in a cylinder ensures that the pressure remains at or below a pressure of 400 kPa. This is crucial as it acts to prevent damage to equipment, potential barotrauma and ventilator variance.

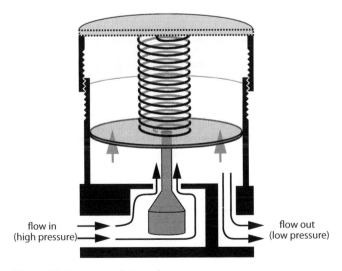

flow in (high pressure)

flow out (low pressure)

Figure 6.9. *A pressure-reducing valve.*

Flow restrictor

Definition
|
| **Flow restrictor:** a flow restrictor drops the pressure in a fluid by the resistance created by a constriction in a pipe.

A flow restrictor acts to reduce the pressure of a gas (or liquid) by a simple constriction in the piping. This is not a particularly sensitive technique because it is dependent on the pressure in the pipeline before the constriction remaining stable – this makes it vulnerable to fluctuations in pressure. It is employed in the gas supply to an anaesthetic machine and is usually situated between the pipeline supply and the anaesthetic machine, lowering gas pressure from the supply pressure of 400 kPa down to a pressure in the range of 100–200 kPa.

Worked example

Question
A company producing CPAP valves have redesigned a 10 cmH$_2$O valve, doubling the area of the diaphragm with the spring remaining unchanged. How might this affect the pressure rating of the valve?

Key points
- The force, F, needed to open the valve is dictated by the spring and this is the same in the redesigned and original valve.
- As the area of the diaphragm is doubled in the new valve then $A_{new} = 2 \cdot A_{old}$
- A valve rated as 10 cmH$_2$O implies that the valve opens (or blows off) when a pressure at, or greater than, 10 cmH$_2$O is applied to it.

Step 1
From Equation 2.3 the pressure needed to open the original valve is related to area and force:

for the old valve
$$F = P_{old} \cdot A_{old}$$

for the new valve
$$F = P_{new} \cdot A_{new}$$

Step 2
As the force is the same to open both valves then from Step 1

$$F = P_{old} \cdot A_{old} = P_{new} \cdot A_{new}$$

Rearranging

$$P_{new} = P_{old} \left(\frac{A_{old}}{A_{new}} \right)$$

Step 3
As $A_{new} = 2 \cdot A_{old}$; the original valve opened at 10 cmH$_2$O, so substituting this into the equation above:

$$P_{new} = \frac{10}{2} = 5\,cmH_2O$$

Answer
The redesigned valve with a diaphragm of twice the surface area of the original now opens at 5 cmH$_2$O, half that of the original.

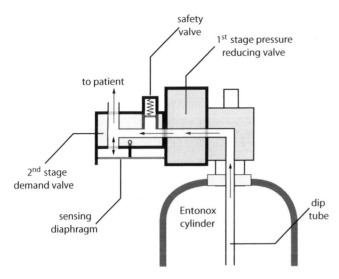

Figure 6.10. *The Entonox valve.*

Two-stage pressure regulator: Entonox

Entonox has a two-valve system to regulate the delivery of the gas; they are both the same design of valve (*Figure 6.10*). Entonox valve = reducing valve + demand valve. There is also a third valve, a pressure-relieving (safety) valve in case of malfunction.

6.5 The siphon effect and air entrainment

The siphon phenomenon (*Figure 6.11*) is, sadly, often used as a method of stealing petrol from a car's petrol tank. A siphon is an inverted 'U'-shaped tube with two arms of unequal length. Liquid can be made to flow 'uphill' powered by the force of liquid falling down the other side. A siphon works because gravity pulling down on the taller column of liquid causes reduced pressure at the top of

> **Definition**
>
> **Siphon effect:** a phenomenon where a liquid from one vessel is drawn off via a tube to another vessel at a lower level.

the siphon. This reduced pressure means gravity pulling down on the shorter column of liquid is not sufficient to keep the liquid stationary. It therefore flows up and over the top of the siphon. Although atmospheric pressure is needed to 'drive' the water upwards, surface tension also plays a part as a siphon has been demonstrated to work in a vacuum, albeit not as effectively.

Consequences of the siphon effect on infusions

There is a potential problem with intravenous infusion held in a glass bottle, such as paracetamol. Because the bottle is not collapsible, a negative pressure is created within the bottle as liquid flows from the bottle into the vein (*Figure 6.12*). Without any form of vent, this negative pressure will soon equilibrate with the pressure in the vein, arresting drug delivery. A vent in the bottle enables air to replace the liquid, so the pressure in the bottle remains at atmospheric pressure, but because of the relatively low pressure of the peripheral venous system, once the bottle is empty, air can continue to infuse down the giving set and into the patient, putting them at risk of an air embolus.

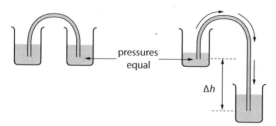

Figure 6.11. *The siphon effect. (a) At equilibrium there is no flow between the beakers. (b) The siphon effect means that the liquid will flow from the higher beaker to the lower one.*

Elevated syringe drivers

Consider a syringe driver that has been positioned at a significant height above the patient delivering an infusion (*Figure 6.12*). The weight of the column of fluid (hydrostatic pressure) has the potential to overcome the friction between a poorly secured plunger and its barrel, so that the syringe could gradually empty. Furthermore, a crack in the syringe, or a loose connection, could result in entrainment of air through the crack as the infusate is siphoned into the patient.

Anti-free-flow mechanism in infusion devices

An infusion device is said to be in free-flow when the infusate flows into the patient under the force of gravity, free of any inhibitions. As a safeguard, the default position of all infusion devices should inhibit the flow of fluid. In practice this means that the default position for the syringe driver has the

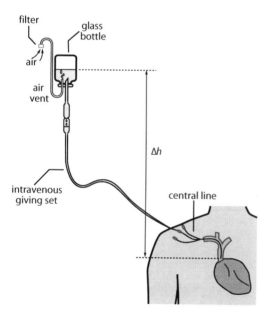

Figure 6.12. *A patient receiving paracetamol intravenously. When the glass bottle is empty, the patient can receive an air embolus.*

arm holding the plunger clamped and the default position for the volumetric pump has the tubing occluded. Anti-siphon valves are used to reduce the risk of free flow, and the insertion of a one-way valve aims to prevent back flow.

6.6 Blood pressure

Blood pressure is created by periodic contractions of the myocardium of the ventricles. This generates sufficient pressure to drive the flow of blood through the circulation. The **mean arterial pressure** (MAP) is not simply the average of the systolic and diastolic pressure, but is the pressure averaged over one cardiac cycle. Because the time spent in diastole is greater than the time spent in systole, the MAP is normally slightly closer to the diastolic pressure than the systolic pressure. Although arterial wave traces vary from patient to patient, a typical example is shown in the graph in *Figure 6.13*.

The shape and size of an arterial waveform is used to calculate several clinical variables including the systolic and diastolic pressures, pulse pressure and MAP. In addition to heart rate, certain arrhythmias are apparent from the waveform shape and size. Other cardiac variables such as myocardial contractility (from the angle of the upstroke) and stroke volume index (from the area under the waveform) can be estimated.

Units

Blood pressure is usually measured in mmHg. Sometimes central venous pressure (CVP) is quoted in traditional units of cmH_2O.

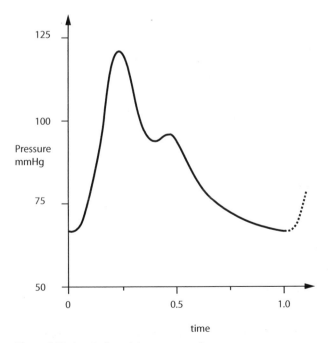

Figure 6.13. *A typical arterial pressure waveform.*

6.7 Non-invasive blood pressure measurement

The auscultatory method and Korotkoff's sounds

Arterial blood pressure can be measured non-invasively with a sphygmomanometer and stethoscope. When a pressure cuff is wrapped around a patient's arm and inflated to a pressure exceeding systolic pressure, the brachial artery is completely occluded and blood flow ceases. As the pressure cuff deflates to below systolic pressure the blood starts to flow through the artery in brief spurts. There is only flow when the pressure generated by the left ventricle is greater than that of the cuff occluding the arm, so each pulse generates a discernable sound because the blood flows in a highly turbulent on–off fashion. These distinct sounds were categorized into five phases by a Russian physician, Nicolai Korotkoff, and can be heard when a stethoscope is placed above the antecubital fossa. The five phases of Korotkoff's sounds are summarized in *Table 6.2*.

Whilst the cuff is deflating, the sounds heard are reflective of the nature of the flow through the artery. In the last phase the diastolic pressure is greater than the cuff pressure and there is no discernible noise as the flow has returned to a stable laminar flow.

The pressure inside the cuff is measured by a sphygmomanometer, which comprises, in addition to the cuff itself, a manometer (either a mechanical Bourdon gauge or a fluid manometer column), an inflating bulb to elevate the cuff pressure, and a deflating valve. The cuff, which should be slightly larger than the diameter of the arm, is inflated to generate a pressure around the arm. The standard adult cuff fits an arm with a circumference of 25–35 cm but other sizes are available. An oversized cuff tends to cause overestimation of blood pressure and vice versa.

Abnormally low and high pressures should be viewed with suspicion, because readings are less reliable at the extremes. Arrhythmias such as atrial fibrillation can distort readings, as can the external pressure from equipment or the surgeon leaning on the inflating cuff. The brachial artery, sphygmomanometer and heart should be on the same horizontal level, otherwise the reading becomes inaccurate. For instance, if blood pressure is taken at head height, the systolic and diastolic pressure readings will be approximately 35 mmHg lower compared to readings taken at heart level, due to differences in hydrostatic pressure in the artery. The inflation and deflation of the cuff rarely harm the patient, but bruising, petechial haemorrhage and ulnar nerve palsy have all been reported.

Table 6.2. *Korotkoff's sounds.*

Phase	Sound	Reason
Phase 1	Clear repetitive tapping	Short bursts of blood flow: systolic pressure
Phase 2	Soft swishing	Low flow of blood
Phase 3	Crisp	Increased blood flow
Phase 4	Thumping/blowing	Occurs at about 10 mmHg above diastolic
Phase 5	Silence	Steady laminar flow resumes: diastolic pressure

Oscillometry

Most non-invasive blood pressure (NIBP) measuring devices are based on the oscillometry technique, first outlined by von Recklinghausen in 1931. His **oscillotonometer** was based on a pair of cuffs: a proximal cuff to occlude the artery and a distal cuff connected to a sensitive pressure gauge. The oscillations caused by blood pulsing under the proximal cuff could be recorded by

> **Definition**
>
> **Oscillometer:** an instrument for measuring the changes in pulsations in the arteries, especially of the extremities.

observing the needle of the gauge. Modern oscillometers are automated electronic systems that can be set to measure the blood pressure at fixed intervals from a single cuff (used for both occlusion and measurement).

When a measurement is required the cuff is inflated by an air pump controlled by a microprocessor. The cuff is slowly deflated through a bleed valve, while a pressure sensor monitors both the cuff pressure and the small oscillations, which begin as soon as the cuff pressure becomes sub-systolic. The maximal amplitude occurs when the cuff pressure is equal to the mean pressure. The oscillations do not disappear at exactly the diastolic pressure, so the diastolic pressure is calculated using the following equation:

$$\text{MAP} \simeq \text{diastolic} + \frac{\text{systolic} - \text{diastolic}}{3}$$

6.7

The pressure is calculated and then shown on a digital display on the front of the monitor. Oscillometric NIBP monitors are not continuous and the frequency of measurement is limited by the measurement time. Most monitors can measure no more often than once every 30 seconds. NIBP monitoring is susceptible to the inaccuracies associated with other cuff-based measurement techniques. Furthermore, NIBP is less accurate than invasive blood pressure monitoring using an arterial catheter (see *Section 6.8*).

Plethysmographic and Penaz volume clamp technique

The Finapres uses the Penaz technique which is similar in basic principle to the oscillometric technique, except that it allows continuous monitoring of blood pressure, i.e. the blood pressure is reported every heartbeat, or at least every few seconds. A small cuff is wrapped around a finger (*Figure 6.14*) and, instead of a pressure sensor, an infrared light-emitting diode and a photo-detector are placed within the cuff. The volume of blood in the arteries may then be monitored;

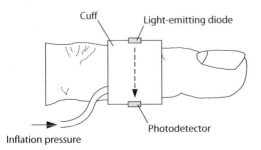

Figure 6.14. *The Penaz technique.*

larger volumes of blood cause greater absorption of light and there is a resulting fall in detected light levels.

A microprocessor-controlled pump inflates the cuff until the mean arterial pressure is reached and this is determined by observing a maximum in the photoplethysmographic pulse signal. The pressure in the cuff is then varied by a rapidly responding feedback system which maintains the volume of blood in the arteries at a constant level. The pressure in the cuff then approximately matches the mean arterial blood pressure.

While the Penaz technique is considered accurate in vasodilated patients and those with normal circulation, it is less accurate in hypotensive patients or those with compromised peripheral blood flow. Small changes in positioning and tightness of the finger cuff can lead to wide variation in readings, even from a single patient. For these reasons, the use of the Penaz technique for blood pressure monitoring is limited in clinical practice.

6.8 Invasive blood pressure monitoring

A direct measurement of blood pressure can be made by connecting an arterial cannula to a pressure transducer via a fluid-filled catheter. Intravascular transducers are now rarely used due to their prohibitive cost and complexity.

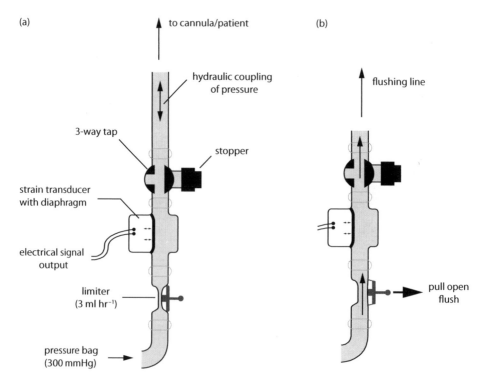

Figure 6.15. *Invasive blood pressure transducer housing. (a) Normal measurement mode. (b) Pulling the flush lever allows a saline (or saline–heparin) bolus to be administered.*

Blood pressure sensors

The sensor elements used for invasive blood pressure measurement in modern clinical systems are usually based on four **strain gauges**: these are thin wafers of semiconductor material bonded to a membrane that is connected to a catheter. The strain gauges are wired together to form a **Wheatstone bridge resistor network** (see *Chapter 18*) which allows measurement of very small variations in pressure. The catheter–sensor system, which is filled with a saline–heparin solution, transmits pressure from the intravascular cannula to the transducer membrane. The transducer should be placed as close to the level of the cannula as possible, to minimize the effect of hydrostatic pressures in the catheter (similarly, the catheter itself should be placed close to the level of the heart). The pressure transducer and catheter are fragile devices with high failure rates so are manufactured as disposable single-use items. This has the added advantage of eliminating the risk of cross-contamination.

The sensor housing is made from clear plastic so that air bubbles are easily seen. Saline (or heparinized saline) flows continuously, at a rate of 3–5 ml per hour, from an intravenous bag through clear IV tubing, past the sensor and out of the tip of the in-dwelling catheter to prevent clotting at the catheter tip. A three-way stopcock between the transducer and the catheter allows sampling of arterial blood from the catheter. After sampling, a lever can open or close the flush valve for rapid flushing of the catheter, as shown in *Figure 6.15*. The electrical connection to the silicon chip is isolated from the saline by a compliant silicone elastomer gel. This allows the pressure to be transmitted from the liquid to the chip, but prevents electric shock from the sensor to the patient. It also prevents the high currents that occur during defibrillation from destroying the chip.

Zeroing the sensor

The sensors are manufactured to have a similar response (i.e. the voltage across the Wheatstone bridge network changes by the same amount for a given pressure rise, for different sensors). However, the 'zero pressure' resistance can differ by a large amount. Before use the sensor is zeroed by turning the stopcock adjacent to the chip so that there is nothing but liquid between the chip and the air (see *Figure 6.16*). The chip is then recording the atmospheric pressure, which is taken as zero. A control

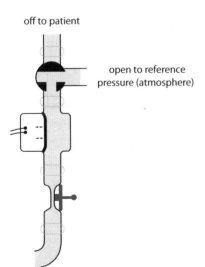

off to patient

open to reference
pressure (atmosphere)

Figure 6.16. *To zero the transducer, the 3-way tap is turned so that the transducer senses atmospheric pressure.*

on the monitor is activated to indicate that the sensor is 'open to air' and the BP reading is zeroed. The stopcock is then returned to its original position ('open to patient').

Blood pressure, like all pressures in the body, is measured as a gauge pressure relative to atmospheric pressure. When a pressure transducer is set to zero it is simply defining the reference point for the gauge pressure as atmospheric pressure; that is why the transducer is open to room air whilst 'zeroing'. Finally, there is no reason to 're-zero' if the vertical height of the transducer is altered: pressure does decrease with altitude; however, it does so very gradually and the difference in atmospheric pressure between the floor and the ceiling of any ward or theatre is negligible.

Distortion of blood pressure waveform

Accurate measurements of blood pressure are important in clinical measurement and physiological research. The physical properties of a blood pressure catheter and sensor can cause distortion of the measured waveform; in other words the recorded pressure waveform does not exactly match the true pressure at all times during the cardiac cycle.

Dynamic changes in the blood pressure in the artery are transmitted by small movements of the saline in the catheter and these cause the movement of the pressure sensor diaphragm. The diaphragm itself is a springy mechanical system with a certain mass and has a tendency to oscillate at its natural frequency, just like a mass on a spring. There is a certain amount of damping of this oscillation caused by resistance to fluid flow and inertia of the liquid. Too much, or too little damping causes distortion as follows.

- If there is too little damping (the under-damped case), oscillation of the sensor diaphragm appears as high-frequency waves superimposed on the pressure signal. This can cause overestimation of systolic pressure (and overestimation of the diastolic pressure) as shown in *Figure 6.17*. The effect on the mean measured blood pressure is not as great.
- In the over-damped case, the sensor response is sluggish, so the blood pressure waveform is excessively smoothed and attenuated, leading to underestimation of systolic pressure (and overestimation of diastolic pressure) and potentially serious clinical error. Over-damping can occur if the catheter is too long (as resistance and inertia of the saline is proportional to the catheter length) or too thin (as resistance will be higher). An air bubble in the catheter can also lead to a dramatic increase in damping. Since the air bubble is compressible, some of the pressure change is absorbed and not transmitted along the catheter, resulting in a smoothing of the pressure waveform.

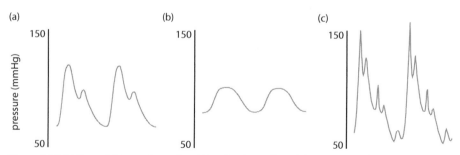

Figure 6.17. *(a) Normal, (b) over-damped and (c) under-damped arterial pressure waveforms.*

Blood pressure transducer and catheter systems are designed to be 'critically damped' to produce the best possible reproduction of the blood pressure signal on the monitor screen.

Summary

- Gauge pressure is the difference between absolute pressure and a reference pressure.
- Blood pressure and other pressures in the body are always measured relative to atmospheric pressure.
- Manometers and Bourdon gauges are simple devices for measuring gauge pressure.
- A barometer is a specific type of manometer for measurement of atmospheric pressure.
- Pressure-regulating valves are constructed from spring-loaded diaphragms and have been designed in various configurations for use in a range of applications.
- Non-invasive blood pressure measurement techniques include oscillometry and the Penaz technique.
- Fluid-filled catheters and transducers can cause distortion of arterial pressure waveforms unless critically damped.

Single best answer questions

For each of these questions, only one option is correct.

1. What is the primary reason for the pressure transducer being at the level of the right atrium when measuring central venous pressure?
   (a) To avoid interference from the arterial pressure.
   (b) To avoid erroneous readings from hydrostatic pressure in the tubing.
   (c) The atmospheric pressure in the room changes significantly with height.
   (d) There is less distortion from pulsation in the heart's chambers.
   (e) Electrical interference from pacemakers is minimized with correct levelling.

2. Which one of the following could be responsible for excessive damping?
   (a) Short tubing from the cannula to the transducer.
   (b) Large radius tubing leading to the transducer.
   (c) Small gauge cannula inserted.
   (d) Repeated flushing of lines.
   (e) Priming that avoids bubbles in the circuit.

3. Which one of the following is true of the Penaz technique?
   (a) The cuff exerts a constant pressure.
   (b) It utilizes a red light source and photodetector.
   (c) It reports blood pressure every 30 seconds.
   (d) It has poor accuracy in hypertensive patients.
   (e) It records mean blood pressure.

4. Which one of the following statements is true?
   (a) Hydrostatic pressure in the short arm is greater than in the long arm.
   (b) Atmospheric pressure drives the liquid up the short arm.
   (c) The siphon can be any length, as long as the receiving vessel is lower than the supplying vessel.
   (d) Surface tension is needed to pull the liquid up the short arm.
   (e) The siphon will work just as effectively in a vacuum.

Multiple choice questions

For each of these questions, more than one option may be correct.

1. The pressure exerted by a spring-loaded diaphragm in a pressure relief valve is proportional to:
   (a) extension
   (b) surface area
   (c) spring constant
   (d) inverse of spring constant
   (e) inverse of extension

2. Which of the following could result from careless positioning of the three-way tap on a pressure transducer housing?
   (a) Exsanguination of the patient.
   (b) Reported blood pressure of zero.
   (c) Damped waveform.
   (d) Excessive delivery of saline–heparin solution to the patient.
   (e) Entrainment of air into an artery.

3. Which are equal to atmospheric pressure at sea level?
   (a) 760 mmHg
   (b) 103.1 kPa
   (c) 1000 mBar
   (d) 1033 cmH$_2$O
   (e) 7.5 psi

4. A mercury barometer is measuring a rising barometric pressure. Which of the following statements are true?
   (a) The length of the mercury column decreases.
   (b) The pressure at the closed ends of the tube falls.
   (c) The hydrostatic pressure of the mercury increases.
   (d) The hydrostatic pressure of the mercury balances the pressure on the reservoir.
   (e) The temperature has no effect on the length of the column.

Chapter 7
Humidity

Having read this chapter you will be able to:
- Define humidity.
- Describe the difference between absolute and relative humidity.
- Appreciate how water vapour affects gas composition in the respiratory tract.
- Understand the importance of humidification in anaesthesia.
- Understand the equipment used to measure and humidify gas mixtures.

7.1 Water vapour content of air

Humidity is simply the amount of water vapour present in the air; it plays a crucial role in the earth's hydrologic cycle, acting as a reservoir for about 1% of the earth's total water content. The presence of water in our atmosphere and its physical interaction with the environment gives rise to many familiar and observable phenomena, from clouds to the sweat that keeps us cool.

> **Definition**
>
> **Saturated vapour pressure:** the saturated vapour pressure of a liquid is the maximum pressure exerted by the evaporated molecules above the liquid at equilibrium.

Understanding how the atmospheric composition of gaseous water varies with temperature and pressure is fundamental to how we measure humidity. At any given temperature there is a maximum amount of water that can be held in gaseous form; this is the **saturated vapour pressure** and varies in a familiar fashion with temperature (see *Figure 7.1*) – the higher the temperature, the greater the vapour pressure.

From *Figure 7.1* it could be deduced that warm air has a greater capacity for holding water than cold air. Whilst this is demonstrably true and nicely explains the process of dew formation (condensation of water as air cools), it is technically inaccurate. It is not in fact the temperature of *air* that is important, but the temperature of the *water*. Because the water vapour is a small constituent component of the air, its temperature and the air temperature will necessarily be very close. When the temperature of water increases, the water molecules gain more energy, allowing them to evaporate more readily. When the temperature is decreased, the less energetic molecules start to clump together because condensation now exceeds evaporation and so the equilibrium begins to shift in favour of liquid water formation. The temperature at which this occurs is called the **dew point**. Whilst this is still an over-simplification, this is the basis of why the water in your exhaled breath condenses on a cold day or why your glasses steam up on entering a warm room.

Cloud formation

The formation of clouds is an elegant demonstration of humidity in action. Infrared radiation from the sun warms water on the earth's surface, increasing its energy and increasing its tendency to move from the liquid to gaseous phase. Around large bodies of water (the oceans) this achieves the saturated vapour pressure for the given temperature.

As described in the *Worked example* in *Section 9.2*, the greater the partial pressure of water in the air, the less dense it is and so the more humid air will rise. As air rises the effect of the earth's

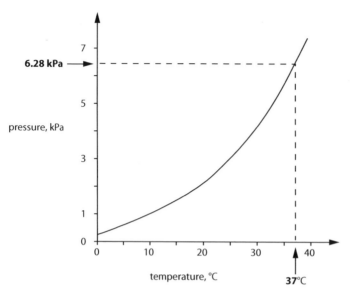

Figure 7.1. *Saturated vapour pressure of water as a function of temperature.*

gravitational field becomes lower, spreading the molecules further apart and decreasing the atmospheric pressure. This process of expansion requires energy and so the air cools. As the saturated air cools down its constituent water molecules now contain less energy and condensation occurs. The water condenses out (onto dust and other hygroscopic particles present in the air) and becomes visible as cloud. The humidity of the air decreases as the water condenses out and the air becomes denser. It therefore stops rising and an evaporation / condensation equilibrium is reached between the surrounding air and the floating body of water in the form of a cloud.

7.2 Absolute and relative humidity

Definitions

Absolute humidity: the mass of the water molecules present (per unit volume).
Relative humidity: the percentage of actual humidity relative to the maximum humidity possible (the saturation point) at a given temperature.

Absolute humidity

Absolute humidity is the mass of water molecules per unit volume, commonly expressed as grams per cubic metre. So if all the air in one cubic metre was trapped and all the water condensed out, the resulting weight would be the absolute humidity per cubic metre. Although absolute humidity is simple to understand, it has limited practical application, because it is difficult to measure, and its effects vary greatly according to the ambient temperature.

Relative humidity

A more commonly used expression of humidity is relative humidity. This is expressed as the ratio of water vapour present in air compared to the maximum amount of water vapour the air could hold. As discussed in the previous section, relative humidity will obviously vary with temperature because the amount of water held by the air is temperature dependent. A relative humidity of 100% means that the air is saturated with moisture. Relative humidity is usually expressed as a percentage as follows:

$$\text{relative humidity} = \frac{\text{actual vapour density}}{\text{saturation vapour density}} \times 100\%$$

7.1 Learn

Units. Absolute humidity is expressed in units of density, i.e. g·m⁻³. Relative humidity is usually expressed as a percentage.

7.3 Measuring humidity

The science of humidity measurement is known as **psychrometry** and a device for measuring humidity is known as a **hygrometer**. Several types of hygrometer are commonly used depending on the required accuracy and specific application. Humidity is difficult to measure directly, so hygrometers usually measure another physical quantity that changes in response to moisture in the air.

Wet and dry bulb hygrometer

This apparatus consists of two glass thermometers, one measuring the ambient temperature and the other with its bulb surrounded by a water-saturated wick, as shown in *Figure 7.2*. The water in the wick will evaporate from around the bulb of the thermometer at a rate determined by the surrounding air temperature and relative humidity, given a constant and regular airflow around the bulb. When the system reaches equilibrium the evaporating water will have caused a temperature drop in the wet thermometer due to the latent heat of vaporization. The degree of temperature drop relative to the ambient temperature recorded by the dry bulb can then be referenced against psychrometric charts to give the relative humidity. A psychrometric chart is essentially a graphical representation of the calculations required to determine the humidity of a sample from the two temperatures recorded by the wet and dry thermometers.

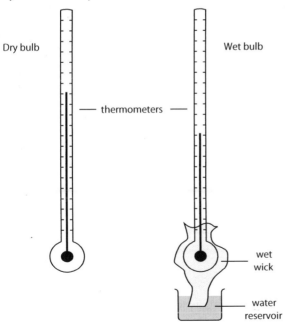

Figure 7.2. *A wet–dry bulb hygrometer.*

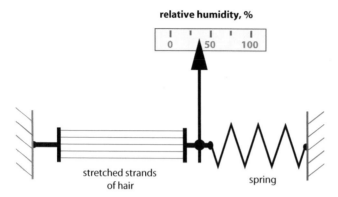

Figure 7.3. *A hair hygrometer.*

Hair tension hygrometers

The cytokeratin molecules that make up a human hair are held together by two types of interactions: disulphide bridges and hydrogen bonds. Whilst the strong sulphur–sulphur bonds are not affected by exposure to water, the hydrogen bonds readily absorb water, causing them to lengthen or 'relax'.

Since the eighteenth century it has been known that hair lengthens in a consistent fashion with the addition of water. Water is readily accepted by the hair's hydrogen bonds at a rate determined by the surrounding relative humidity. A hair under tension and exposed to the environment can therefore easily be calibrated to give a reading of the relative humidity (see *Figure 7.3*). This approach is commonly used in domestic analogue hygrometers such as those found in cigar humidors.

Dew point hygrometers

The dew point is the temperature at which the water in a sample of moist air is at its saturated vapour pressure (see *Section 7.1*). In other words, any further cooling below that temperature will result in condensation. If the ambient temperature and saturated vapour pressure (at that temperature) are known, relative humidity can be calculated from the dew point using psychrometric charts. A high relative humidity would make the dew point closer to the current air temperature: if the dew point is equal to the current temperature, then this indicates 100% humidity.

The most basic device of this kind is a Regnault's hygrometer which consists of a silver tube (good thermal conductivity) containing ether. Air is bubbled through the ether, causing it to vaporize (latent heat of vaporization) and therefore cool the tube. The temperature at which condensation begins to form on the outside surface of the tube is the dew point. Although the Regnault's hygrometer is a mid-nineteenth century device, accurate electronic hygrometers used today are based on the same principle. These substitute a chilled mirror for a glass tube of ether and use electronic sensors to detect condensation on the mirror's surface.

Meteorological humidity measurement using satellites

Meteorologists are concerned with measuring the amount of water vapour present in the atmosphere so that they can make predictions about the prevailing weather patterns. They can also tell us how comfortable we will be feeling in hot weather by using temperature and relative humidity measurements to derive a 'feels-like' temperature. Satellites use infrared radiation that is absorbed by water in the troposphere to derive the measurement of absolute humidity.

7.4 Humidity and human physiology

Sweating

Sweating is the primary means of cooling body temperature in humans. Sweat is composed mainly of water and is excreted by the sweat glands in our skin. The water then evaporates into the air at a rate proportional to the surrounding relative humidity. This is an energy-requiring process (latent heat of vaporization) and this energy is supplied as heat by the skin, so exerting an overall cooling effect.

We are very sensitive to ambient humidity, because residing in a fully saturated environment would render this all-important cooling mechanism useless. For example, if exposed to an environment with an ambient temperature of 24°C with a relative humidity of 0%, we perceive the temperature to be 21°C; in the same ambient temperature but with a relative humidity of 100% we suddenly feel as though the temperature has gone up to 27°C. A relative humidity of 45–55% is the range we find most comfortable.

Respiration

The nose is the organ of humidification, specifically the inferior turbinates. As cold air passes over the inferior turbinates it is warmed to 36°C. Additional water vapour is added from the moist lining of the nasal mucosa. By the time the air reaches the large bronchi the mixture is fully saturated at 44 mg/L, giving a partial pressure of approximately 6 kPa.

The problems associated with administering medical gases are principally twofold.

- First, the gases are manufactured to be as dry as possible to eliminate ice and water damage to valves and regulators.
- Secondly, when anaesthetized, artificial airways (ETT or LMA) bypass the normal physiological humidification mechanisms.

Moisture in the respiratory tract is important for ciliary function and mucous transport; prolonged exposure to dry gas causes secretions to become tenacious and harder to move which can result in mucous plugging and subsequent hypoventilation. Dry gas also removes more moisture from the epithelial lining in an attempt to improve humidity. This cools the respiratory mucosa with a detrimental effect on the cilia, inhibiting their activity. Prolonged exposure results in keratinization of the mucosal surface and total loss of cilia.

Heat loss due to respiration can be calculated. Consider both the heat loss from warming inspired air (ventilation × specific heat capacity of air × temperature rise) and the heat loss from humidifying dry air (ventilation × water required × specific latent heat of vaporization). In the context of an anaesthetized adult this figure is relatively insignificant (roughly 10% of total heat loss) compared to the more important causes of heat loss, namely radiation, convection and evaporation. In neonates, however, this does start to become significant due to their higher rates of ventilation and their increased surface area to volume ratio.

7.5 Humidification of inhaled air

Heat and moisture exchange filter (HMEF)

The HMEF is the most commonly used humidifier in regular anaesthetic practice. This neat piece of equipment (*Figure 7.4*) has the advantages of being inexpensive (and therefore disposable), passive,

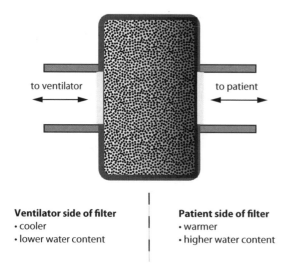

Ventilator side of filter
• cooler
• lower water content

Patient side of filter
• warmer
• higher water content

Figure 7.4. *Heat and moisture exchange filter (HMEF).*

and efficient enough to provide adequate humidification of dry gases for up to 24 hours. The heat and moisture exchange works by creating a sealed unit, near the patient end of the breathing system, containing a hygroscopic material such as calcium chloride or silica gel. As the warm and moist gas from the patient reaches the HMEF, the moisture from the gas condenses onto the hygroscopic surface, simultaneously heating the element via the latent heat of condensation (see *Section 1.2*). With the next inspiration of dry cold gas over the moist element this process is reversed, warming and humidifying the gas the patient receives.

With good materials and design this process is about 80% efficient and minimizes problems caused by moisture and heat loss. The addition of a 0.2 µm filter renders the interface impermeable to bacteria and viruses, thereby avoiding contamination of ventilators and breathing circuits. The disadvantages are that because it is a passive device, the HMEF is not 100% efficient and the patient will therefore lose heat and moisture over time, although as demonstrated above this is negligible. Also, the filter itself has a volume that adds dead space to the circuit and adds resistance. The added dead space can range from 8 mL in a paediatric HMEF to 100 mL in an adult, while the additional resistance can be up to 2.0 cmH$_2$O. Whilst this does not normally cause a significant problem, in certain clinical situations, such as with neonates and those with grossly impaired respiratory mechanics, these effects can become problematic. A more commonly experienced problem is the hygroscopic material and filter acting as a dam to secretions, greatly increasing the work of breathing. This is easily remedied by vigilance and replacement.

Water bath humidifiers

Another commonly employed method for humidifying dry gas is the use of a water bath. These come in two main varieties, active and passive. Whilst an active water bath can achieve 100% efficiency and can also be used to heat the patient, they remain bulky and complex compared to the HMEF and their use is therefore generally restricted to patients requiring longer-term ventilation or oxygen therapy.

Passive water baths simply consist of a chamber of water through which the inspired gas is bubbled to achieve full saturation. Various refinements are used to optimize the bubble size and increase the surface area of exposed gas. The disadvantage of this system is that the temperature of the water limits the maximum achievable humidity. This effect is exacerbated by the cooling of the water bath secondary to the latent heat of vaporization as the water is vaporized. This is remedied by an active system incorporating a heating element and thermostat. The system is designed to keep the water bath at a specific temperature (40–60°C). This increases the temperature of the gas mixture and therefore the achievable humidity. This system is capable of delivering fully saturated gas at 37°C at high flow rates which represents a significant advantage over the HMEF.

All water baths need to include a water trap in their design and this is particularly important for active systems, because the cooling of the gas as it moves away from the hot bath to the patient will result in condensation appearing in the breathing circuit. This can easily accumulate into a small pool in a redundant loop of tubing (*Figure 7.5*) and could result in wet drowning. This risk may be minimized by heating the tubing and preventing condensation forming. The temperature of the water bath is also important. Water baths at around 40°C minimize the risk of scalding the patient's airways with overly heated gas, but run the risk of creating an ideal environment for microbial growth. By

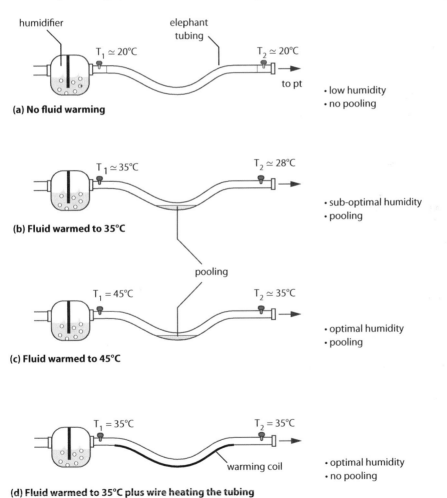

(a) No fluid warming

- low humidity
- no pooling

(b) Fluid warmed to 35°C

- sub-optimal humidity
- pooling

(c) Fluid warmed to 45°C

- optimal humidity
- pooling

(d) Fluid warmed to 35°C plus wire heating the tubing

- optimal humidity
- no pooling

Figure 7.5. *Water bath humidifiers: overcoming the problems of cooling and condensation in elephant tubing.*

heating the water to 60°C the risk of bacterial contamination is reduced but the gas temperature must now be very carefully monitored. A thermistor on a feedback loop to the water bath's thermostat can adjust the temperature of the water, and therefore inspired gas, to ensure that the patient does not suffer from airway scalding.

7.6 Nebulizers

Definition
Nebulizers: these generate an aerosol of either micro-droplets or particles of solid, enabling delivery of medication to the lungs.

Aerosols are small particles of liquids or solids suspended in a carrying gas. They are encountered every day and include dusts, bacteria, yeast, water droplets and smoke particles. Medical aerosols can be produced by a nebulizer where the stability and penetration of an aerosol are crucial to therapy. The stability of the aerosol is dependent on the liquid or solid's ability to remain in suspension and the depth reached by the aerosol on inhalation, and is dependent on its stability. These are both determined by the particle size.

For liquid medication to enter the alveoli the droplets must be smaller than the diameter of the terminal bronchioles. Droplet sizes are usually quoted in microns (1 μm = 1×10^{-6} m) and fall within the size range of 0.005 μm to 50 μm in diameter. For droplet sizes below 5 μm, gravity exerts a negligible effect.

Particles or droplets in the range 5 to 10 μm tend to deposit in the upper airways, with material below 5 μm penetrating further into the lungs. Below 3 μm, the droplets enter the alveoli and become therapeutically beneficial. Droplets below 1 μm are ideal but significantly smaller than this and particles will be exhaled without having a therapeutic effect.

Medication must remain intact rather than changing into the gaseous state. This is the essential difference between vaporizers that generate a vapour and nebulizers that produce liquid droplets. The temperature for an aerosol generated by a nebulizer must not exceed 37°C and the process must not alter the structure of the medication being carried.

Jet or gas driven nebulizer (also known as atomizers)

A high flow of gas is driven over a capillary tube that is immersed into the fluid to be nebulized. High-pressure air is driven through a small orifice, generating negative pressure as a result of the Venturi effect (a full explanation of the Venturi effect is given in *Chapter 8*). These nebulizers are simple and low cost, but small variations in gas flow rate can result in inconsistent delivery of aerosol to the patient.

Ultrasound driven nebulizer

The ultrasound nebulizer incorporates a ceramic piezoelectric transducer that changes electrical energy into mechanical energy (pressure oscillations). The transducer sits at the bottom of the chamber and vibrates at a frequency of 1.5 MHz. The vibrations are transmitted through the water and focused on a flexible diaphragm that vibrates in sympathy. The diaphragm is in contact with the solution to be nebulized and violently shakes the solution into particles. At low frequencies, larger particles are produced, but at higher frequencies, a fine mist is generated. At very high power settings the chemical makeup of some medications can be disrupted.

Ultrasonic nebulizers tend to produce a more consistent particle size than jet nebulizers and, as a result, produce a much greater deposition into the lungs. There has been concern expressed over the long-term use of ultrasonic nebulization because the quantity of fluid deposited on the lungs over time might inadvertently affect surface tension stability in the alveoli.

Summary

- Absolute humidity is the mass of water in a gas mixture in $g \cdot m^{-3}$.
- Relative humidity is the ratio of the mass of water present relative to the mass of water required to saturate the sample.
- Saturated vapour pressure (SVP) rises with temperature.
- Absolute humidity is measured by drying a known volume of air and then weighing the water that condenses out.
- A hygrometer is a device for measuring humidity.
- Three types of hygrometer are: hair tension (simple, least accurate), wet and dry bulb (relatively simple, moderately accurate), dew point, e.g. Regnault's (complex but most accurate).
- Normal physiological humidification mechanisms achieve 100% saturation by the time inhaled air reaches the large bronchi.
- Breathing dry gases for long periods of time damages the mucociliary transport system, essential for maintenance and defence.
- The passive heat and moisture exchange filter (HMEF) is commonly employed and has the advantage of being cheap, disposable and relatively efficient.
- To achieve 100% relative humidity for patients receiving long-term ventilation an active water bath system must be used.
- Nebulizers deliver micro-droplets and particles of solids suspended in a gas to deliver medication to the alveoli.

Single best answer questions

For each of these questions, choose the single best answer.

1. Regarding humidity, which is true?
   (a) Relative humidity is proportional to absolute humidity.
   (b) Absolute humidity is independent of temperature.
   (c) Absolute humidity increases with temperature.
   (d) The amount of water in the air depends on the air temperature.
   (e) Hair hygrometers measure absolute humidity.

2. As humidity rises:
   (a) human hair tends to contract in length
   (b) the temperature difference between wet-bulb and dry-bulb thermometers increases
   (c) the saturation vapour pressure of water decreases
   (d) the dew point decreases
   (e) the density of the air increases

Multiple choice questions

For each of these questions, mark every answer either true or false.

1. Concerning humidity, which of the following statements are true?
   (a) Relative humidity is the ratio of the mass of water vapour present in a sample compared to the mass of water vapour in the environment.
   (b) The saturated vapour pressure of air at any given temperature is equivalent to a relative humidity of 100% at the same temperature.
   (c) Temperature is directly proportional to saturated vapour pressure.
   (d) Higher relative humidity increases the risk of sparks due to the build-up of static electricity.
   (e) The density of air is indirectly proportional to its relative humidity.

2. Concerning the HMEF, which of the following statements are true?
   (a) HMEF stands for humidification and moisture exchange filter.
   (b) It contains a filter of 30 μm diameter.
   (c) It needs an external power supply.
   (d) It is reusable.
   (e) It is not 100% efficient and the patient will therefore lose heat and moisture over time.

3. In adults:
   (a) heating alone humidifies air in the nose
   (b) heat loss from respiration may be significant

   (c) heat loss from sweating is impossible if the relative humidity is 100%
   (d) the partial pressure of water in the alveoli is 8 kPa
   (e) the partial pressure of water in the alveoli changes with altitude

4. The dew point of water:
   (a) is dependent on temperature only
   (b) increases with increasing relative humidity
   (c) decreases with increasing absolute humidity
   (d) is the air temperature at which condensation forms for a given humidity
   (e) is the air temperature at which condensation forms for a given vapour pressure

5. Which of the following are true with regard to cloud formation?
   (a) Humid air rises because it is less dense than dry air.
   (b) As the humid air rises it contracts.
   (c) Droplets form around tiny particles in the air.
   (d) Expanding air releases energy to the surroundings.
   (e) The cloud stops rising as the air becomes denser.

Chapter 8
Measurement of gas flow

Having read this chapter you will be able to:
- Calculate the flow of fluid through a tube or other system.
- Explain the difference between laminar and turbulent flow.
- Understand how the Reynolds number determines flow characteristics.
- Understand Bernoulli's principle and the Venturi effect.
- Explain how a rotameter works and understand its limitations.
- Understand the principle behind pneumotachometers and other flowmeters.

8.1 Flow

Flow is simply the movement of a gas or a liquid through a tube or other system. Flow $\dot{Q}$ is defined as the volume of fluid passing a point in unit time:

$$\dot{Q} = \frac{\Delta V}{\Delta t}$$

8.1 Learn

where ΔV is the change in volume
Δt is the time interval over which the flow is measured

Flow is represented by the symbol $\dot{Q}$ which is the rate of change of quantity Q, where the small dot above the symbol indicates a rate of change of the quantity. Measurement of gas flow has applications in many areas of medicine, particularly in anaesthesia and respiratory physiology. Blood flow measurement is explored in *Chapter 16*. 'Quantity' Q usually refers to volume, so $\dot{Q}$ is technically referred to as volume-flow. In some applications it is more conventional to express mass-flow instead. In this text, unless otherwise stated, 'flow' means 'volume-flow'. The units of volume-flow are usually expressed in $L \cdot s^{-1}$ (or $mL \cdot s^{-1}$).

Conservation of flow

Consider a wide river containing a narrow section (e.g. a sluice). The water can be seen to move much faster in the narrow section than in the wider part. Flow remains constant, but the velocity of the various sections changes according to cross-sectional area, in order to conserve a constant flow rate. Now consider a cylindrical tube whose cross-sectional area changes, as shown in *Figure 8.1*.

For a tube of varying diameter, at two different points (1 and 2):

$$\dot{Q} = A_1 \cdot v_1 = A_2 \cdot v_2$$

8.2

where A is the cross-sectional area
v is the velocity of the fluid at each point

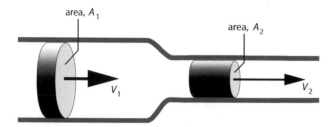

Figure 8.1. *The conservation of flow: the velocity is seen to increase as a fluid flows through a constriction. Flow is conserved at all points.*

The relation between flow and velocity is fundamental to many applications; for example, the calculation of cardiac output (see *Chapter 16*). Doppler ultrasound systems are able to measure aortic velocity, and so to convert this value to flow the cross-sectional area of the aorta must be known.

Worked example

Question
Calculate the mean velocity of blood flowing through the aorta of radius 1.5 cm at a flow rate of 6.0 L·min⁻¹.

Key points
- Convert to SI units, 6.0 L·m⁻¹ = 0.1 L·s⁻¹ = 0.0001 m³·s⁻¹ and 1.5 cm = 0.015 m.

Step 1
From Equation 8.2:

$$\dot{Q} = A \times v, \text{ rearranging}: \ v = \frac{\dot{Q}}{A}$$

the area, A, of a circle is $\pi \cdot r^2$ where r is the radius

$$v = \frac{\dot{Q}}{\pi \cdot r^2} = \frac{0.0001 \text{ m}^3 \cdot \text{s}^{-1}}{\pi \cdot (0.015 \text{ m})^2}$$

$$v = \frac{1 \times 10^{-4}}{7.1 \times 10^{-4}} = 0.14 \text{ m} \cdot \text{s}^{-1}$$

Answer
The mean blood velocity in the aorta is 0.14 m·s⁻¹ (usually stated as 14 cm·s⁻¹).

8.2 Laminar flow

Definition

Laminar flow: orderly movement of a fluid that complies with a model in which parallel layers have different velocities relative to each other.

When watching a steadily flowing river, the flow of water may be seen to be fastest in the middle, while near the banks of the river the water flows more slowly. This behaviour is also observed in fluid travelling slowly along a wide straight cylindrical tube. At relatively low flow velocities the flow can be modelled on layers or cylinders of flow at differing rates, the fastest velocity occurring in the centre of the tube and the slowest at the edge where there

(a)

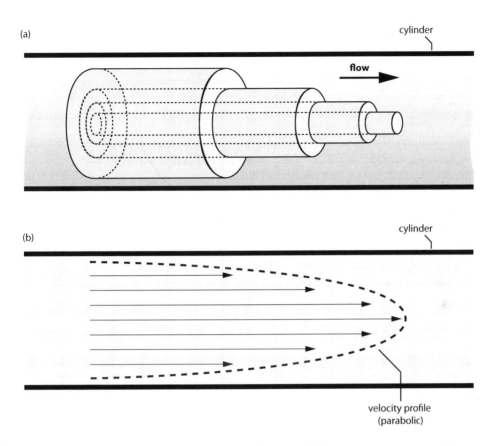

(b)

Figure 8.2. *Laminar flow through a tube with a (a) 3D or (b) 2D view: fluid travels in concentric layers of velocity.*

is friction between the wall of the tube and the fluid. This distinctive velocity profile (*Figure 8.2*) is maintained as long as laminar flow exists, i.e. in the absence of eddies or turbulence. Calculations or measurements of velocity usually refer to the mean velocity, since a range of velocities is occurring simultaneously.

Resistance and laminar flow: Ohm's law

Flow occurs when there is a difference in pressure between two points, otherwise known as a pressure gradient, or a pressure drop. A fluid moves from a zone of higher pressure to a zone of lower pressure, 'driven' by the pressure difference. Any resistance to the flow, for example, a significant constriction in a tube, will not prevent flow, but will restrict the flow rate for a given pressure difference. If resistance is increased, a greater **driving pressure** is needed to maintain a fixed flow rate. A resistance to flow always shows a pressure difference (or pressure 'drop') across it if flow is present, as shown in *Figure 8.3*.

Clinical example

Systemic vascular resistance
Patients with vascular disease usually have associated hypertension. This is because the heart must work harder to produce a 'driving' blood pressure to maintain sufficient blood flow through a raised systemic resistance.

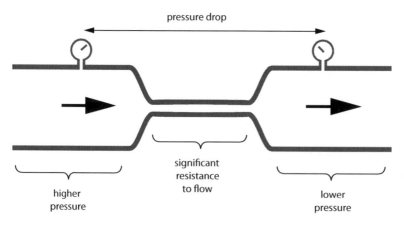

Figure 8.3. *Flow is driven by a pressure difference across a resistance.*

For laminar flow, the flow rate is directly proportional to the pressure driving the flow. Ohm's law applied to the flow of a fluid expresses this, so the flow rate though a tube, assuming laminar flow exists is:

$$\dot{Q} = \frac{\Delta P}{R}$$

8.3 **Learn**

where ΔP is the driving pressure
            R is the flow resistance of the tube

The equation is analogous to Ohm's law for electricity (see *Chapter 18*). *Figure 8.4* illustrates that flow is proportional to pressure. The gradient of the graph is the resistance.

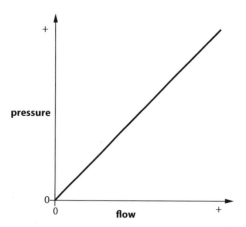

Figure 8.4. *Driving pressure against flow-rate for laminar flow: the driving pressure is proportional to the flow rate.*

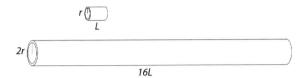

Figure 8.5. The two tubes have the same resistance to laminar flow.

Calculating laminar flow resistance

The resistance of a tube depends on the dimensions of the tube and the properties of the fluid flowing through it. A thinner tube has a much higher resistance to flow than a thicker one; for example, a 15G cannula has significantly higher resistance than its 14G counterpart. Viscous liquids also produce high resistance to flow; for example, a 50% glucose solution flows more slowly through narrow tubing than does water. The resistance of a tube may be calculated for a given fluid using the **Hagen–Poiseuille law**. This law assumes that the liquid is incompressible, viscous and that flow is laminar.

$$R = \frac{8\mu L}{\pi r^4}$$

8.4

where L is the length of the tube
            μ is the (dynamic) viscosity
            r is the tube radius

Clearly the resistance is directly proportional to the length L of the tube. Substituting into Ohm's law (Equation 8.3), then

$$\dot{Q} = \frac{\pi r^4}{8\mu L} \cdot \Delta P$$

8.5 Learn

where ΔP is the driving pressure

The flow is proportional to the fourth power of the radius so, for example, doubling the radius causes a 16-fold increase in flow! The two tubes in *Figure 8.5* have the same resistance to laminar flow; the larger tube has a radius twice that of the smaller one, but is 16 times longer.

8.3 Turbulent flow

The flow pattern of a river running over rapids is very different to the steadily flowing river discussed earlier. The water's path of travel becomes far less predictable than for laminar flow. This is an example of turbulent flow. An intermediate example is water flowing near the bank of a steadily flowing river, which often tends to meander, turning round in gentle circles. This is an example of eddies, the forerunner to full-blown turbulence.

> **Definition**
>
> **Turbulent flow:** movement of a fluid in which small-scale currents in the fluid move in irregular patterns, while the overall flow is in one direction.

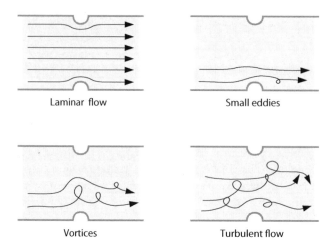

Laminar flow   Small eddies

Vortices   Turbulent flow

Figure 8.6. *In a tube containing obstacles, laminar flow occurs at low flow rates, but as the flow increases, eddies form near the obstacles. As the flow rate increases further, vortices and finally fully developed turbulent flow develop.*

Consider again the flow in the tube as it increases to a higher rate. As can be seen in *Figure 8.6*, eddies and vortices tend to develop close to obstacles or other irregularities in the tube wall such as sharp angles or bifurcations. As the flow rate increases further, these eddies will turn into vortices and finally into fully developed turbulent flow and the laminar model breaks down.

Reynolds number

Fluid dynamics, the study of the flow of fluid, rapidly becomes highly complex. However, in well-controlled circumstances the point at which flow changes from laminar to turbulent flow can be estimated using the Reynolds number, *Re*, which is named after Osborne Reynolds (1842–1912) of Manchester University, one of the first Professors of Engineering. The Reynolds number allows us to predict whether turbulent or laminar flow would occur in a given system. The Reynolds number is a dimensionless quantity, i.e. it has no units.

$$Re = \frac{2 \cdot r \cdot v \cdot \rho}{\mu}$$

8.6 Learn

where r is the tube radius (m)
v is the velocity (m·s^{-1})
ρ is the fluid density (kg·m^3)
μ is the viscosity (N·m^{-3}·s)

When the Reynolds number is less than 2000, flow is predominantly laminar, and when it is greater that 4000, turbulent flow dominates. Between 2000 and 4000, the flow is called transitional, e.g. laminar flow with eddies and/or vortices. As a rule, as the velocity increases, laminar flow turns into transitional and then turbulent flow, because of the increasing Reynolds number. High density, low viscosity and a large radius all tend to produce more turbulence if other variables are constant.

In medicine, turbulence generates sound waves such as ejection murmurs and carotid bruits, as well as the Korotkoff sounds observed when using a cuff to measure blood pressure (see *Section*

Worked example

Question
Calculate whether laminar or turbulent flow would dominate if water flows through a tube of radius 1 cm at a speed of 0.2 m·s⁻¹ and dynamic viscosity 8.9×10^{-4} N·m⁻³·s (density, 1000 kg·m⁻³).

Step 1
Calculate the Reynolds number from Equation 8.6.

$$Re = \frac{2 \cdot r \cdot v \cdot \rho}{\mu}$$

$$Re = \frac{2 \cdot (0.01\,\text{m}) \cdot (0.2\,\text{m} \cdot \text{s}^{-1}) \cdot (1000\,\text{kg} \cdot \text{m}^{-3})}{(8.9 \times 10^{-4} \text{N} \cdot \text{m}^{-3} \cdot \text{s})}$$

$$Re = \frac{4}{8.9 \times 10^{-4}} = 4494$$

Answer
Since the Reynolds number is greater than 4000, turbulent flow is the dominant flow pattern.

6.7). Pumping up the cuff to a pressure greater than the diastolic pressure causes partial occlusion of the brachial artery, because the radius of the artery is reduced. The blood velocity increases since flow is maintained unless the cuff pressure approaches the systolic pressure. Both reduced radius and increased velocity cause an increase in the Reynolds number, so turbulence develops which is audible through the stethoscope.

In the lungs, turbulent flow dominates in the large airways, which has the effect of purging the trachea and larger bronchi with fresh air each time a breath is taken. In the small airways, the air moves more slowly so the Reynolds number is small and laminar flow dominates. This ensures airflow to the alveoli occurs with minimal energy expenditure.

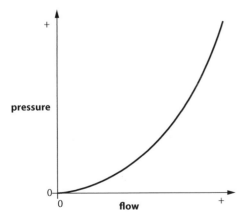

Figure 8.7. *Driving pressure against flow-rate for turbulent flow.*

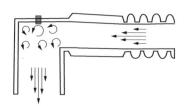

Good fluid dynamics   **Poor fluid dynamics**

Figure 8.8. *A well-designed catheter mount should produce laminar flow. By contrast, turbulent flow can occur in poorly designed connectors, yielding a higher resistance for a given flow.*

Resistance and turbulent flow

The faster and most economical way to get from one place to another is usually directly, in a straight line. Turbulent flow is not linear and fluid does not travel in a straight line. The rate of flow has increased so much that this is no longer possible; this makes the fluid travel faster but via a less direct route. For turbulent flow, the rate of flow is proportional to the square root of the pressure:

$$\dot{Q} \propto \sqrt{\Delta P}, \text{ or } \dot{Q}^2 \propto \Delta P$$

8.7

This is in contrast to laminar flow where flow-rate is directly proportional to pressure (see Equation 8.3). It can be seen from *Figure 8.7* that when turbulent flow develops, the resistance to flow (the gradient) is not constant, but increases with increasing flow rate.

Poorly designed respiratory connectors can cause unnecessary turbulence and hence extra resistance in a breathing circuit, as shown in *Figure 8.8*. Eddies form where sharp angles occur, for example, at a right-angled joint.

8.4 Bernoulli's principle

Bernoulli's principle explains the Venturi effect, the principle used by Venturi masks for producing diluted gas mixtures. Put very simply, the principle states that fluid moving rapidly, e.g. through a constriction, exerts less pressure than a static fluid (see *Figure 8.9*).

The energy of a flowing fluid exists in two forms: kinetic energy (as a result of its velocity) and potential energy (as a result of its pressure). As the velocity increases at a constriction, the kinetic energy increases. The total energy must remain constant, so the potential energy must fall. The potential energy of a gas is proportional to the pressure it exerts and so the pressure exerted on the wall of the tube therefore decreases with increasing velocity.

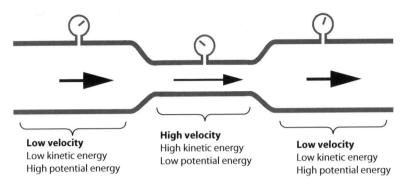

Low velocity
Low kinetic energy
High potential energy

High velocity
High kinetic energy
Low potential energy

Low velocity
Low kinetic energy
High potential energy

Figure 8.9. *According to Bernoulli's principle, a fluid moving at high velocity through a tube exerts less pressure on the walls of the tube than a static or slowly-moving fluid.*

The most dramatic demonstration of Bernoulli's principle is the action of an aerofoil. The shape of an aeroplane wing is designed so that air flowing over the top of the wing travels faster than the air flowing under the wing, and so there is less pressure on the top than on the bottom, resulting in lift.

The unnerving experience of your car being pulled towards a lorry as you overtake it is explained by the Bernoulli principle (*Figure 8.10*). The narrow passageway for the air to travel between the two vehicles means the air travels faster but at a lower pressure. The pressure from the outside of the vehicles is greater and acts to push them together.

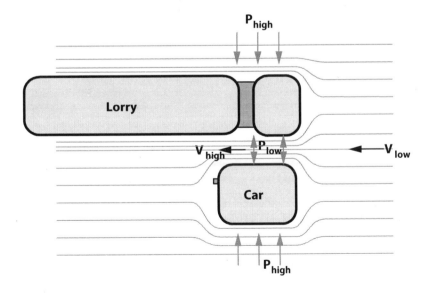

Figure 8.10. *Reduced pressure between two moving vehicles occurring as a result of Bernoulli's principle.*

8.5 The Venturi effect

If the constricted tube shown in *Figure 8.9* contained a hole at the constriction, then air from the outside could be entrained, provided that the pressure inside the constriction was sub-atmospheric. This is known as **jet entrainment**. A nebulizer (e.g. a bronchodilator) works on a similar principle, except that liquid is entrained and is broken down into tiny droplets by the force of the moving gas in the tube. This is also how a carburettor in a car engine works: fuel is entrained and mixed with rapidly moving air before being ignited in the engine.

Venturi mask

The Venturi mask delivers a set concentration of oxygen to a patient from a 100% oxygen supply without complicated gas mixing apparatus. The mask contains a Venturi valve, a simple device moulded from plastic (*Figure 8.11*) which makes use of the **Venturi effect**, a special case of the Bernoulli principle. Oxygen (from a cylinder or other source) is supplied to the valve through plastic tubing and passes through the centre of the valve. The oxygen passes through a small constriction, so its velocity increases (through flow conservation) and air is entrained through holes in the sides of the valve adjacent to the constriction, and so mixes with the oxygen. The air is entrained because the high velocity of oxygen causes a reduction in pressure inside the valve due to the Bernoulli principle. A Venturi valve is also referred to as a **high airflow with oxygen enrichment** (HAFOE) valve.

The **entrainment ratio** is simply the ratio of entrained flow to driving flow:

$$\text{Entrainment Ratio} = \frac{\text{Entrained Flow}}{\text{Driving Flow}} \qquad \textbf{8.8}$$

In practice the entrainment ratio is not constant at all flow rates, and a partially obstructed air inlet can result in delivery of higher oxygen concentration, i.e. a reduced entrainment ratio.

The percentage of oxygen delivered depends on the rate of entrainment, which is determined by the size of the holes in the facemask valve and to a lesser extent by the rate of flow of oxygen. Different colours of valve are engineered to deliver a fixed percentage of oxygen, e.g. a red HAFOE valve delivers 40% O_2 concentration. Note that the quoted figure is accurate for a fixed oxygen flow rate only. *Table 8.1* gives a list of available HAFOE valves and their colours.

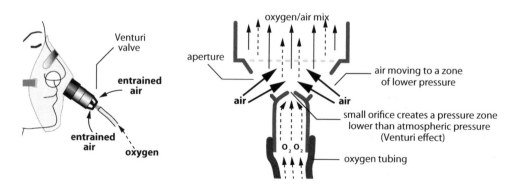

Figure 8.11. *A Venturi mask showing a high airflow oxygen entrainment (HAFOE) valve.*

Table 8.1. *High Air Flow Oxygen Entrainment (HAFOE) valves.*

Delivered O₂%	Fresh gas flow (L·min⁻¹) [rate of flow of oxygen to mask]	Colour for Venturi valve attached to oxygen mask
24% (largest aperture)	2	Blue
28%	4	White
31%	6	Orange
35%	8	Yellow
40%	10	Red
60% (smallest apertures)	15	Green

8.6 The Coanda effect

If a spoon is placed partially in the path of water flowing from a kitchen tap the direction of the flow appears to alter so as to 'stick' to the curved surface of the spoon, as shown in *Figure 8.12*. This tendency of a fluid stream to be attracted to a nearby surface is known as the Coanda effect. The effect can be dramatic, resulting in a significant deviation of flow.

As has already been seen with the Venturi effect, when the water leaves the tap at speed, the flowing fluid entrains fluid (in this case air) into the stream of flow. When there is an obstruction, such as the spoon's surface, this entrainment is dramatically reduced on the spoon side. There is a drop in pressure on the spoon side of the jet and this causes a deflection in the flow towards the spoon.

If a gas is flowing down a tube with a bifurcation or fork, then the gas might not split along each path. Because of the Coanda effect, gas tends to 'hug' one wall more than the other. This phenomenon can manifest itself in the uneven distribution of inhaled gas in the alveoli. Similarly it can lead to ischaemia in apparently normal coronary arteries where the flow of blood is unevenly distributed.

> **Definition**
>
> **Coanda effect:** states that a fluid or gas stream will hug a convex contour when directed at a tangent to that surface.

The Coanda effect is put to good use in a **switching-flow ventilator valve**. This is a carefully designed valve whose shape causes gas to flow from an oxygen supply or ventilator to a patient during inspiration. The gas hugs the wall of the valve and bypasses an open vent on the opposite side of the wall. During expiration, air from the patient is redirected to the vent, because the flow pressure from the gas supply forces the gas to the opposite side of the tube. This type of valve has no moving parts, so is reliable and can be produced very cheaply. This technique is sometimes referred to as **fluid logic.**

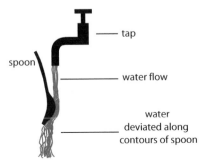

tap

spoon

water flow

water deviated along contours of spoon

Figure 8.12. *Water flowing over the contours of a spoon demonstrates the Coanda effect.*

8.7 Volume and flow measurement

Gas flow measurement

Continuous and reliable indication of the flow of oxygen and other gases is invaluable to anaesthetists. The **variable orifice flowmeter** (*Figure 8.13*), also known by the trade name of Rotameter, provides a failsafe measurement of gas flow. This type of flowmeter is a simple design with the important benefit of not requiring a power supply. A control knob allows precise adjustment of gas flow through a needle-valve. Above this, a vertical glass tube, tapered so it is wider at the top than the bottom, contains a bobbin which is supported by the upward flow of gas through the tube. When flow commences, the bobbin rises until the downward pull of gravity is balanced by the upward force of gas. This upward force decreases the further the bobbin rises, because the gas escapes around the bobbin more easily as the tube gets wider. The position of the bobbin is thus dependent on the rate of gas flow. Common designs feature a flat-topped bobbin so the flow rate is read off from the top of the bobbin onto a scale. Flutes in the bobbin cause it to rotate which reduces the risk of the bobbin sticking to the sides of the tube. Alternatively a spherical bobbin may be used and the flow rate is read from the bobbin's centre.

Variable orifice flowmeters are calibrated for a particular gas, since the gas density and viscosity both affect the bobbin's position. Most variable orifice flowmeters can read over a wide range of flow rates, and this is achieved either by using a variable taper, or by using high-flow and low-flow devices in series.

Measurement of respiratory flow

The flow rate obtained during special breathing manoeuvres performed as part of a lung function test is a useful measurement, as it indicates whether a patient has any ventilatory obstruction or restriction. The lung volume can also be found from the time-integral of the flow rate, and this calculation is done in real-time by a computer connected to a flowmeter.

Modern spirometers are able to measure respiratory flow rate and volume simultaneously. The most popular approach is to measure flow rate at the mouth and record it on an electronic data

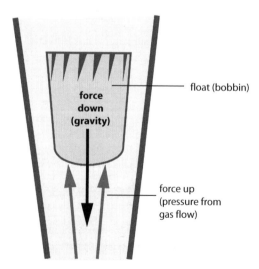

force down (gravity)

float (bobbin)

force up (pressure from gas flow)

Figure 8.13. *Variable orifice flowmeter (or Rotameter).*

acquisition system. Respiratory volumes are obtained by numerical integration of the respiratory flow signal, since

$$F = \frac{dV}{dt}, \quad \text{so} \quad V = \int F \, dt \qquad \qquad \textbf{8.9}$$

Figure 8.14 shows graphs of volume and flow against time on the same time axis for a forced inspiration followed by a forced expiration. According to Equation 8.9, the differential of the **volume–time curve** (gradient of the curve) produces the flow at a given time. This can be plotted as a **flow–time curve** as shown. Similarly, the area under the flow–time curve gives the inspired and expired volumes. Commonly used respiratory volume flowmeters fall into two categories: rotating-vane and differential pressure flowmeters.

Rotating-vane flowmeter

This type of sensor has a small turbine in the flow path, as shown in *Figure 8.15*. The rotation of the turbine can be related to the volume flow of gas. Interruption of a light beam by the turbine is

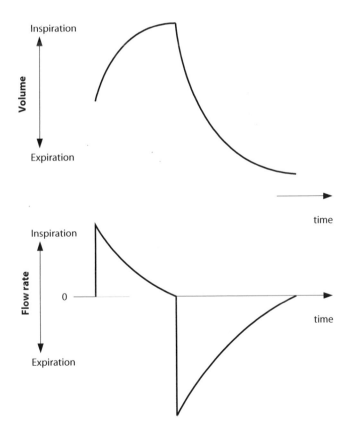

Figure 8.14. *Graphs of volume against time and flow against time on **the same time axis** for a forced inspiration followed by a forced expiration.*

sensed and converted to a voltage which is proportional to flow and this is displayed continuously. The volume of gas breathed in or out is found by integrating the volume flow with respect to time. Because of the small but significant inertia of the vane, these systems are most accurate at low respiratory flow rates. Nevertheless they are commonly found in the mouthpieces of lung function equipment.

Differential pressure flowmeter – pneumotachometer

The pneomotachometer (or pneumotachograph) is basically a circular tube containing a fine metal mesh which provides a small resistance to flow (*Figure 8.16*). During breathing, the flow causes a small pressure difference on either side of the mesh. The pressure difference is measured by a pair of pressure sensors connected by small tubes placed in the wall of the tube on either side of the mesh.

The pneumotachometer has the advantage of requiring no moving parts so is reliable. The calculated flow rate is proportional to the pressure difference according to Ohm's law which assumes that only laminar flow occurs in the tube. Pneumotachometers are designed with a large diameter at the point of measurement, which keeps the flow velocity down, resulting in laminar flow, as predicted by the Reynolds number equation (see Equation 8.6).

The prevention of water vapour condensation in a pneumotachometer is of particular importance. The capillary tubes and screen pores are easily blocked by liquid water, which decreases their surface area, thereby increasing their resistance. This problem is avoided by heating the resistance element, usually by placing an electrical resistance heater around it.

Differential pressure flowmeters - pitot tube flowmeter

This is a variation of the pneumotachometer, but there is no need for a flow resistor. Instead the two pressure sensors are connected to a pair of tubes, such that the end of one tube faces forward into the path of fluid flow and is parallel to the flow, while the other faces backwards, away from the flow, as shown in *Figure 8.17*. The symmetrical design allows flow measurement in either direction.

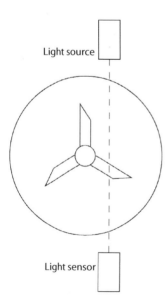

Figure 8.15. *A rotating-vane respiratory flowmeter.*

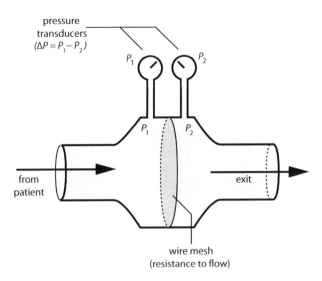

Figure 8.16. *A pneumotachometer.*

The tubes are connected to the pressure sensors, so there is no flow in the tubes. However, the air in the flow-facing tube is compressed, causing a pressure increase. The compression arises because the kinetic energy of the moving air (proportional to the square of the velocity) is converted into potential energy (proportional to pressure) in the tube. The pressure difference is therefore equal to the square of the velocity. Note also that flow is not measured directly, and the velocity varies across the tube. It therefore has to be assumed that at a fixed point in the tube, the velocity is proportional to the flow rate.

Wright peak flow meter

The Wright peak flow meter (*Figure 8.18*) is a simple low-cost device which records the maximal expired flow. Air from the patient pushes against a diaphragm which moves in the direction of air flow. The movement of the diaphragm is opposed by a spring, but causes a narrow slot to open through which the expired air escapes, reducing pressure on the diaphragm. A sliding marker indicating the peak flow rate is pushed by the diaphragm, which continues to move along the tube until the spring force overcomes the air pressure.

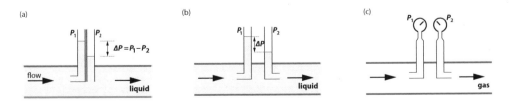

Figure 8.17. *A range of pitot tube flowmeters. (a) A classic pitot tube; (b) a pitot tube that has been adapted for two-way flow measurement; and (c) a pitot tube adapted for gas flow.*

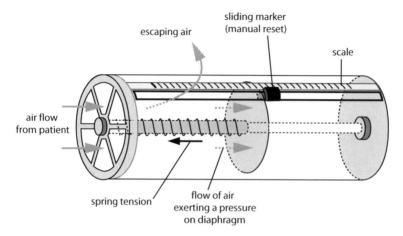

Figure 8.18. *Wright peak flow meter.*

Benedict–Roth spirometer

An alternative approach to calculating volume changes by integrating the flow rate is to measure the volume directly. This basic technique has been in use since the nineteenth century, and involves collecting the gas passing through the airway opening. The device used for this measurement is known as a spirometer. The widespread and historical use of this device has given rise to use of the term **spirometry** to mean the measurement of changes in lung volume for testing of pulmonary function, regardless of whether a spirometer, flowmeter plus integrator, or other technique is used.

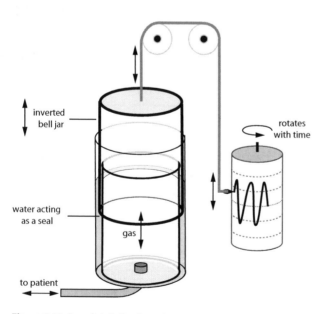

Figure 8.19. *Benedict–Roth spirometer.*

The Benedict–Roth spirometer (see *Figure 8.19*), is basically an expandable compartment consisting of a movable, statically counterbalanced, rigid chamber or 'bell', a stationary base and a dynamic seal between them. The bell can move up and down freely, so the pressure inside the bell is close to atmospheric pressure. The seal is often water but dry seals have also been used. Changes in the internal volume, V_s, of the spirometer are proportional to the displacement of the bell. This motion is traditionally recorded on a rotating drum but any displacement sensor may be used.

The Benedict–Roth spirometer generally underestimates expired volumes due to contraction of exhaled air and condensation of water vapour as the air cools inside the spirometer.

Summary

- Flow can be either laminar or turbulent depending on various conditions.
- Laminar flow occurs when a fluid flows at low flow rates through smooth tubes.
- Obstacles and bifurcations can cause eddies, vortices or full-blown turbulence.
- The transition to turbulent flow also depends on velocity, tube radius, density and viscosity according to the Reynolds number.
- If the Reynolds number is less than 2000, flow is predominantly laminar, but if it is greater than 4000, turbulence dominates.
- Laminar flow is proportional to driving pressure, and turbulent flow is proportional to the square root of the driving pressure.
- A fast-moving fluid exerts less pressure than a static fluid according to the Bernoulli principle.
- The Bernoulli principle produces the Venturi effect and the Coanda effect, both of which are used in anaesthetic apparatus.
- Measurement of respiratory gas flow can be achieved by a pneumotachometer, a pitot flowmeter and a rotating-vane flowmeter.
- Respiratory volumes can be measured by integrating flow rate or using a Benedict–Roth spirometer.

Single best answer questions

For each of these questions, choose the single best answer.

1. In the large airways of the lung:
   (a) laminar flow occurs as this requires less driving pressure
   (b) turbulence occurs due to low velocities
   (c) turbulence occurs which produces a higher flow rate for a given pressure
   (d) turbulence occurs due to large tube diameter
   (e) there is a mixture of turbulent and laminar flow

2. The Reynolds number increases if which of the following decreases?
   (a) viscosity
   (b) tube radius
   (c) flow
   (d) velocity
   (e) density

3. Which statement best describes the Bernoulli principle?
    (a) Moving air molecules have a smaller component of velocity perpendicular to flow.
    (b) Moving air exerts lower pressure because raised kinetic energy requires a drop in potential energy.
    (c) The pressure on a thin-walled tube is lower due to its lower surface area.
    (d) Static air exerts more pressure because its molecules have higher thermal kinetic energy.
    (e) Moving air exerts less pressure due to frictional forces acting on the walls, parallel to the direction of flow.

Multiple choice questions

For each of these questions, mark every answer either true or false.

1. Which of the following statements are true of Venturi masks?
    (a) Oxygen is entrained through holes in the sides.
    (b) They rely on the Coanda effect to mix air and oxygen.
    (c) The oxygen concentration is not affected by flow rate.
    (d) Larger holes result in lower delivered oxygen concentration.
    (e) They have no moving parts.

2. A rotating-vane flowmeter:
    (a) is suitable for high respiratory flow rates
    (b) is not affected by condensation
    (c) measures volume directly
    (d) is not suitable for lung function testing
    (e) measures flow in both directions

3. Which of the following statements are true?
    (a) Laminar flow is proportional to the square of driving pressure.
    (b) Resistance to laminar flow remains constant at all flow rates.
    (c) Pressure is proportional to the square of turbulent flow.
    (d) A Reynolds number of 2500 describes transitional flow.
    (e) Ohm's law applies to both laminar and turbulent flow.

Chapter 9
The gas laws

Having read this chapter you will be able to:
- Explain the physics behind breathing.
- Work out the partial pressure of oxygen in a hyperbaric chamber.
- Understand the physics behind anaesthesia at altitude.
- Get to grips with the laws affecting gas storage in cylinders.

9.1 The ideal gas

The gas laws allow us to predict how gases will behave under different conditions such as altered temperature and pressure. They are based on the concept of an **ideal gas** whose molecules act like minuscule rubber balls as they undergo elastic collisions. An ideal gas behaves in the following way:
- The molecules are assumed to be so far apart that there is no attraction between them.
- The volume of the molecules themselves is negligible.
- The molecules are in random motion, obeying Newton's laws of motion.

Of course ideal gases do not really exist in nature. The behaviour of real gases, however, approximates ideal gases in all but the most extreme conditions, such as at very low temperatures or high pressures. The gas laws allow us to predict and calculate macroscopic properties such as volume, temperature and pressure, and these provide average values for an entire volume of gas. At a molecular level there are considerable fluctuations around the mean values; the properties of an individual molecule are its kinetic energy, momentum and velocity.

Standard temperature and pressure

When do the gas laws hold true? In general they are more accurate at room temperatures and atmospheric pressures, but they are less accurate when a gas is on the verge of becoming a liquid (condensation), at very high pressures, and also at very low temperatures. The phrase 'at standard temperature and pressure' or 'at **STP**' is often used to succinctly inform the reader that the discussion applies to normal conditions, and STP is usually taken to mean 0°C at atmospheric pressure at sea level.

> **Definition**
>
> **Standard temperature and pressure (STP):** this refers to conditions where the temperature is 273.15 K (or 0°C) and the atmospheric pressure is 101.3 kPa (or 760 mmHg).

9.2 Avogadro's law and Avogadro's constant

Figure 9.1 shows three balloons all containing exactly the same volume of gas, all at the same temperature and pressure. One balloon is filled with helium, one with oxygen and the other xenon. All three balloons contain exactly the same number

> **Definition**
>
> **Avogadro's law (hypothesis):** equal volumes of gases, at the same temperature and pressure, contain the same number of molecules.

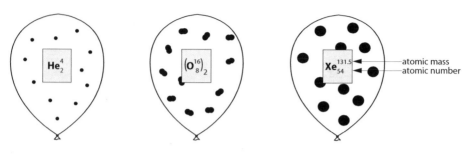

Figure 9.1. *According to Avogadro's law, all three balloons containing the same volume of gas contain the same number of molecules.*

of molecules. This is in keeping with Avogadro's law that the volume a gas occupies is not related to the size of the molecules that make up the gas.

The amount of a substance is measured in **moles**: it is one of the seven base units of the SI system of units. The constant that quantifies how many molecules make up one mole is named after the Italian scientist Avogadro. The **Avogadro constant** is 6.02×10^{23} molecules per mole and is so large that if there were that many pineapples they would fill the volume of the Earth. For a solid, such as carbon, one mole is roughly the amount of lead in a pencil and for an ideal gas one mole at STP occupies 22.4 litres.

The relationship between the number of molecules in a sample and the number of moles present is:

$$\text{number of molecules} = \text{number of moles} \times \text{Avogadro's number} \qquad \textbf{9.1}$$

The molar mass (the mass of one mole) of a substance is simply the molecular mass expressed in grams; e.g. one mole of water has a mass of 18 g (water has a molecular mass of 18). In other words:

$$\text{mass of a substance} = \text{molar mass} \times \text{number of moles} \qquad \textbf{9.2}$$

Worked example

Question
How many moles are there in 11 g of nitrous oxide and how many molecules are present?

Key points
- The molecule nitrous oxide (N_2O) has two nitrogen atoms and one oxygen atom.
- Molecular mass of oxygen is 16 and for nitrogen it is 14.

Step 1
- The molar mass of nitrous oxide is equal to the molecular mass, expressed in grams.
- Molecular mass $= (14 \times 2) + 16 = 44$, so molar mass $= 44$ g.

Step 2
- The number of moles can be calculated by rearranging Equation 9.2:

$$\text{number of moles} = \frac{\text{mass of substance}}{\text{molar mass}}$$

$$= \frac{11}{44} = 0.25 \, \text{mole}$$

Step 3
- Using Equation 8.1 the number of molecules can be found.

$$\text{number of molecules} = \text{number of moles} \times \text{Avogadro's number}$$

$$= 0.25 \times (6.02 \times 10^{23}) = 1.51 \times 10^{23} \, \text{molecules}$$

Answer
There are 0.25 moles and 1.51×10^{23} molecules in 11 g of nitrous oxide.

Worked example

Question
What is the mass of 0.2 moles of the volatile gas isoflurane?

Key points
- Isoflurane has a chemical formula of $C_3H_2ClF_5O$ giving it a molar mass of 184.5 g·mol⁻¹.

Step 1
- Using Equation 8.2 the mass can be calculated:

$$\text{mass of a substance} = \text{molar mass} \times \text{number of moles}$$
$$= 184.5 \times 0.2 = 36.9 \, \text{g}$$

Answer
The mass of 0.2 moles of isoflurane is 36.9 g.

Worked example

Question
Why is humid air less dense than dry air?

Key points
- Humid air contains water vapour which is gaseous H_2O molecules.
- Examining equal volumes of dry air and another of humid air (at the same temperature and pressure) then Avogadro's law states that they contain equal numbers of molecules.

Step 1

- Estimate the mass of one mole of air.
- Molar mass of oxygen, $M_{O_2} = 32$ (~one-fifth of air)
- Molar mass of nitrogen, $M_{N_2} = 28$ (~four-fifths of air)

$$\text{Approximation of the molar mass of air, } M_{air} \simeq \left(\frac{1}{5} \times M_{O_2}\right) + \left(\frac{4}{5} \times M_{N_2}\right)$$

$$\simeq \left(\frac{1}{5} \times 32\right) + \left(\frac{4}{5} \times 28\right) = 6.4 + 22.4 \text{ g·mol}^{-1}$$

$$M_{air} \simeq 28.8 \text{ g·mol}^{-1}$$

Step 2

- Molar mass of water, $M_{H_2O} = 18$ g·mol^{-1}.

Answer

$M_{H_2O} < M_{air}$, so substituting a water molecule for a molecule of air will decrease the mass of one mole of the gas. As it is the number of particles rather than the mass that determines volume then the volume will remain unchanged and instead it is the density that will be lowered with greater humidity.

Note

The precise molar mass of air is slightly higher at 28.9 g if the exact percentages of oxygen and nitrogen are used and heavier minor constituents of air such as argon are taken into account.

9.3 Partial pressure

Definition

Dalton's law: for a gas the total pressure is simply all the partial pressures added together.

Imagine that a box contains a mixture of two gases, oxygen and helium. The pressure on the walls of the box arises from the two types of molecules each colliding with the walls. The pressures generated by each gas individually are known as the partial pressures, and these are related to the number of molecules of each gas. So there will be a partial pressure for helium (P_{He}) and for oxygen (P_{O_2}). If the helium gas were to be removed the new total pressure would be equal to the previous partial pressure of the oxygen.

The total partial pressure P_T can be calculated by using **Dalton's law**:

$$P_T = P_1 + P_2 + P_3$$

9.3 Learn

where P_1, P_2 and P_3 are the partial pressures of the gases present

Air is a mixture of several gases. The partial pressure of each constituent gas is equal to the atmospheric pressure, as shown in *Figure 9.2*.

The partial pressure of water vapour in ambient air is not fixed but varies according to local conditions and this is discussed in *Chapter 7*. It is usually taken as 1.3 kPa unless otherwise stipulated. The partial pressure of water vapour in the alveoli does not alter. The airways deliver

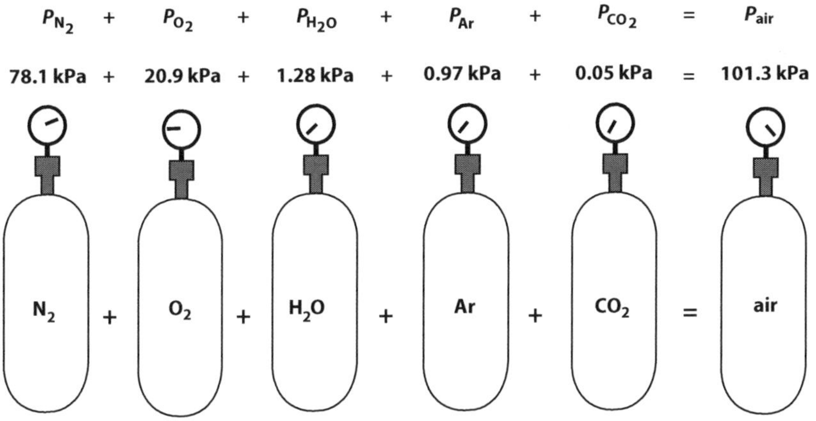

$$P_{N_2} \ + \ P_{O_2} \ + \ P_{H_2O} \ + \ P_{Ar} \ + \ P_{CO_2} \ = \ P_{air}$$

$$78.1\ kPa \ + \ 20.9\ kPa \ + \ 1.28\ kPa \ + \ 0.97\ kPa \ + \ 0.05\ kPa \ = \ 101.3\ kPa$$

N_2 + O_2 + H_2O + Ar + CO_2 = air

Figure 9.2. *Applying Dalton's law of partial pressures to air. The atmospheric pressure is the sum of the partial pressures of the components of air.*

the maximum partial pressure possible, 6.3 kPa, which is the saturated vapour pressure (SVP) for water vapour at 37°C. This value is independent of the total air pressure. The *Worked example* below demonstrates that when air is humidified, the water vapour 'displaces' a fraction of the other gases in the air, since the total pressure does not increase (see *Figure 9.3*). Reduction in oxygen partial pressure can have severe consequences at high altitude, where the partial pressure of oxygen is very low.

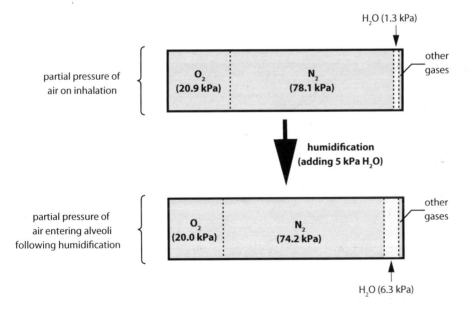

partial pressure of air on inhalation

H_2O (1.3 kPa)

O_2 (20.9 kPa) N_2 (78.1 kPa) other gases

humidification (adding 5 kPa H_2O)

partial pressure of air entering alveoli following humidification

O_2 (20.0 kPa) N_2 (74.2 kPa) other gases

H_2O (6.3 kPa)

Figure 9.3. *Partial pressures of inhaled air: humidification during inhalation changes the partial pressure of the constituents of air. Note that at sea level both before and after humidification the total pressure (atmospheric pressure) remains constant at 101.3 kPa.*

Worked example

Question

The process of humidification of inhaled gas by the airways increases the partial pressure of water vapour as it approaches the alveoli. Under normal conditions the partial pressure of water vapour in air is 1.3 kPa but it rises by 5 kPa to a total of 6.3 kPa following humidification. How much does this alter the partial pressure and the concentration of oxygen entering the alveoli?

Key points

- The airways add water vapour to inhaled air, achieving saturated water vapour pressure, which at 37°C is 6.3 kPa.
- The overall pressure remains the same so the partial pressures of the original constituents of air are diluted to make room for the extra water vapour.
- Dry air contains 20.9% oxygen (fractional concentration = 0.209).

Step 1

- Applying Dalton's law (Equation 9.3), the *reduced share* of pressure to be divided between the constituents of air following humidification is:

$$\text{Reduced share of pressure} = \text{atmospheric pressure} - \text{partial pressure of added water vapour}$$
$$= 101.3 - 5.0 \text{ kPa}$$
$$= 96.3 \text{ kPa}$$

Step 2

- Now we can calculate the altered partial pressure of oxygen following humidification.

$$\text{altered partial pressure of oxygen} = \text{reduced share of pressure} \times \text{fraction of oxygen}$$
$$= 96.3 \times 0.209 = 20.1 \text{ kPa}$$

Step 3

- From this the percentage of oxygen entering the alveoli can be calculated:

$$\text{altered percentage of oxygen} = \frac{\text{partial pressure of oxygen}}{\text{total pressure}} \times 100\%$$

$$= \frac{\text{altered partial pressure of oxygen}}{\text{atmospheric pressure}} \times 100\%$$

$$= \frac{20.1}{101.3} \times 100 = 19.9\%$$

Answer

Inspired oxygen concentration is reduced from 20.9% in air to 19.9% with a partial pressure of 20.1 kPa on entering the alveoli, resulting in a drop of 1% in concentration.

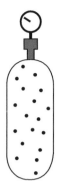
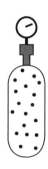

Figure 9.4. Boyle's law: the two cylinders both contain equal numbers of molecules but the gas in the smaller cylinder is at a higher pressure.

9.4 Boyle's law

Imagine a box containing gas molecules. The molecules collide with the walls of the box and are felt by the walls as pressure. If you were to halve the volume of the box and no gas escapes, the pressure doubles since the molecules bump into the walls twice as often. In other words the pressure is proportional to the volume of the gas as long as the temperature is unchanged:

> **Definition**
>
> **Boyle's law (the first ideal gas law):** the volume of a gas is inversely proportional to its pressure (at a fixed temperature).

$$P \, \alpha \, \frac{1}{V}$$

Figure 9.4 shows two gas cylinders containing equal amounts of gas. The smaller cylinder is at a higher pressure as a result of more frequent collisions per unit area of cylinder wall, as predicted by Boyle's law. This can be seen simply with a bicycle pump: if you place your finger over the nozzle of the pump, the plunger is easy to push in at first, but as you compress the air further it gets more difficult to push against the increasing pressure.

Figure 9.5 shows a graph of pressure against volume for gases at two temperatures. The curves shown are known as **isothermals** (constant temperature). The gas at the higher temperature has a higher pressure for a given volume and vice versa. The product of pressure and volume are constant at constant temperature.

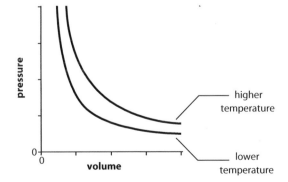

Figure 9.5. Boyle's law: the inverse relationship between pressure and volume produces lines on the graph that are known as isothermals.

Clinical examples

Gas in a cylinder
When a gas cylinder is filled the number of gas molecules held in the cylinder increases and so the density of the gas increases. The gas is being forced from a larger to a smaller container and Boyle's law determines that the pressure will rise in the cylinder. An oxygen cylinder at a pressure one hundred times that of atmospheric pressure is capable of releasing one hundred times the cylinder's volume of oxygen.

Work of breathing
The expansion of the thoracic cavity and resultant increase in volume of the lungs leads to a negative pressure in the lungs according to Boyle's law. This creates a pressure gradient compared to the air outside of the nose and mouth resulting in air flowing into the lungs.

Diving
When a diver descends and ascends the pressure in the body increases and decreases accordingly and any trapped gas, such as in a dental cavity, will contract on descent and expand on ascent.

Worked example

Question
A partly used 'E' oxygen cylinder has a pressure of 100 bar with an internal volume of 4.5 litres. If oxygen was required at a flow of 2.5 L·min^{-1}, roughly how long would the cylinder last?

Key points
- We need to find the volume (V_B) that the gas in the cylinder would expand to if it were at atmospheric pressure (P_B).
- In SI units 1 bar = 100 kPa so the pressure in the cylinder, P_{cyl}, is 1×10^4 kPa and P_B is simply atmospheric pressure, 101.3 kPa.
- The question is only demanding a rough 'back of the envelope' calculation, so it is acceptable to approximate P_B to 100 kPa as this makes the calculations more straightforward.

Step 1
- Calculate the volume the oxygen would occupy at P_B (1 atm) using Boyle's law (Equation 9.5)

$$P_{cyl} \cdot V_{cyl} = P_B \cdot V_B$$

rearranging

$$V_B = \frac{P_{cyl} \cdot V_{cyl}}{P_B}$$

$$V_B = \frac{100 \times 4.5}{1} = 450 \text{ litres}$$

Step 2
- We know both the volume and the rate of flow of oxygen (2.5 L·min^{-1}).

rate of flow is the volume flowing per unit time:

$$\text{flow rate} = \frac{\text{volume}}{\text{time}}$$

rearranging

$$\text{time} = \frac{\text{volume}}{\text{flow rate}} = \frac{450}{2.5} = 180\,\text{min}$$

Answer

The oxygen would empty after 180 minutes.

Notes

- The pressure gauges on most gas cylinders are not particularly accurate and a substantial margin of error should be anticipated.
- Strictly speaking, the volume of oxygen at atmospheric pressure should have been corrected by subtracting the volume of the cylinder itself. This is because when the cylinder is 'empty' it still has a gas left in it at a pressure equal to the atmosphere.

9.5 Charles's law

Imagine a gas enclosed in an expandable box. If the gas in the box is then heated the box expands. The molecules of the gas, when hotter, bounce around faster, pushing back the sides of the box and increasing the volume they are enclosed by. The volume is proportional to the temperature.

Alternatively consider two identical balloons that a child takes home from a party; one is left in the garden exposed to the midday sun and the other balloon is put in a large fridge (*Figure 9.6*). There are the same number of molecules in each balloon, but the balloon warming in the sun expands to a greater volume while the balloon in the fridge shrinks in volume. The higher the temperature of gas molecules, the faster they move and this generates greater pressure.

At constant pressure, Charles's law states that the volume of a gas expands steadily with increasing temperature. The volume is in fact proportional to the absolute temperature, as shown in *Figure 9.7*. As the temperature approaches absolute zero, the ideal gas model breaks down (absolute zero is 0 K (–273°C) and is the temperature at which theoretically all motion of molecules ceases).

> **Definition**
>
> **Charles's law (the second ideal gas law):** at a given pressure the temperature is directly proportional to the volume of a gas.

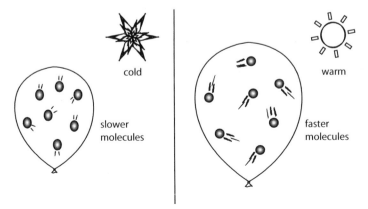

Figure 9.6. *Charles's law: the faster molecules in the warmer balloon force the balloon to expand.*

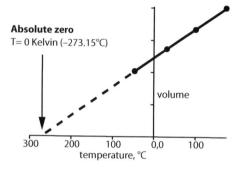

Absolute zero
T= 0 Kelvin (−273.15°C)

volume

300   200   100   0,0   100
temperature, °C

Figure 9.7. *Charles's law: the volume of a gas at constant pressure is proportional to absolute temperature.*

$$V \propto T$$

9.5 **Learn**

Charles's law explains why a hot air balloon rises: if a gas is heated it expands and the molecules gain in energy, so move faster. The expanding air in the balloon causes some air to escape at the base. The remaining hot air is less dense relative to the colder air outside of the balloon, so that the balloon becomes lighter than air and floats upwards.

Clinical examples

Bourdon thermometer
The Bourdon thermometer is based on expansion of gas in a tube that is linked to a dial to allow temperature to be monitored (see *Chapter 4*).

Exacerbation of the bends
A post-dive hot bath or a strenuous workout is not recommended because a rise in temperature of the body can result in the expansion of small bubbles of nitrogen that may be present in the tissues.

9.6 The pressure law: Gay-Lussac's law

Definition

The pressure law (Gay-Lussac's law; the third ideal gas law): the pressure of a gas is directly proportional to its temperature (within a fixed volume).

If you were to heat the gas in a non-expandable box until its temperature doubled, the pressure inside the box would also double, because the molecules would move faster and bump into the walls more often. The pressure is proportional to the temperature of a gas; this works out if the temperature is measured relative to absolute zero (−273°C).

This can be applied to two identical cylinders: one of the cylinders has been left out in the sun and the other has been stored in a cool room. As the temperature rises in the cylinder exposed to the sun, the gas molecules gain kinetic energy, i.e. they move at faster speeds. The faster molecules generate more pressure meaning that the pressure in the hotter cylinder increases. The opposite is true for the cylinder dropping in temperature, and its pressure drops.

The pressure law is also known as the third ideal gas law, or Gay-Lussac's law after its discoverer, Joseph Louis Gay-Lussac. At constant volume, pressure is proportional to absolute temperature:

$$P \propto T$$

9.6 **Learn**

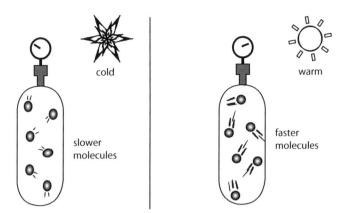

Figure 9.8. *The pressure law: as the gas increases in temperature so does the speed with which the gas molecules move, generating higher pressures in a fixed volume.*

Figure 9.9 shows a graph of pressure against temperature in a fixed volume. The pressure and temperature are directly proportional, generating a straight line. The plotted line, if extended to the temperature axis, intersects it at absolute zero (−273.15°C or, in SI units, 0 K). Of course, below the boiling point of the gas, the pressure law does not apply because the gas condenses to become a liquid.

Clinical example

Filling ratios
The degree to which a cylinder should be filled is partly dependent on the pressure law. The filling ratios for gas cylinders must take into account the rise in pressure in a cylinder associated with a rise in temperature. If the pressure reaches a critical level the cylinder will rupture at its weakest point and explode. For this reason cylinders should be filled at the ambient temperature at which they are going to be stored and used. Scuba diving tanks are often filled in a water bath set to the temperature appropriate to the location of the dive (see Chapter 13).

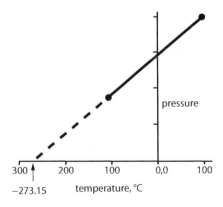

Figure 9.9. *The pressure law, also known as Gay-Lussac's law, has pressure directly proportional to temperature at a fixed volume.*

9.7 The combined gas laws

The gas laws (Boyle's law, Charles's law and the pressure law) may be combined into one equation called the combined gas law. A condition for the combined gas equation is that the amount of gas must remain constant. The combined gas law simply states that the product of pressure and volume is proportional to the absolute temperature:

$$P \cdot V \propto T$$

9.7

or, for the same gas under two different sets of conditions:

$$\frac{P_1 \cdot V_1}{T_1} = \frac{P_2 \cdot V_2}{T_2}$$

9.8 Learn

Worked example

Question

A bubble is discharged from the tank of a diver at 40 m depth in the sea, at a water temperature of 10°C. The bubble is initially 20 mL in volume; what size will the bubble be on reaching the surface where the water temperature is 20°C?

Key points
- Assume that for every 10 metres in depth descended the pressure increases by the equivalent of the atmospheric pressure at the surface (P_B).
- The temperature must be in kelvin (0 K = −273°C) and the volume in m³ (1 mL = 1×10^{-6} m³).

Step 1
- Calculate the pressure at 40 m depth:
  Pressure at 40 m depth, P_{40m} = pressure at surface + pressure due to water above
  For every 10 m descent the pressure is increased by another atmospheric pressure P_B

$$P_{40m} = P_B + \left(\frac{\text{depth dived}}{10} \times P_B \right) = P_B + \left(\frac{40}{10} \times P_B \right)$$

$$P_{40m} = 5P_B$$

Step 2
- Using the combined gas law (Equation 9.8)

$$\frac{P_B \cdot V_{surface}}{T_{surface}} = \frac{P_{40m} \cdot V_{40m}}{T_{40m}}$$

- Rearranging to isolate $V_{surface}$, the volume of the bubble at the surface:

$$V_{surface} = \frac{P_{40m} \cdot V_{40m} \cdot T_{surface}}{P_B \cdot T_{40m}}$$

- In Step 1 it was shown that $P_{40m} = 5P_B$

$$V_{surface} = \frac{5 \times P_B \times 20 \times 293}{P_B \times 283} = \frac{5 \times 20 \times 293}{283}$$

$$V_{surface} = 104 \, \text{mL}$$

Answer

The volume of the bubble has increased more than five fold to 104 mL.

9.8 The universal gas law

Avogadro's law (*Section 9.2*) tells us that, at constant pressure and temperature, the volume is proportional to the number of particles. Applying this to the combined gas law produces the universal gas equation:

$$P \cdot V = n \cdot R \cdot T$$

9.9 **Learn**

where n is the number of moles of the gas

             R is a number called the universal gas constant (R is equal to 8.31 J·K^{-1}·mol^{-1})

The universal gas equation (Equation 9.9) is very useful because it allows a volume to be calculated from a pressure of a gas (or vice versa) if the amount of gas and the temperature are known. *Figure 9.10* shows a flow diagram which summarizes how the universal gas equation is derived from the three gas laws.

Clinical example

Gas cylinders
The universal gas law can be used to calculate the amount of gas in a cylinder if the pressure is known (see *Chapter 13*).

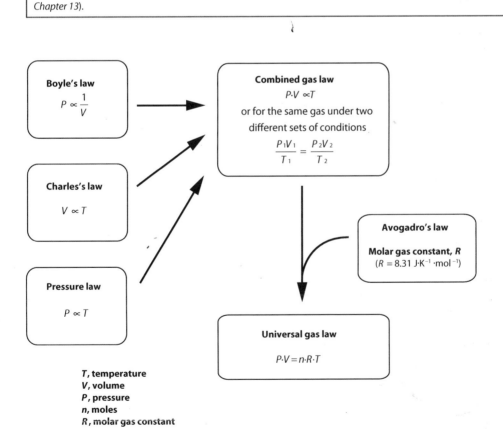

Figure 9.10. *The gas laws combine to form the universal gas law that takes the amount of a gas into account.*

Worked example

Question

How much volume would 32 g of oxygen occupy when at 0°C and at sea level?

Key points

- Oxygen is a gas unless under extreme conditions and the universal gas law allows gas volume to be calculated.
- All values need to be in SI units so temperature becomes 273 K and pressure at sea level can be assumed to be 101.3 kPa – this is standard temperature and pressure (STP). The SI unit for volume is the cubic metre (1 m³ = 1000 L)
- Oxygen has an atomic mass of 16 but as a gas it is diatomic (O_2) making the molecular mass 32.

Step 1

- Calculate the amount of oxygen in moles using Equation 8.2. Mass of oxygen gas is 32 g and the molar mass of oxygen is 32 g·mol⁻¹.

$$\text{amount in moles, } n = \frac{\text{mass of gas}}{\text{molar mass}}$$

$$n = \frac{32}{32} = 1 \text{ mole}$$

Step 2

- The volume is calculated using the universal gas law (Equation 9.9):

$$P \cdot V = n \cdot R \cdot T$$

for one mole, $n = 1$ so rearranging:

$$V = \frac{R \cdot T}{P}$$

where $R = 8.31\,\text{J·K}^{-1}\text{·mol}^{-1}$, $T = 273\,\text{K}$, $P = 101.3 \times 10^3\,\text{Pa}$

$$V = \frac{8.31 \times 273}{101.3 \times 10^3} = 0.0224 \,\text{m}^3 = 22.4\,\text{L}$$

Answer

The volume of one mole of a gas (oxygen in this case) is 22.4 litres at STP.

Notes

- If there is a constant in an equation check that the units for the constant match the units for the other variables in the equation. In this case R (8.31 J·K⁻¹·mol⁻¹) contains K (kelvin) which would strongly suggest that the temperature should be in kelvin.
- Take care with the units for volume; it is the most common source of error when using the universal gas law.

Summary

- The notion of an ideal gas is helpful to predict behaviour of real gases under known conditions, and this behaviour is expressed in the gas laws.
- Very large molecules, or gases at the extremes of temperature and pressure, do not obey the gas laws as closely.
- The gas laws relate pressure, volume and temperature along with the number of moles of a substance.
- The partial pressures of the individual constituents of a gas add up to the total pressure of a gas mixture.
- When the lungs expand the volume increases and the pressure drops: this is Boyle's law. The pressure in the lungs becomes sub-atmospheric causing gas to move into the lungs, driven by the pressure difference.
- Pressure in cylinders increases with temperature, and with a sufficient rise can lead to explosion: this is the pressure law.

Single best answer question

For this question, choose the single best answer.

1. A fixed mass of an ideal gas initially has a volume, V, and an absolute temperature, T. Its initial pressure may be doubled by changing its volume and temperature to:

    (a) $\frac{1}{2} \cdot V$ & $4 \cdot T$
    (b) $\frac{1}{4} \cdot V$ & $\frac{1}{2} \cdot T$
    (c) $2 \cdot V$ & $\frac{1}{4} \cdot T$
    (d) $4 \cdot V$ & $2 \cdot T$
    (e) none of the above

Multiple choice questions

For each of these questions, mark every answer either true or false.

1. A child at a party holds two balloons of identical size, one filled with air and the other with helium. According to the gas laws, which of these statements is true?

    (a) There are far more molecules in the helium balloon as helium atoms have a lower atomic mass.
    (b) The balloons hold equal numbers of molecules.
    (c) The helium balloon has a lower density because it contains fewer molecules.
    (d) They are not acting as ideal gases so the gas laws do not apply.
    (e) The pressure in the balloon filled with air is considerably greater due to the larger molecules.

2. Concerning oxygen, which of the following statements are true?

    (a) Oxygen is not an ideal gas due to its large molecular size.
    (b) The diatomic nature of the gas molecule means that the ideal gas laws are a poor guide to the gas's behaviour.
    (c) The percentage of oxygen in air does not significantly alter at altitude.
    (d) The partial pressure of oxygen does not significantly differ with altitude.
    (e) Boyle's law is applicable to oxygen stored at high pressure in a cylinder.

3. At STP which of the following are true?
   (a) The percentage of oxygen molecules is just over one-fifth of air.
   (b) The pressure in SI units is 101 Pa.
   (c) The temperature in SI units is 373 K.
   (d) The pressure is notably higher than that usually found at sea level.
   (e) Observations for gases made at STP are always applicable to clinical practice.

4. If the concentration of oxygen in air remains constant but the atmospheric pressure halves, which of the following are true?
   (a) Less gas is inhaled because of Boyle's law, seriously compromising ventilation.
   (b) The partial pressure of all the gases in air doubles.

   (c) The partial pressure of oxygen will be a quarter of what it was at STP.
   (d) There will be a lower partial pressure of oxygen, dropping the concentration gradient across the alveolar membrane.
   (e) Though important at higher pressures, Dalton's law is not useful at lower pressures.

Chapter 10
Diffusion, osmosis and solubility

Having read this chapter you will be able to:
- Explain the concepts of diffusion and osmosis.
- Distinguish between a solvent, solute and solution.
- Understand the partition coefficient.
- Appreciate the role of pressure and temperature in solubility.
- Explain colligative properties and Raoult's law.

10.1 Diffusion

Imagine a tank of water divided by a glass partition. If coloured dye is added to one side of the tank, the liquid on that side will gradually turn coloured as the dye disperses. The dye (the **solute**) diffuses throughout the water (the **solvent**) to form a **solution**. Eventually the water on one side of the tank will be a uniform colour. If the partition is removed slowly without disturbing the water, the coloured water will slowly diffuse until both sides of the tank are coloured, albeit a lighter shade. The speed of this

> **Definition**
>
> **Diffusion:** the process by which there is movement of a substance from an area of high concentration of that substance to an area of lower concentration.

diffusion of the dye within the water depends on the motion of the water molecules, which are not bound in a fixed manner to one another and are in a constant state of motion; this motion ensures that the dye spreads indefinitely.

As a rule, gases are much less dense than liquids so there is more space between the molecules; this results in fewer collisions, so gas molecules can cover much greater distances in a given time. Diffusion occurs much faster in gases than in liquids, as verified when someone lets off a stink bomb in a large room. The kinetic energy of the molecules increases with temperature, so warmer gases or liquids show faster diffusion rates than when cold.

Diffusion involves the movement of molecules, as does flow, but there is a fundamental difference between the two processes. Flow of fluids may be thought of as bulk transportation driven by differences in pressures between two points. Diffusion on the other hand is a **passive process** driven by random motion of molecules in all directions; however, net movement from a region of high to low concentration is observed over time. To help understand this, imagine the partitioned tank from before, but this time the water on both sides contains equal concentrations of dye. Now when the partition is removed, although diffusion still takes place, there will be no *net* diffusion from one liquid to another.

Diffusion through a permeable membrane

Gas or liquids will diffuse from one side of a membrane to the other, as long as the membrane is **permeable** to the gas or liquid (i.e. lets the molecules pass through). *Figure 10.1* illustrates diffusion of a solute and a solvent through a permeable membrane. Many membranes including latex are permeable only to certain (usually smaller) molecules, and these are called **semi-permeable**

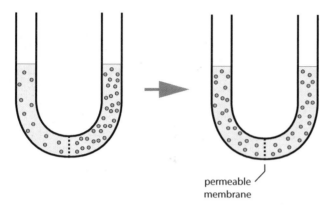

permeable
membrane

Figure 10.1. *A U-tube contains water (solvent) with a salt dissolved in it (solute). A permeable membrane allows both solvents and solutes to move and reach equilibrium.*

membranes. Capillary walls are semi-permeable membranes, allowing gases to diffuse through the walls, but are impermeable to plasma and blood cells. Diffusion thus plays an important role in the process of respiration. Diffusion of gases through membranes is also fundamental to understanding how the blood takes up inhaled anaesthetic gases, and how they pass through the blood–brain barrier.

Fick's law of diffusion

The diffusion of a gas through a membrane is described by Fick's law of diffusion. This applies to any membrane with some permeability to gas molecules, including tissues such as the alveolar membrane. The law states that the rate of transfer of a gas through the membrane is proportional to the tissue area and the difference in gas partial pressure between the two sides, and inversely proportional to the tissue thickness:

$$\text{rate of diffusion} \propto \frac{\text{surface area} \times \text{concentration gradient}}{\text{membrane thickness}}$$

10.1 Learn

Diffusion constant

The diffusion constant allows the diffusion rate to be calculated for any membrane and is dependent on the permeability of the membrane to the gas that is diffusing through it. The diffusion constant is also affected by the properties of the gas, namely its density and, in the case of diffusion into a liquid, the solubility of the gas.

Fick's diffusion equation includes the diffusion constant. The diffusion rate $\dot{V}_{gas}$ is given by:

$$\dot{V}_{gas} = D \cdot \frac{A}{T} \cdot (P_1 - P_2)$$

10.2 Learn

where A is the surface area

D is the diffusion constant

T is the thickness to diffuse through

P_1 and P_2 are the partial pressures of the gases on either side of the membrane

Graham's law of diffusion

For a party some balloons are blown up with air, and some are filled from a helium cylinder. The morning after the party the helium balloons are markedly more deflated than those that hold air. The reason for the difference in the rate of diffusion through the wall of the balloon is simply that helium molecules are physically smaller than most molecules in air (predominantly

> **Definition**
>
> **Graham's law of diffusion:**
> the rates at which gases diffuse are inversely proportional to the square root of their densities.

nitrogen molecules). Because density is much easier to measure than molecular size, Graham's law is based on density, stating that lower density gases diffuse more quickly. From Avogadro's law, equal numbers of molecules of different gases take up equal volumes, therefore density is proportional to molecular weight, which is closely related to the size of the molecules.

$$\text{rate of diffusion} \propto \frac{1}{\sqrt{\text{density}}} \qquad \textbf{10.3}$$

From Avogadro's law (*Section 9.2*) the density is directly proportional to the molecular weight of the molecules in a gas, so:

$$\text{rate of diffusion} \propto \frac{1}{\sqrt{\text{molecular mass}}} \qquad \textbf{10.4}$$

When a gas diffuses through a membrane into a liquid, the rate of diffusion is proportional to the solubility of the gas in the liquid. Each gas has different solubilities in different liquids, although we are usually concerned with the water solubility (which applies to blood too), so

$$\text{rate of diffusion} \propto \text{solubility of the gas} \qquad \textbf{10.5}$$

The diffusion constant depends only on these two factors, being proportional to the solubility of the gas in the tissue but inversely proportional to the square root of the molecular weight:

$$D = \frac{\text{solubility of the gas}}{\sqrt{\text{molecular mass}}} \qquad \textbf{10.6 Learn}$$

Carbon dioxide diffuses much more rapidly than oxygen through the alveolar membrane since it has a much higher solubility but a similar molecular weight. Despite its low molecular weight, helium hardly diffuses at all because its solubility is very low.

From Fick's law of diffusion, a faster diffusion rate is gained by

- a large surface area
- a large concentration gradient (or gas tension)
- a small thickness to diffuse through
- high solubility in medium diffusing through
- low molecular weight/density

10.2 Diffusion of respiratory and anaesthetic gases

Although diffusion is a passive process, the net flow of gas molecules seems to be 'driven' by a concentration (or partial pressure) gradient on either side of a semi-permeable membrane. Gas exchange occurs through a series of diffusion stages coupled with blood transport around the

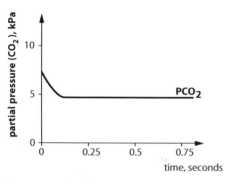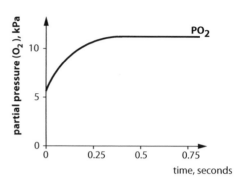

Figure 10.2. *Partial pressure in blood as it passes through the pulmonary capillaries.*

circulation system. The respiratory system is heavily dependent on diffusion to transport oxygen to the cell and carbon dioxide away from the cells. If the alveolar wall thickens, for example due to disease processes such as fibrosing alveolitis, diffusion will become impaired.

In healthy lungs, the respiratory membrane is 0.5–1.0 μm thick. In a resting subject, the time taken for a blood cell to pass through the pulmonary capillaries, the transit time, is 0.75 seconds. Carbon dioxide diffusion is complete in 0.1 seconds, after which the partial pressure gradient reduces to near to zero, whereas oxygen diffusion completes in approximately 0.3–0.4 seconds, as shown in *Figure 10.2*. This means that diffusion is complete halfway through the red blood cell's journey through the capillary.

Oxygen passing from inhaled air to tissue diffuses through the alveolar wall into the capillary blood because the partial pressure is much higher in the alveoli than in the blood (because the blood is supplied to the pulmonary capillaries by the pulmonary artery, which contains deoxygenated blood). The oxygen dissolves momentarily in the plasma, then quickly diffuses into the red blood cells, again 'driven' by a concentration gradient due to the high concentration of deoxyhaemoglobin in the red cell. Once the red cell reaches the systemic tissue (e.g. the muscles), the oxygen diffuses back through the erythrocyte wall and through the capillary into the interstitial fluid and eventually to the muscle cell. The oxygen is again driven by a concentration gradient, this time between the oxygenated red blood cells and oxygen-starved muscle cells.

Reduction in the effective surface area of the alveolar membrane, for example through emphysema or lobectomy, also leads to compromised diffusion, although the effect is rarely clinically obvious at rest. Poor pulmonary circulation will also cause impaired gas exchange, as the crucial partial pressure gradient across the membrane is not maintained.

The diffusion characteristics across the alveoli of most volatile anaesthetic agents are similar to those of carbon dioxide. If a patient is adequately oxygenated, then provided that a sufficient inhaled concentration of anaesthetic agent is present, the patient's blood concentration of anaesthetic should not be a concern.

Rubber absorbing volatile gases

Rubber is liable to absorb volatile gases by diffusion and this creates a problem for components constructed from rubber in the breathing system. If there are rubber components in the system they can act as a storage reservoir for the volatile gases, releasing volatile vapours long after the gas has been switched off. Historically, systems contained considerable amounts of rubber but this is now

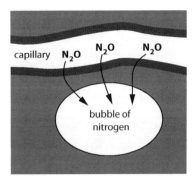

Figure 10.3. *The partial pressure of nitrous oxide in the nitrogen bubble is zero prior to induction, but as nitrous oxide carried in blood enters the capillaries it diffuses along a concentration gradient, enlarging the bubble.*

much less of a problem because the system is mainly latex-free; it is now being made up of silicone and PVC components and much of this is single patient use, being disposed of immediately following the procedure.

Clinical example

Nitrous oxide and the bends
A small amount of nitrogen dissolves in the blood of divers at depth. This is because nitrogen is very slightly soluble, and this solubility increases at higher pressures (*Section 10.4*). Bubbles of nitrogen subsequently form in the blood of divers subjected to rapid decompression because the nitrogen comes out of solution. This is known as the bends, and is a painful and potentially lethal condition. Nitrous oxide should be avoided when anaesthetizing anyone known to have recently been diving to significant depths, because nitrous oxide is more soluble than nitrogen and readily diffuses across the alveolar membrane during induction of anaesthesia. The bubbles of nitrogen can be expanded further by the diffusion of nitrous oxide from blood to join the nitrogen already present, as shown in *Figure 10.3*, dangerously exacerbating the symptoms.

10.3 Lung function test of pulmonary diffusing capacity

The **diffusing capacity** of the lung is a useful clinical variable for assessing how effectively the lung allows diffusion of oxygen into the blood. It is measured by making the patient inhale gas containing a small quantity of carbon monoxide (CO) and measuring how much is taken up by the blood in the pulmonary capillaries while the gas is held in the lung. This is achieved by measuring the difference between the CO concentration in the inspired and expired gas. Carbon monoxide is used as a marker gas because it is highly soluble in blood, so the uptake of the gas is not flow-limited.

Fick's law of diffusion (Equation 10.2) states that the amount of gas transferred across a sheet of tissue is proportional to the area, a diffusion constant and the difference in partial pressure, and inversely proportional to the thickness. For a complex structure like the blood–gas barrier of the lung, it is not possible to measure the area and thickness in a living patient and so instead the Fick equation is re-written

$$\dot{V}_{gas} = D_L \cdot (P_1 - P_2)$$

10.7

where D_L is called the *diffusing capacity of the lung* and is very similar to the diffusion constant in Equation 10.2, but incorporates the area and thickness as well as the diffusion properties of the tissue and the gas concerned. Thus the diffusing capacity for carbon monoxide (CO) is given by

$$D_L = \frac{\dot{V}_{CO}}{(P_1 - P_2)}$$

10.8

where P_1 and P_2 are the partial pressures of alveolar gas and capillary blood, respectively

The partial pressure of CO in blood is extremely small and can be neglected, so the diffusing capacity is simply given by:

$$D_L = \frac{\dot{V}_{CO}}{(P_{ACO})}$$

10.9

Where P_{ACO} is the alveolar partial pressure of carbon monoxide. In words, the diffusing capacity of the lung for CO is the volume of CO transferred in millilitres per minute per kPa of alveolar partial pressure.

Measurement technique

Several techniques for making the measurement are available. The *single breath method* is the most frequently used in clinical practice and has a long history of progressive refinement. There are many variations on the exact method used, which yield broadly similar results.

The patient is first required to exhale maximally, then draws in a vital-capacity breath of a gas mixture containing about 0.3% carbon monoxide and about 10% helium. The breath is held for 10 seconds and a gas sample is then taken after the exhalation of the first 0.75 litres, which is sufficient to wash out the patient's dead space. The end-expiratory partial pressure of carbon monoxide is measured directly using an infrared gas analyser. It is assumed that no significant amount of helium has passed into the blood because helium is almost completely insoluble. Therefore, the ratio of the concentration of helium in the inspired gas to the concentration in the end-expiratory gas, multiplied by the inspired volume (vital capacity) gives the total alveolar volume during the period of breath holding.

From the measured data, the diffusing capacity, adjusted for the patient's haemoglobin concentration, can then be calculated and normalized for the alveolar volume measured at the same time with helium. These calculations are now usually performed automatically by computer, which also compares the values with predicted 'normal' values based on the patient's gender, height, age, etc.

10.4 Osmosis

Definition

Osmosis: the diffusion of a solvent across a membrane while the solute remains.

Consider a beaker of water where a drop of blood has been added. The red blood cells swell as water passes into them and this continues until they burst. Why does haemolysis occur? The outer membrane of the red blood cell is a semi-permeable membrane that allows smaller molecules to pass through it but not larger ones. For a red blood cell that contains electrolytes such as potassium and sodium cations, the water molecules pass through the membrane until the concentration of electrolytes is equal on either side (or until the cell bursts!). The concentration gradient causes the molecules to move from a more dilute to a more concentrated solution. Osmosis is also the mechanism that is at work

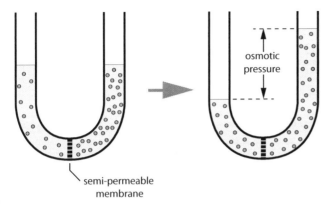

Figure 10.4. *Osmosis. Water (solvent) passes through a semi-permeable membrane from a solution of low concentration to higher concentration.*

when slugs are killed by pouring salt on them. In effect the skin of gastropods is a water-permeable membrane (unlike ours), so the salt draws water from the slug's body.

Osmosis can be quantified in terms of **osmotic pressure**; the required pressure to stop the flow from one side of the membrane to the other. If pure water, or two **isotonic** solutions, are placed either side of a water-permeable membrane (*Figure 10.4*), water molecules pass in and out in each direction at the same rate, i.e. there is no net flow of water through the membrane. Osmosis is important in biological systems because, as we have seen, they contain semi-permeable membranes, and these membranes are generally impermeable to organic solutes with large molecules, such as starch, but are permeable to water. Water molecules travel through the cell walls by diffusion and osmosis therefore provides the primary means by which water is transported into and out of cells.

> **Definitions**
>
> **Isotonic solutions:** two or more solutions that have the same concentration of a solute.
> **Hypertonic solution:** has a higher concentration of a solute in comparison to another solution.
> **Hypotonic solution:** has a lower concentration of a solute in comparison to the other solution.

10.5 Solubility

Solubility is the ability of a substance to dissolve, such as a lump of sugar dissolving in a cup of hot tea. The substance that is being dissolved is known as the solute and the substance into which the solute is dissolved in known as the solvent; in totality the solute and the solvent are referred to as the solution. So, applying this to the tea: the sugar is the solute, the water is the solvent and the cup of sweetened tea is the solution. Incidentally, whilst stirring accelerates the rate the sugar dissolves, if left alone the sugar would dissolve of its own accord: the amount of sugar which could dissolve (the solubility) is unchanged by mechanical agitation. However, if the tea cooled the solubility would be affected; much less sugar can be dissolved in cold water than in hot.

> **Definition**
>
> **Solubility:** the amount (in moles) of a solute that can be dissolved in unit volume of solvent under specified conditions.

Generally gases are soluble in liquids and as solutes they are either in the form of molecules or ions dependent on the solute, solvent and conditions. For instance, for water (a good solvent) some solutes dissolve as neutral molecules while others dissociate and dissolve as ions, carrying a charge, creating an electrolyte solution.

Solubility, pressure and temperature: Henry's law

Nitrogen has limited solubility in blood and so does not take part in respiratory gas exchange. However, nitrogen becomes a serious factor in respiration for divers, bringing on confusion and 'the bends'. As the pressure increases during a diving descent so does the partial pressure of nitrogen and as a result the amount of nitrogen dissolved into the blood becomes significant. This is a consequence of Henry's law: the degree a gas dissolves into a fluid increases proportionally to the rise in partial pressure.

> **Definition**
>
> **Henry's law:** at a constant temperature, the amount of a given gas that dissolves in a given type and volume of liquid is directly proportional to the partial pressure of that gas in equilibrium with that liquid.

Henry's law is given by the following equation:

$$C_X = k_H \cdot P_X$$

10.10

where C_X is the concentration of the gas
k_H is the **Henry's law constant**
P_X is the partial pressure of the gas in solution

The Henry's law constant depends on the gas, the solvent and the temperature. Solubility falls as temperature rises, and this is another point of concern for a diver. As discussed in the last section, a diver's body will cool during a dive in a cold sea and if, following a hasty ascent, the diver decides to have a hot bath, the danger of nitrogen coming out of solution is exacerbated. Henry's law requires that the temperature remains constant, otherwise the amount of gas dissolved will change.

A bottle of fizzy drink neatly illustrates the effect of both temperature and pressure on solubility. When the bottle top is unscrewed pressure is released. The liquid is now at a lower pressure and as a result gas comes out of solution. If it is a hot day and the drink is poured into a glass the liquid's

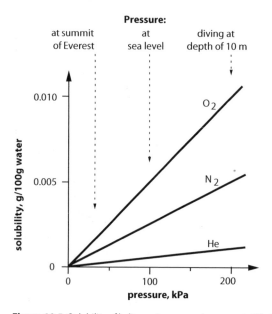

Figure 10.5. *Solubility of helium, nitrogen and oxygen at differing partial pressures, at a temperature of 25°C.*

temperature rises and as a result more gas comes out of solution: this produces lots of froth but leaves the drink rather 'flat'.

Solubility coefficients for gases and liquids

The solubility of solids in liquids is measured in term of moles, the units for measuring the amount of a substance per unit volume, and is applicable to gases as well as solids. As solubility varies with temperature any coefficient of solubility is only specific to a specific temperature. *Figure 10.5* shows how the solubility coefficient in water varies with pressure for three different gases.

Worked example

Question
Carbon dioxide is a bigger molecule than oxygen yet it diffuses at a greater rate through the respiratory membrane. Why?

Answer
In the gaseous state oxygen diffuses quicker than carbon dioxide because it has lower molecular weight (Graham's law). However, carbon dioxide is considerably more soluble in the fluid on the respiratory membrane and this is why it diffuses faster through the membrane.

10.6 Partition coefficient

A bottle of olive oil can be used to estimate the potency of an anaesthetic agent. The solubility of anaesthetic gas in the oil indicates the anaesthetic effect, because the high percentage of fat in the brain means that the oil is a good model of the brain's absorption ability. The Meyer–Overton graph (*Figure 10.6*) shows how the potency of an anaesthetic, quantified by its minimum alveolar concentration (MAC), is related to the oil/gas partition coefficient.

The **partition coefficient** measures the tendency of a solute to dissolve in two different immiscible solvents (phases). The partition coefficient is written as $\lambda(a,b)$ where a and b are the locations of where the solutes are travelling to and from, respectively. The partition coefficient does not have units and is temperature dependent. The partition coefficient can also be calculated for a liquid/gas interface. Pulmonary gas uptake is a function of the blood solubility of a vapour, indicated by the blood/

Definitions

Partition coefficient: the ratio of concentrations of a substance in two phases of a mixture of two immiscible solvents.
Blood/gas coefficient: the ratio of the concentration of an anaesthetic agent in blood to that in the same volume of gas in contact with that blood at equilibrium.
Oil/gas coefficient: the ratio of the concentration of an anaesthetic agent in oil (adipose tissue) to that in the same volume of gas in contact with that oil, at equilibrium.

air partition coefficient, λ(blood, gas). Because partition coefficients are temperature dependent, the blood/gas partition coefficient must be calculated at body temperature. An anaesthetic agent with λ(blood, gas) = 0.5 inhaled at 8% concentration would produce a 4% concentration in the arterial blood; this concentration is found simply by multiplying the concentration in air by the partition coefficient.

Figure 10.7a shows what happens if a volume of 100% nitrous oxide gas at atmospheric pressure is allowed to reach equilibrium with blood. λ(blood, gas) for nitrous oxide is 0.47 at 37°C, so 100 mL of blood at equilibrium with the gas will contain 47 mL of dissolved nitrous oxide. Note that the

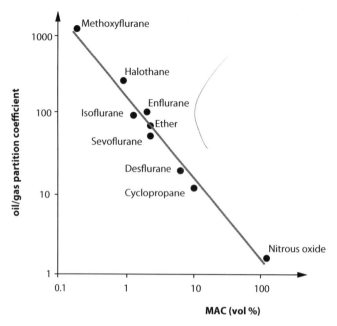

Figure 10.6. *The Meyer–Overton graph relating the oil/gas partition to MAC. Note that both scales are logarithmic.*

partial pressures of nitrous oxide in the gas and the blood are both 101 kPa according to Dalton's law (Equation 9.3).

Figure 10.7b shows a similar situation if the nitrous oxide is equilibrated with 100 mL oil and 100 mL blood. Since nitrous oxide is more soluble in oil than in blood, the oil will contain more N_2O than the blood at equilibrium. The partition coefficient, λ(blood, oil) is equal to 0.34, so once equilibrium is reached, the amount of N_2O in the oil is greater than in the blood (actually 140 mL).

Intuitively, an anaesthetic that was highly soluble in blood would appear to be an ideal inhaled anaesthetic agent. However, such a compound, although it transfers quickly from the lungs to the blood, does so at the expense of exerting a lower partial pressure once dissolved. The agent stays in solution rather than passing to the brain tissue. A lower partial pressure gradient means a lower

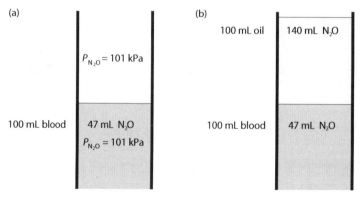

Figure 10.7. *Effect of partition coefficients on the volume of nitrous oxide dissolved in various solvents exposed to 100% N_2O at atmospheric pressure. (a) The blood/gas partition coefficient = 0.47, so 47 mL of N_2O dissolves in the blood; (b) the blood/oil partition coefficient = 0.34, so more N_2O dissolves in the oil than in the blood.*

rate of diffusion from the blood to the brain (Equation 10.2). The higher the blood/gas partition coefficient, the longer the time for the anaesthetic to work and, just as importantly, the longer the time for the anaesthetic to exit the body. So in fact a low solubility is the desired trait.

Definition

Minimum alveolar concentration: the MAC is the concentration of vapour in the lungs required to prevent a reflex response to a skin incision (pain) in 50% of patients; it is a measure of anaesthetic potency.

10.7 Colligative properties of solutions

A lorry gritting the roads is a common sight in winter, helping to stop the roads from becoming hazardous with ice. The grit contains salt and works by lowering the freezing point (equal to the melting point). The freezing point of water becomes lower than 0°C as more particles are added until the point at which the salt stops dissolving.

Colligative properties, such as vapour pressure, osmotic pressure and variations in boiling and freezing point, are properties of solutions that depend simply on the number of molecules of solute in a given volume of solvent rather than the properties (e.g. size, mass or the identities) of the solute molecules. In contrast, non-colligative properties depend on the identity of both the dissolved species and the solvent. An example of a colligative property is the lowering of the freezing point of a liquid by addition of a non-volatile solute. The amount by which the freezing point drops is related to the number of molecules (equal to the amount of substance) added. Another example is the lowering of vapour pressure by adding a solute. The more solute particles on the liquid's surface the fewer solvent particles on the surface, so evaporation is impeded (*Figure 10.8*). The amount that the vapour pressure rises is proportional to the molar concentration of the solute according to Raoult's law. The resulting solution has a higher boiling point than the original solvent.

Definition

Raoult's law: the rise in vapour pressure of a solvent is proportional to the molar concentration of the solute.

Osmometer: freezing point change

Osmotic pressure is measured by an osmometer and is used for testing body fluids such as urine and plasma. It is also used to find the relative molecular mass of compounds, particularly larger molecules. Measuring osmotic pressure directly is hampered by the difficulty in manufacturing a perfect semi-permeable membrane that does not let small ions diffuse through. Instead it can be measured via a colligative property: the freezing point is related to the osmotic pressure.

The osmometer consists of a sample chamber, a stirrer and a temperature probe along with a cooling chamber. The sample is super-cooled whilst being continuously stirred to a temperature lower than the expected freezing point. Whilst being vigorous stirred it freezes in a slush-like state: equilibrium between ice and liquid. This is the freezing point, and the temperature is recorded.

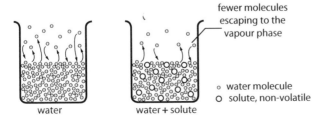

Figure 10.8. *Vapour pressure is reduced when solute particles decrease the surface area available to the water molecules.*

The changes in the freezing point are small so a highly sensitive thermistor is used to measure temperature.

Osmometer: vapour pressure change and the sweat test

According to Raoult's law the change in vapour pressure with the addition of a solute (such as a salt) to a solvent (such as water) is proportional to the concentration of solute present. So it is then possible to work out the content of salt present in sweat by measuring the vapour pressure of a sample. This can then be compared to the values for water containing no salts and the concentration of salts in the sample calculated. This is the principle behind the sweat test used to identify the higher salt content present in the sweat of cystic fibrosis sufferers.

Summary

- Diffusion through a permeable membrane is an important mechanism in respiratory gas exchange.
- Fick's law of diffusion states that the thickness of the membrane and partial pressure gradient affect the rate of diffusion.
- The diffusion constant affects the rate of diffusion and is proportional to the solubility and the molecular weight of the gas.
- Lung function tests of diffusing capacity take into account the diffusion constant as well as the surface area and thickness of the alveolar membrane.
- Osmosis is the transfer of a solvent across a semi-permeable membrane.
- The partition coefficient of an anaesthetic agent between water and oil has an effect on its potency.
- Colligative properties are those that depend only on the concentration of a solute and not the properties of the solute molecules themselves.

Single best answer questions

For these questions, choose the single best answer.

1. Which of the following explains the reduction in diffusing capacity caused by fibrosing alveolitis?
   (a) The thickness of the alveolar membrane is decreased.
   (b) The area of the alveolar membrane is decreased.
   (c) The pulmonary blood flow is reduced.
   (d) The thickness of the alveolar membrane increases.
   (e) The partial pressure gradient across the membrane is reduced.

2. Inhaled helium does not diffuse into blood because:
   (a) it has too low a density
   (b) it has a low viscosity
   (c) it is insoluble
   (d) the alveolar membrane is impermeable to helium
   (e) it is inert

3. Which one of the following is true of inhaled anaesthetic agents?
   (a) A high oil/water partition coefficient results in a potent anaesthetic effect.
   (b) A low oil/water partition coefficient results in a potent anaesthetic effect.
   (c) A high solubility in water results in a potent anaesthetic effect.
   (d) A high solubility in water results in a less potent anaesthetic effect.
   (e) A high solubility in oil results in a more potent anaesthetic effect.

4. Regarding osmosis, which one of the following statements is true?
   (a) Osmosis involves movement of uncharged small solute molecules through a membrane.
   (b) Movement of solvent molecules through a membrane ceases when osmotic pressure is zero.
   (c) Osmosis is driven by attraction between solvent molecules.
   (d) The osmotic pressure within a blood cell placed in distilled water decreases with time.
   (e) Oxygen transfer from the plasma to the red blood cell requires osmosis.

5. Which one of the following statements is true?
   (a) Carbon dioxide is used to measure diffusing capacity because it diffuses across the membrane and is not abundant in blood.
   (b) The diffusing capacity of the lungs is dependent on the membrane surface area.
   (c) Helium is used to measure the diffusing capacity.
   (d) The diffusing capacity is not affected by haemoglobin concentration and cardiac output.
   (e) The diffusing capacity of the lungs is not affected by lung volume.

Multiple choice questions

For each of these questions, mark every answer either true or false.

1. The diffusion constant is proportional to:
   (a) the solubility of the gas
   (b) the inverse of the solubility of the gas
   (c) the inverse of the square root of the molecular weight of the gas
   (d) the inverse of the square of the molecular weight of the gas
   (e) the inverse of the molecular weight of the gas

2. Adding salt to ice causes what effect?
   (a) The ice melts because the freezing point is lowered.
   (b) The ice melts because the melting point is raised.
   (c) The ice melts because the latent heat of fusion is increased.
   (d) The ice melts because the melting point is lowered.
   (e) The ice melts because the vapour pressure is decreased.

3. Which of the following is not a colligative property?
   (a) Osmotic pressure.
   (b) Partition coefficient of a solute between oil and water.
   (c) Increase in boiling point by addition of a solute.
   (d) Rate of diffusion of molecules through a membrane.
   (e) Reduction in vapour pressure by addition of a solute.

4. Regarding gas exchange in the lung, which of the following statements are true?
   (a) Blood transits a capillary in approximately 0.75 s at rest.
   (b) During exercise the capillary transit time is reduced, so equilibrium between blood and alveolar gas cannot take place.
   (c) Oxygen diffuses more slowly than carbon dioxide due to its lower solubility.
   (d) Oxygen and carbon dioxide diffuse at roughly the same rate due to their similar molecular weights.
   (e) Thickening of the alveolar membrane has a greater proportional effect on oxygen transfer than carbon dioxide transfer.

5. Which of the following statements are true regarding Henry's law?
   (a) Nitrogen has very limited solubility in blood.
   (b) The solubility increases at depth due to higher partial pressure.
   (c) The bends occur on decompression due to formation of nitrogen bubbles in the blood.
   (d) The bends can be prevented by inhaling nitrous oxide during decompression.
   (e) Solubility of gases increases at higher temperatures.

Chapter 11

Measuring gas and vapour concentrations

Having read this chapter you will be able to:
- Explain the basics of an infrared gas analyser.
- Explain the difference between main-stream and side-stream sampling.
- Understand how paramagnetic and fuel cell oxygen analysers work.
- Understand the principle of the sensing electrodes used in blood gas analysis.
- Know the basics of gas chromatography, mass spectrometry and Raman spectroscopy.

11.1 Respiratory gas monitoring

The need to promptly assess the presence and concentrations of gases in the clinical setting is critical to anaesthesia, and so anaesthetic rooms and operating theatres have monitors for measuring respiratory gas concentrations. Modern instruments can measure the respiratory gases oxygen and carbon dioxide as well as anaesthetic gases such as nitrous oxide and volatile agents. The analyser usually contains two sensing modules, one for oxygen and one for everything else. The oxygen sensor exploits oxygen's paramagnetic properties, while the sensor for other gases works on the principle of infrared absorption.

Respiratory gas monitors must have rapid response times since the concentration of gas measured at the mouth or nose varies rapidly over one respiratory cycle. The carbon dioxide concentration, for example, varies from a maximum near the end of expiration (the end-tidal concentration) to a minimum of just above zero (the atmospheric concentration, approximately 0.1%) during inspiration.

There are two techniques to sample the gas in the breathing circuit: **main-stream** and **side-stream** sampling. For main-stream sampling, a detector clips on to a dedicated tubing section and a data cable communicates between the detector and the anaesthetic monitoring system, as shown in *Figure 11.1a*. In principle, monitors using main-stream sampling can respond immediately to changes in concentration, producing a real-time measurement. In the past the sensors were large, heavy, bulky, hot with prolonged use, and easy to damage, though recent designs have improved matters. They increase dead space slightly, but this is not clinically significant other than in paediatrics or in patients with reduced lung volumes. Main-stream monitoring does not usually allow oxygen monitoring, since the size of the sensor is restricted.

The side-stream sampling method uses a thin sampling tube linking the circuit to a detector module in the anaesthetic monitoring system, as shown in *Figure 11.1b*. A small fan generates a small negative pressure at the module end of the tubing drawing off a constant flow of gas from the circuit, typically 150–200 mL·min^{-1}. A water trap placed just before the module prevents condensation entering the analyser. This setup has the advantage that the breathing tube remains free of a bulky sensor, while the measurement module can be large enough to incorporate an oxygen analyser in series with the infrared analyser. However, the gases in the sample tubing can mix leading to less precise data, the tubing is also vulnerable to occlusion, and the sampling tube introduces a time lag of a few seconds before the concentration is displayed.

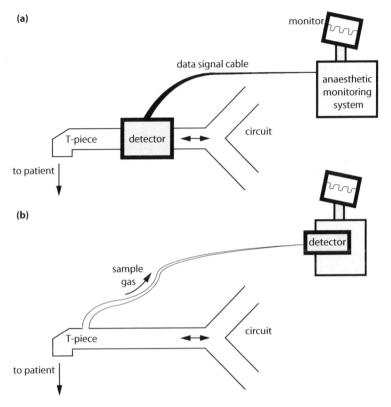

(a)

monitor

data signal cable

anaesthetic
monitoring
system

T-piece — detector — circuit

to patient

(b)

detector

sample
gas

T-piece — circuit

to patient

Figure 11.1. *(a) Main-stream and (b) side-stream sampling.*

11.2 Infrared absorption spectroscopy for gases

Light appears to pass through air with ease, but some gases do absorb significant amounts of electromagnetic radiation. It is the make-up of the gas molecules that dictate their ability to absorb. Polyatomic gases such as nitrous oxide, carbon dioxide and water vapour absorb infrared electromagnetic waves, whereas individual atoms, and in general elementary gases such as oxygen, nitrogen and helium, do not.

Beer's law (*Section 15.4*) applies to gases as well as liquids and states that the concentration of gas present is directly proportional to the absorbance of electromagnetic waves. Crucially, at particularly wavelengths this can be significant enough to measure. *Figure 11.2* shows the absorption spectrum of carbon dioxide and nitrous oxide. Carbon dioxide selectively absorbs specific wavelengths of infrared light at a peak wavelength of 4.28 μm. To calculate the percentage of carbon dioxide:

$$\text{percentage of CO}_2 = \frac{\text{partial pressure of carbon dioxide}}{\text{atmospheric pressure}} \times 100\% \qquad \textbf{11.1}$$

Mixtures of gases are known to produce certain variations of absorption wavelength due to interactive forces between molecules. This so-called **collision broadening effect** not only broadens the absorption peak but can also cause a shift in the peak absorption wavelength. Nitrous oxide and carbon dioxide are well known to interact with each other altering the wavelength of absorbance.

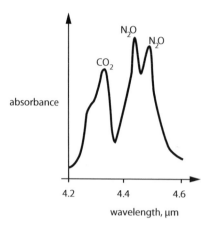

Figure 11.2. *Absorption spectra of carbon dioxide and nitrous oxide.*

Gas analysers must account for this effect when calculating $EtCO_2$ (end-tidal CO_2) if nitrous oxide is also known to be present in the expired gas.

The infrared analyser (see *Figure 11.3*) produces infrared radiation by heating a wire and this radiation is then filtered to select a single wavelength which the gas of interest is known to absorb. The sample chamber has windows made from material that allows infrared light to pass through, such as sapphire (glass cannot be used as it absorbs infrared), and a photodetector measures the intensity of the radiation passing though the chamber. Some systems have a parallel chamber containing air as the control gas with an assumption of no carbon dioxide being present in the air, allowing compensation for changes in intensity of the light source.

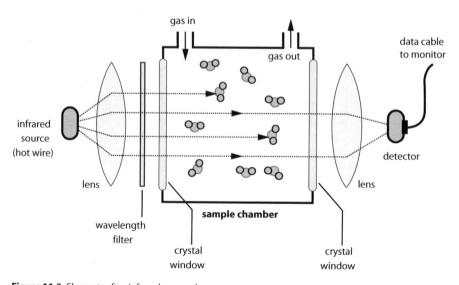

Figure 11.3. *Elements of an infrared gas analyser.*

11.3 Capnography

A capnometer is a device for measuring exhaled carbon dioxide concentration. Most devices are capable of displaying a **capnograph** (or **capnogram**), a waveform graph of concentration against time over each respiratory cycle; the instrument itself is now often referred to as a capnograph. The end-tidal carbon dioxide concentration is calculated automatically from the capnograph trace and an updated value is shown, usually once per breath. Units are given in percent volume (e.g. 5%) or as a volume ratio (e.g. 0.05). Alternatively, the user can choose to display the partial pressure (see *Section 9.3*) of CO_2 in the exhaled gas, in units of mmHg or kPa.

A nominal capnograph trace is shown in *Figure 11.4*. The value increases when expiration begins. There is a slight lag, called the **rise time,** caused mostly by mixing of gas in the sample chamber which results in an S-shaped **expiratory upstroke** (between points A and B on the graph). The expiratory plateau (B to C) has a slight upward slope due to continued diffusion of CO_2 across the alveolar membrane during expiration. End-tidal concentration ($EtCO_2$) is taken as the maximum value (dotted line). Inspiration is marked by a downstroke (C to D) followed by a flat baseline plateau (D to E) that continues until the end of inspiration. For breath-by-breath monitoring, a capnogram is displayed over a short timescale, while for trend monitoring, several minutes (or hours) of data are displayed.

11.4 Paramagnetic oxygen analysers

Gaseous oxygen is weakly attracted to a magnetic field. Oxygen molecules have paramagnetic properties because the electrons in their outer shells are unpaired. At very, very low temperatures (–183°C) oxygen exists as a liquid and can be suspended in a magnetic field due to its strong paramagnetic properties when so cold. At normal temperature, though weak, oxygen's paramagnetic properties can be exploited to measure its concentration in a gas.

> **Definition**
>
> **Paramagnetic oxygen analyser:** measures the concentration of oxygen in a gas by exploiting the weak paramagnetic properties that are present in oxygen but not in the other major components of air.

Null-deflection paramagnetic oxygen analyser

The **null-deflection paramagnetic oxygen analyser** comprises a sample chamber containing a beam connected to two nitrogen-containing spheres. This 'dumb-bell' is suspended by a torsion balance as shown in *Figure 11.5*. When no oxygen is present, the spheres come to rest over the poles of a

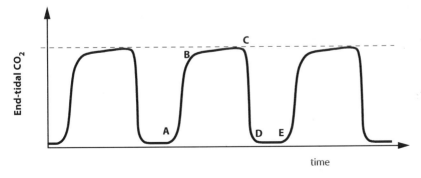

Figure 11.4. *A nominal capnograph trace. A–B is the expiratory upstroke, B–C is the expiratory plateau, C is the end-tidal concentration, C–D is on inspiration, and D–E is the baseline.*

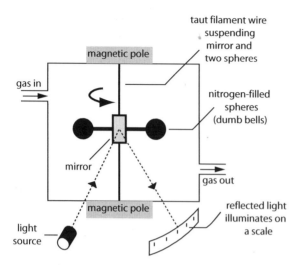

Figure 11.5. *Null-deflection paramagnetic oxygen analyser.*

strong magnet, but when oxygen is present it displaces (or pushes) the weakly diamagnetic nitrogen filling the suspended spheres away from the magnet, causing rotation of the beam. The movement of spheres moves a mirror attached to the beam which reflects a spot of light onto a scale which can be read by the user. This type of analyser is highly accurate, although it is vulnerable to interference from water vapour, vibrations and variations in ventilation pressure, especially at high flow rates. Another drawback is that the analyser has a very slow response time, somewhere in the region of 10 seconds. For these reasons, the null-deflection analyser is unsuitable for real-time expired gas monitoring, so its use is confined to measuring oxygen concentration in respiratory gas supplies.

Pulsed-field paramagnetic oxygen analyser

The pulsed-field paramagnetic oxygen analyser (*Figure 11.6*) overcomes the problem of the slow response times experienced with the null-deflection analyser. The pulsed-field analyser also relies

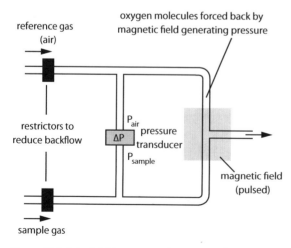

Figure 11.6. *Pulsed-field paramagnetic oxygen analyser.*

on paramagnetism, but a completely different measurement method is utilized. Air is drawn from the breathing circuit and is mixed with a reference gas, normally room air, within the analyser. A magnetic field is switched on which attracts oxygen molecules. This causes oxygen to accumulate in the region of the field, causing an increased pressure on one side of a double-sided pressure transducer. The pressure difference is a reflection of the difference in partial pressures between the sample and the reference gas. In practice, the magnetic field is turned on and off repeatedly creating an alternating pressure typically at a frequency of around 100 Hz.

11.5 Electrochemical cells

An electrochemical cell (see *Figure 11.7*) is a device that produces electrical current from a chemical reaction. When connected to a circuit as shown, metal atoms within the anode are oxidized and lose electrons forming cations (positively charged ions) that migrate towards the cathode. A current flows within the cell from the cathode, through the external circuit (the bulb in the diagram), to the anode. There are many types of cell constructed from an enormous range of metals and electrolyte solutions. Lead-acid car batteries, alkaline batteries and rechargeable Ni-Cad batteries are examples of different kinds of electrochemical cell.

> **Definition**
>
> **Cations and anions:** an ion is a molecule that contains an imbalance of charges: the number of protons does not equal the number of electrons. Positively charged ions are called cations and negatively charged ions, anions.

The galvanic fuel cell

The galvanic fuel cell is a type of electrochemical cell where oxygen is the missing ingredient for an electrochemical reaction to take place. The fuel cell is thus an ideal means of detecting the presence

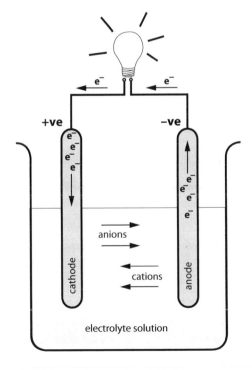

Figure 11.7. *A general electrochemical cell.*

of oxygen and the current generated gives an indication of its concentration. This device has the added advantage that it does not need an external power supply. It is similar to the Clark electrode that is discussed in *Section 11.7*. As current flow is directly proportional to the uptake of oxygen at the cathode then, by Henry's law, it is also proportional to the partial pressure of oxygen in the sample gas.

A simplified fuel cell is shown in *Figure 11.8*. It has a gold mesh cathode, a lead anode and, separating the two electrodes, a potassium hydroxide electrolyte solution. When oxygen enters the solution a chemical reaction occurs generating excess hydroxide ions. At the **gold cathode** when oxygen is present:

$$O_2 + 4e^- + 2H_2O \rightarrow 4OH^-$$

11.2 Learn

Hydroxyl ions enter the electrolyte solution of potassium hydroxide and migrate to the lead anode. At the **lead anode**:

$$Pb + 2OH^- \rightarrow PbO + H_2O + 2e^-$$

11.3 Learn

A current is thus generated as the electrons flow.

The fuel cell has a response time of up to 30 seconds and a thermistor compensates for the variations in current that occur with temperature change. It does have a limited life span because the anode gradually decreases in size over time. Nitrous oxide can affect the fuel cell as it diffuses into the cell, and then reacts with lead to produce nitrogen, changing partial pressures and potentially damaging the cell. There are adapted fuel cells that are used only if nitrous oxide is given. Fuel cell oxygen analysers are routinely used in anaesthetic machines to monitor the oxygen concentration in the supply gas. They are also ideal for use in scuba diving, as they are lightweight, reliable and portable.

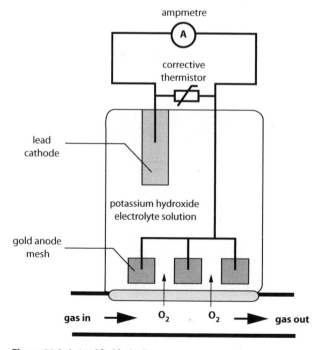

Figure 11.8. *A simplified fuel cell.*

11.6 Electrodes used in arterial blood gas analysis

The arterial blood gas analyser can be thought of as a collection of sensors, electrolyte solutions and electronic circuitry. The prime sensors are the **Clark electrode** (oxygen), the **Severinghaus electrode** (carbon dioxide) and the **Sanz electrode** (pH). They give quick and relatively accurate measurements of gas partial pressures in the plasma and the plasma pH.

Arterial sampling syringes have heparin or a similar anticoagulant added to prevent blood clots inside the analyser causing a blockage. Samples should be bubble-free and analysed immediately after drawing from the patient. An air bubble in the sample causes gases in the blood to rapidly equilibrate with the air in the bubble causing erroneous measurements. Blood gas samples are analysed at a standard temperature of 37°C irrespective of the patient's actual temperature. This method is known as α-stat (measuring at the patient's actual temperature is known as pH-stat).

The membranes and glass employed in the various designs of electrodes provide a physical barrier that protects electrodes from becoming coated with proteins from the blood that would otherwise prevent them from functioning. After a time, the membrane itself becomes coated with proteins, which can cause erroneous results. This is prevented by regularly changing the sensor membranes.

Measuring the partial pressure of oxygen: the Clark electrode

The Clark electrode (also called the polarographic electrode) allows the partial pressure of oxygen in blood to be measured. It is named after Leland Clark, who designed the electrode whilst building the first bubble oxygenator for cardiac surgery. The anode is a silver wire coated in silver chloride, the cathode is made from platinum, and they are connected by a potassium chloride solution (see *Figure 11.9*). A small fixed voltage of the order of 0.6 V is applied across the electrodes. At the cathode oxygen, electrons and water react to deliver hydroxide ions:

$$O_2 + 4e^- + 2H_2O \rightarrow 4OH^-$$ **11.4**

The current depends on the supply of oxygen molecules to allow the generation of the charge-carrying hydroxide ions. This current is a direct reflection of the partial pressure of oxygen in the sample allowing accurate measurement.

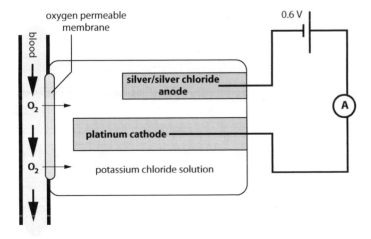

Figure 11.9. *The Clark electrode (simplified).*

Measuring the pH: the Sanz electrode

The Sanz electrode (*Figure 11.10*) measures the pH in the blood. A glass permeable to hydrogen ions separates the blood sample and a buffer solution. Because hydrogen ions consist of a proton with no electron they are extremely small and the glass will let them pass, while remaining impermeable to other ions, atoms and molecules. The hydrogen ion concentration within the measuring electrode is maintained at a constant value by the buffer solution and this means that the potential across the glass is dependent solely upon the concentration of positively charged hydrogen ions in the blood sample channel. The reference electrode is the silver/silver chloride electrode which is suspended in a saturated potassium chloride solution. The potential difference between the two electrodes indicates the concentration of hydrogen ions.

Measuring the partial pressure of carbon dioxide: the Severinghaus electrode

The Severinghaus electrode (*Figure 11.11*) measures the partial pressure of carbon dioxide in blood. There is a dilute bicarbonate buffer and as carbon dioxide diffuses through the membrane it reacts with the water molecules to form carbonic acid. This in turn dissociates to form bicarbonate ions and, crucially, hydrogen ions. The following occurs:

$$CO_2 + H_2O \leftrightarrow H_2CO_3 \leftrightarrow H^+ + HCO_3^-$$

11.5 Learn

This change in pH is proportional to the concentration of the dissolved carbon dioxide in the blood. The glass electrode measures this change in concentration of hydrogen ions and indirectly the partial pressure of carbon dioxide is measured. The silver/silver chloride electrode acts as a reference electrode.

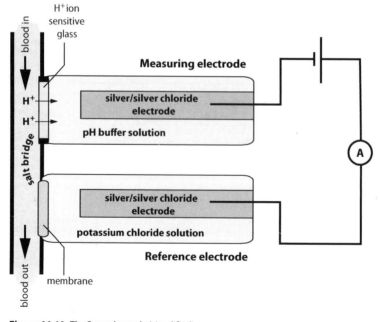

Figure 11.10. *The Sanz electrode (simplified).*

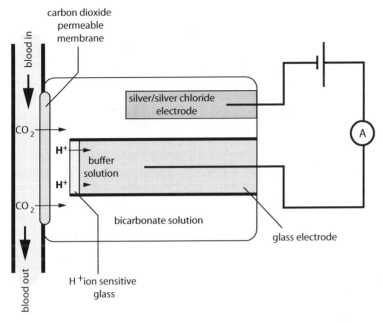

Figure 11.11. *The Severinghaus electrode (simplified).*

Measuring the concentration of other ions

The basic form of the pH electrode can be adapted to measure other ions such potassium, calcium and sodium ions. The reference electrode remains, but the measuring electrode is changed such that it is sensitive to another ion, rather than hydrogen ions.

11.7 Other gas monitoring techniques

Gas chromatography

Chromatography is a technique applicable to both gases and liquids and is based on the separation of compounds in a **chromatography column** prior to analysis. Drugs in solution can be analysed but first they must be mixed with a volatile compound prior to testing. Gas chromatography can measure the concentration of all the components of a gas mixture and can measure trace elements in the theatre atmosphere, or measure drug concentrations including steroids, phenothiazine and benzodiazepines. There are two phases, a mobile (or moving) phase and a stationary phase, and separation of compounds depends on their partition between the two phases. It can detect very low concentrations though it is time consuming, not capable of sampling continuously, and the gas cannot be returned to the patient.

The mobile phase is a gas that is moved through the column: the phase comprises an inert **carrier gas** into which the volatile sample is injected. Both the sample and carrier gas travel through the column together. The carrier gas is usually helium, hydrogen, or nitrogen.

There are two general types of column, **packed columns** and **capillary columns**. Packed columns contain a finely divided, inert, solid support material (such as kaolin, alumina, silica or activated charcoal) coated with liquid stationary phase. Most packed columns are a few metres in length and have an internal diameter of 2–5 mm. Capillary columns are approximately one-tenth the diameter of packed columns and instead of a support material, have a thin film of liquid stationary phase coating their walls. An alternative design has a thin film of support material onto which the liquid phase has been adsorbed.

The carrier gas is passed through a column at a tightly controlled temperature. The various components move through the column at different rates, according to their degree of attraction to the stationary phase. A detector is positioned at the far end of the column and is able to detect compounds other than the carrier gas. The positions of detection peaks indicate the time taken to travel though the column and are unique to each compound. The height of each peak indicates the concentration.

Mass spectrometry

Mass spectrometry is a technique for measuring low concentrations of gases and though once used in theatres it is now mainly used in research laboratories. A mass spectrometer creates positive ions (positively charged particles) from gas molecules by bombarding them with high speed electrons, knocking out electrons from the outer shells of atoms within the molecules. The ions are then accelerated by passing them through an electric field and then deflected using a strong, fixed magnetic field. Heavier ions are deflected less than lighter ions, so each type of ion is separated according to its charge to mass ratio. An array of detectors is positioned to collect the deflected ions, and their relative abundance is recorded. This charge to mass ratio is unique to each molecule, allowing identification of the molecules. With mass spectrometry the gas cannot be returned to the patient because it undergoes ionization. The benefits of this technique are that it is highly accurate and can measure all gases. However, the machines are cumbersome and are easily damaged.

Raman spectroscopy

When photons of electromagnetic energy interact with atoms they usually bounce off, retaining their energy and also their initial frequency and wavelength. This is comparable to a rubber ball bouncing off a wall and retaining its energy, so called **elastic scattering**. Both the photon and the atom remain unchanged after the collision. A small minority (approximately one in ten million) of impacting photons, however, do not simply bounce off the atom, instead they are absorbed momentarily. The absorbed photon gives energy to the atom, raising one of the atom's electrons to a higher energy level. It then returns to a different energy level than its original state, so a photon is released with a different energy to the initial photon. This type of collision is known as **Raman scattering**, and is generally referred to as **inelastic scattering**.

Because the energy levels in each type of atom are unique, the emitted photons have a signature wavelength for individual molecules. The wavelengths are analysed to produce a **Raman spectrograph**. A Raman spectroscope has an argon laser that produces monochromatic light, which is passed through a sampling chamber and the Raman scattered light is measured at right angles to the laser beam. It is most suitable for carbon dioxide or nitrous oxide detection. It benefits from being small and portable, simple to use, low maintenance and the calibration is robust; it is not so commonly used now, having been replaced with cheaper infrared analysers.

Summary

- Infrared absorption spectroscopy is the most common technique for measuring the concentration of respiratory gases.
- Oxygen is not readily detectable using infrared analysis; instead a paramagnetic analyser must be used.
- The pulsed-field paramagnetic oxygen analyser has a rapid response time so is suitable for measuring oxygen concentration over the respiratory cycle.
- The galvanic fuel cell and the Clark electrode are also able to measure oxygen concentration (or partial pressure).
- The fuel cell is self-powering which is an important advantage because it does not require an external power supply.
- The Severinghaus electrode measures carbon dioxide concentration/partial pressure, and the Sanz electrode measures pH.
- Gas chromatography, mass spectrometry and Raman scattering have been largely replaced by other techniques for routine anaesthetic use.

Single best answer questions

For these questions, choose the single best answer.

1. Which one of the following statements is true of paramagnetic oxygen analysers?
   (a) The null-deflection analyser is not sensitive to flow-rate.
   (b) The null deflection analyser contains a beam with oxygen-filled glass spheres at each end.
   (c) The pulsed-field detector has a slow response time.
   (d) The pulsed-field detector measures pressure changes induced by a magnetic field attracting oxygen molecules.
   (e) The pulsed-field detector measures a higher pressure in the sample path compared to the reference path if the oxygen concentration is less than that of air.

2. Which one of the following statements is true of Raman spectroscopy?
   (a) Roughly 10% of photons undergo inelastic scattering with gas molecules.
   (b) Raman scattered photons always have a lower energy than incident photons.
   (c) Raman scattering is less accurate than infrared spectroscopy.
   (d) All gases are detectable using Raman scattering.
   (e) Photons are detected at an angle of 90° to the laser beam in a Raman spectrograph.

Multiple choice questions

For each of these questions, mark every answer either true or false.

1. Which of the following statements are true of respiratory gas sampling?
   (a) Side-stream sampling minimizes dead space.
   (b) Side-stream sampling has a slower response time.
   (c) Main-stream sampling is less accurate.
   (d) Main-stream sampling allows oxygen and carbon dioxide monitoring.
   (e) Side-stream sampling draws off up to 500 mL of gas per minute from the breathing circuit.

2. Which of the following gases are detectable using infrared absorption?
   (a) Carbon dioxide.
   (b) Oxygen.
   (c) Nitrogen.
   (d) Nitrous oxide.
   (e) Isoflurane.

Chapter 12
Vaporizers

Having read this chapter you will be able to:
- Understand the fundamentals of a variable bypass vaporizer.
- Appreciate the role of the heat sink in a vaporizer.
- Be able to explain temperature compensation mechanisms in variable bypass vaporizers.
- Understand the principles behind a dual circuit vaporizer for delivering desflurane.
- Understand the functioning of a vaporizer at altered atmospheric pressure.

12.1 Introduction to vaporizers

Saturated vapour pressure and concentration

Definition
Vapour: a substance in its gas phase at a temperature below its critical temperature.

When the top is taken off a bottle of vinegar, those nearby soon sense a distinctive smell. Whilst the vinegar is a liquid at room temperature, there are some molecules that escape from the surface layer of the liquid as a gas, diffuse through the air and stimulate our olfactory neurons.

A vapour is simply a substance that exists as a gas below its critical temperature (see *Section 1.3*). Every substance has a critical temperature above which the substance can only exist as a gas, no matter how much pressure is applied.

The critical temperature of water is 374°C (or 647 K). Below this, any gaseous water (steam) that is encountered must therefore technically be described as water vapour. As discussed in *Chapter 7*, air in the lungs is saturated with water vapour. When breath is exhaled into cold winter air, the vapour quickly condenses to the liquid state and the visible cloud is actually a collection of micro-liquid droplets. The water has turned from the gaseous to liquid phase.

The molecules that make up any substance hold a wide range of energies. Temperature is a measure of the average of those energies and some molecules have enough energy to break the intermolecular bonds that keep them in a liquid state and exist above the liquid in a gaseous form.

Above the surface of any liquid, atmospheric pressure is constantly exerting a 101.3 kPa downward pressure. Any vapour that exists above the liquid's surface contributes to this total of 101.3 kPa of pressure. This portion of the 101.3 kPa is termed the partial pressure for that vapour (see *Chapter 9*). If a substance is in an enclosed container the liquid and gas phase will reach equilibrium. The pressure of the vapour measured at equilibrium is therefore a fraction of the total atmospheric pressure and is known as the saturated vapour pressure (SVP).

A vaporizer allows accurate doses in vapour form to be delivered to the patient. Historically, the Schimmelbusch mask was used to deliver an ether anaesthetic: the mask comprising a metal frame housing absorbent material. Ether was dripped on to the material which, being highly volatile (a high SVP at room temperature), created a vapour that was inhaled by the patient. The anaesthetist dripped more ether from the bottle onto the mask as the patient began to stir. This was the earliest form of vaporizer. Since the Schimmelbusch mask a wide variety of vaporizers have been designed, all with a common goal: to deliver a consistent and calculable concentration of anaesthetic vapour to a patient.

12.2 The draw-over vaporizer

The nearest modern day equivalent of the Schimmelbusch mask is the draw-over vaporizer design which is still in use in the military as part of the tri-service apparatus. It has the advantage of being light, and because it has minimal internal resistance it can be positioned within the anaesthetic breathing system itself. The vaporizer is called the Oxford Miniature Vaporizer (OMV) and can be used with a variety of different volatile agents as long as the scale on the dial is changed. This is probably the only remaining example of a 'vaporizer in-circle' (VIC) system in use today. Clarifying whether or not a vaporizer is 'in-circle' or 'out-of-circle' can quickly be worked out by considering whether or not vapour is added to the gas mixture before or after fresh gas enters the patient's breathing system (see *Figure 12.1*).

12.3 Variable bypass vaporizers

The variable bypass vaporizer (or plenum vaporizer) is a reliable and reasonably accurate device. The fresh gas flow is split into a carrier gas that travels through a vaporizing chamber, and a bypass gas that rejoins with the carrier gas after the vaporizing chamber to deliver a set concentration to the patient (*Figure 12.2*).

As fresh gas enters the vaporizer chamber the positive pressure pushes the gas through the vaporizing chamber (or plenum) where anaesthetic agent joins the fresh gas as a vapour. These types of vaporizers are exposed to the high-pressure fresh gas in the anaesthetic machine and have a high internal resistance. This makes them unsuitable for use as a 'vaporizer in-circle'. The **splitting ratio** is the ratio of the flow of gas through the vaporizing chamber to the flow through the bypass channel.

The accuracy of a variable bypass vaporizer is dependent on the vaporizing chamber consistently maintaining the SVP of the volatile agent. If there is a high flow of carrier gas through the vaporizing

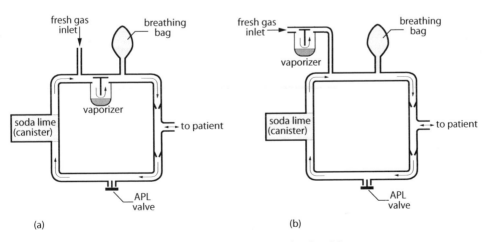

Figure 12.1. *The (a) vaporizer in-circle (VIC) and (b) vaporizer out-of-circle (VOC) set-ups.*

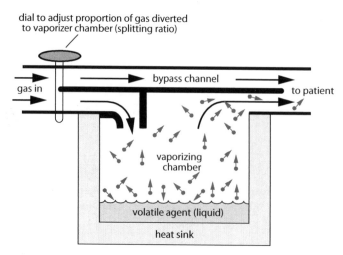

Figure 12.2. *A plenum (or variable bypass) vaporizer.*

chamber, maintaining the SVP is a design challenge, because the vapour from the surface has to be quickly replaced from the liquid reservoir. To maximize evaporation, the most widely used designs employ wicks that soak up the liquid and substantially increase the surface area for liquid to evaporate from (see *Figure 12.3*). In an alternative design, the fresh gas can be introduced beneath the liquid anaesthetic surface where it bubbles up (scintillates).

Boyle's bottle

Boyle's bottle was the earliest type of plenum vaporizer. It was invented by Henry Boyle and featured on his Boyle's machine, widely recognized as the first anaesthetic machine. The volatile anaesthetic is placed in a bottle and the gas is steered by a cowl to flow directly over the surface of the liquid. The control of the splitting ratio is managed entirely manually by varying a plunger to alter the proximity of the incoming gas to the surface of the volatile liquid. The main limitation of the Boyle's bottle was its inability to cope with temperature fluctuations, in particular the loss of heat from the volatile

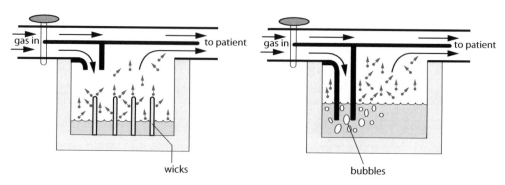

Figure 12.3. *Methods of increasing evaporation rates.*

vaporizing liquid. One method of overcoming this was to place the bottle inside a warm-water bath. Of course the effort required for this, as well as manoeuvering the steering cowl to administer the correct concentration of vapour, required frequent adjustments and hawk-like observation.

12.4 Factors affecting delivered concentration of anaesthetic agent

Evaporative cooling

The temperature of the volatile liquid reflects the average of all the different energies of its molecules. Some will be whizzing around and can easily escape the liquid, but these are the molecules with the most energy. If the molecules with the greatest energy are removed with the carrier gas, the temperature (energy average) of the remaining volatile liquid will fall. This energy required to change state is referred to as latent heat of vaporization and is the energy needed to convert a unit of mass of liquid to a vapour state (see *Chapter 1*).

Definition
Heat sink: used to transfer heat from a material (solid or liquid) to a fluid medium to minimize fluctuations in temperature.

To counter this phenomenon, a **heat sink** is incorporated in a vaporizer. A heat sink is a material with high specific heat capacity that is also a good conductor of heat. It acts as a reservoir of thermal energy to dilute the loss of thermal energy from vaporization. The considerable weight of a vaporizer is largely due to the heat sink.

Temperature and flow dependence

The metal body of a plenum vaporizer conducts heat from the surroundings to the anaesthetic agent. The concentration of anaesthetic agent delivered to the patient increases with increasing

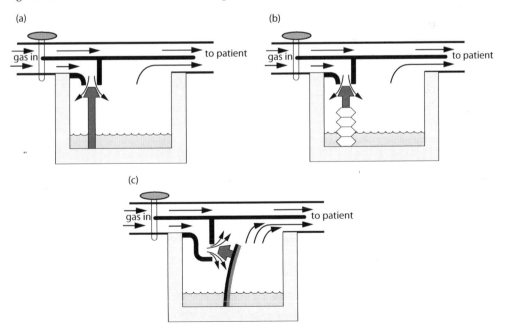

Figure 12.4. *Temperature compensation using (a) a metal rod, (b) liquid bellows, and (c) a bimetallic strip.*

Table 12.1. *Properties of commonly used volatile agents.*

	SVP at 20°C	Boiling point
Halothane	32 kPa	50.2°C
Isoflurane	33 kPa	48.5°C
Sevoflurane	21 kPa	58.6°C
Desflurane	88.5 kPa	22.8°C

temperature, because a higher temperature results in a higher SVP. Because the temperature of the chamber is not constant, variable bypass vaporizers have a mechanism to automatically adjust the proportion of gas flow entering the chamber according to the temperature within the chamber. The higher the temperature, the lower the required splitting ratio, i.e. more gas bypasses the vaporizing chamber.

There are several designs of temperature-compensated vaporizers. In the simplest design, a metal rod expands as it becomes hotter (*Figure 12.4a*), and the tip of the rod reduces the inflow of carrier gas as the temperature rises. A variation of this design uses a bellows filled with liquid that expands with a rise in temperature (*Figure 12.4b*). Finally, a bimetallic strip is the most commonly used method. The strip is constructed from two metals with different coefficients of thermal expansion. The strip bends to a greater or lesser extent depending on the temperature due to the differential expansion of the two metals (*Figure 12.4c*).

Factory calibration of vaporizers

Table 12.1 summarizes the SVPs (at 20°C) and boiling points of the commonly used volatile anaesthetic agents. Because each volatile agent has a different SVP, vaporizers are generally calibrated for one type of agent only. Desflurane is especially volatile, having a high SVP and low boiling point, so requires a special design of vaporizer (see *Section 12.5*). *Figure 12.5* shows a graph of SVP against temperature for the common volatile anaesthetic agents.

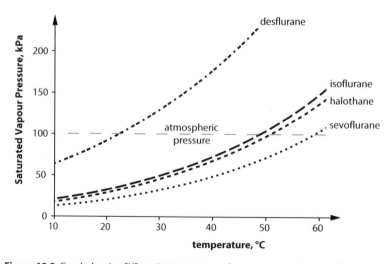

Figure 12.5. *Graph showing SVP against temperature for common volatile anaesthetic agents.*

Frequently there is a non-linearity in the output concentration of volatile agent when the fresh gas flow is varied, particularly at low flows. Each vaporizer has its own characteristics, for example, the early Tec series had marked inaccuracies at flows of 1 L·min⁻¹ and below. Intermittent positive pressure ventilation can cause back flow in the vaporizer chamber; this is usually prevented or limited by a valve (flow restrictor) downstream from the vaporizer.

Independent verification of the vaporizer's output is obtained using an infrared anaesthetic gas analyser in the patient's breathing system. This provides a breath-by-breath measure of the inhaled concentration of vapour and gives valuable information as to the depth of anaesthetic being delivered.

12.5 Direct injection vaporizers

Some anaesthetic machines have been manufactured with direct injection systems that work similarly to the fuel injection system on a car. The anaesthetic is sprayed under pressure into the fresh gas stream. The rate of fresh gas flow into the system is controlled by a graduated throttle valve. The vaporizer is engineered so that the gas flow drives the injection of volatile agent resulting in the spray increasing with increasing gas flow, giving a constant concentration. The direct injection vaporizer avoids the problems caused by the change in vapour pressure with temperature. Some systems have a variable nozzle controlled by a microprocessor that receives feedback from a variety of airflow and pressure control sensors to maintain a constant delivered anaesthetic concentration.

12.6 The dual circuit vaporizer: a vaporizer to deliver desflurane

Desflurane differs from the other volatile agents because it has a very low boiling point of just 22.8°C, so the temperature on a warm summers day would be enough to boil desflurane, potentially delivering a harmful dose to the patient.

In this vaporizer, desflurane is stored at a heightened pressure of 200 kPa, nearly double atmospheric pressure, and a raised temperature of 39°C (see *Figure 12.6*). It is more complex than

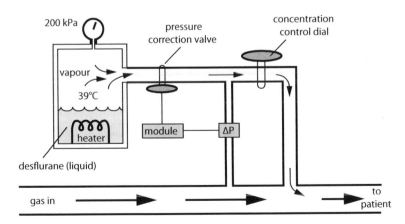

Figure 12.6. *A dual circuit desflurane vaporizer.*

a standard vaporizer because it requires electrical components. The temperature is regulated and a pressure transducer measures the difference in pressure between the fresh gas flow and the vapour flowing out of the vaporizer: this in turn regulates a valve controlling flow out of the vaporizer (the pressure correction valve). A period of time for the vaporizer to warm up is needed prior to use.

12.7 Vaporizers functioning at altered atmospheric pressures

How would a vaporizer function at the low atmospheric pressure experienced half way up Mount Everest? Or how would it function at the high atmospheric pressure generated in a hyperbaric chamber? Three key points need to be considered:
- Though the percentage of a volatile gas is the quoted figure it is actually the partial pressure of the vapour that is clinically relevant. Fick's law of diffusion (*Section 10.1*) shows that it is the difference in partial pressures that determines the diffusion across a membrane.
- SVP is not affected by atmospheric pressure only temperature. So because a vaporizer is dependent on the SVP of the agent and this remains unchanged, the same partial pressure of volatile agent will be delivered.
- The concentration of the volatile agent does change, as this is the vapour pressure of volatile agent (unchanged) relative to the atmospheric pressure (changed). To summarize, for increased atmospheric pressures the concentration of the vapour will drop and vice versa.

If the atmospheric pressure deviated from 101.3 kPa (at sea level), the dial on the vaporizer will not deliver the concentration indicated but it will deliver the same partial pressure of vapour regardless of atmospheric pressure. The alternative of course it to get a vaporizer factory calibrated for the relevant atmospheric pressure!

Summary
- An ideal vaporizer will deliver a known concentration of volatile anaesthetic vapour to the patient in all conditions.
- The saturated vapour pressures are different for each anaesthetic agent; hence some agents are more volatile than others.
- In variable bypass (plenum) vaporizers, the temperature dependence of delivered concentration can be compensated for by automatic adjustment of the splitting ratio.
- Saturated vapour pressure is affected by temperature but is independent of pressure.
- A heat sink is incorporated into a vaporizer to minimize temperature fluctuation.
- Different mechanisms are used for automatic temperature compensation, most commonly the bimetallic strip.
- Desflurane is extremely volatile so requires a special type of vaporizer where the desflurane is kept at an elevated pressure of 200 kPa and a constant temperature of 39°C.
- Direct injection vaporizers allow the delivered concentration of anaesthetic to be precisely controlled electronically.

Single best answer questions

For these questions, choose the single best answer.

1. The definition of a vapour is best stated as:
   (a) a substance in the gaseous state
   (b) a substance in its gas phase at a temperature below its critical temperature
   (c) a substance in its gas phase at a temperature above its critical temperature
   (d) a gas that is visible to the naked eye at SVP
   (e) a gas that is inhaled other than air at SVP

2. The role of the heat sink in a vaporizer can be best described as:
   (a) an active warming system for the vaporizing chamber
   (b) an active cooling system for the vaporizer casing
   (c) a density stabilization mechanism
   (d) transferring heat from a solid or liquid material to a fluid medium to minimize changes in temperature
   (e) a reserve reservoir of anaesthetic agent

3. The reason that desflurane cannot be delivered using a standard draw-over vaporizer is best stated as:
   (a) the cost of the agent
   (b) the large fluctuations in atmospheric pressure
   (c) the low volatility of the agent
   (d) the low boiling point of desflurane
   (e) the high boiling point of desflurane

Multiple choice questions

For each of these questions, mark every answer either true or false.

1. The saturated vapour pressure of a volatile agent is affected by a change in:
   (a) temperature of the liquid
   (b) the atmospheric pressure
   (c) the anaesthetic agent in use
   (d) the design of the vaporizer
   (e) position of the vaporizer in (VIC) or out (VOC) of the circuit

2. Regarding the temperature compensation mechanisms in a vaporizer:
   (a) a heat sink acts to reduce the flow of fresh gas into the vaporizing chamber
   (b) a Tec 6 (Desflurane) utilises a bellows
   (c) a bi-metallic strip has two metals with different coefficient of thermal expansion
   (d) the Boyle's bottles used a water bath to stabilize temperature
   (e) a heat sink does not contribute significantly to the mass of a vaporizer

3. Which of the following statements concerning a vaporizer to deliver desflurane are true?
   (a) A dual circuit vaporizer is commonly used.
   (b) Desflurane might freeze if the vaporizer fails.
   (c) It must overcome the low boiling point of desflurane.
   (d) It requires a power supply.
   (e) It needs time to 'warm-up' prior to use.

Chapter 13
Medical gas supplies

Having read this chapter you will be able to:
- Appreciate the principles for gas stored in cylinders designated for clinical use.
- Understand the safety measures demanded for cylinder storage and their clinical use.
- Explain the issues with liquefied gas in a cylinder.
- Understand piped medical gas and vacuum.
- Appreciate the conditions that can lead to fire and explosions in the clinical setting.

13.1 General principles of compressed gas cylinders

Definition
Compressed gas storage: when gas is pumped into an enclosed space such as a cylinder both the density and pressure increase. Some gases change to a liquid state under pressure within the cylinder.

A gas cylinder (or gas bottle) is a vessel used to store gases at pressures above atmospheric pressure. When a gas cylinder is filled, more and more gas molecules are forced into the confines of the cylinder and Boyle's law (*Section 9.4*) determines that the pressure will rise in the cylinder. The molecules are much closer together than when at atmospheric pressure. For some compounds the proximity of molecules allows bonds to form and as a result there is a change of state from a gas to a liquid. Most notably in anaesthesia, nitrous oxide and carbon dioxide exist as liquids within a cylinder, but when the cylinder valve is opened it is the vapour (gas) above the liquid that is released.

Cylinders are engineered to tolerate pressures 66% above the filling pressures that are specified for the gas they hold, but there are still hazards associated with cylinders, such as fire, explosion, contact burns, attached equipment freezing, and inaccurate pressure gauge readings.

The cylinder valve controls the flow of gas from the cylinder itself. Having first checked that the seal on the cylinder is intact, the cylinder's valve should be briefly opened prior to attachment to any clinical equipment such as the anaesthetic machine. This brief blast of gas should expel any dust and any manufacturing debris present. A Bodok seal is a neoprene washer placed between the gas cylinder and the cylinder yoke ensuring a gas-tight seal.

When attached to equipment the cylinder valve should be turned by two turns to ensure full opening; failure do this can lead to compromised flow, particularly when the cylinder is emptying. When closing the valve the force employed should be firm rather than brutal so as to avoid damaging the valve. For opening and closing of a cylinder valve, remember: 'right is tight, left is loose', alternatively 'clockwise to close'. Gas cylinders are normally used in conjunction with pressure regulators to reduce the pressure from the high levels within the cylinder to a more useable level. Pressure regulators are described in *Chapter 6*.

Cylinder identification

A pin index system on the cylinder valve (see *Figure 13.1*) is designed to ensure the correct gas cylinder is attached to the correct inlet on the pressure regulator or anaesthetic machine. The positions of the holes on the cylinder valve correspond with pins fitted to the yoke attached to the equipment. The

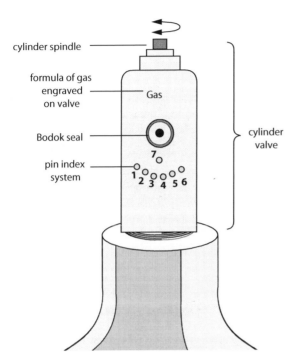

cylinder spindle

formula of gas
engraved
on valve

Gas

Bodok seal

cylinder
valve

pin index
system

Figure 13.1. *The pin index system for a medical gas cylinder.*

pin positions for each gas are unique, so if an attempt is made to fit the wrong gas cylinder to the equipment, a tight seal will not be made, as the pins cannot locate correctly.

Above the pin system an engraved chemical formula of the gas held within the cylinder should be visible. Along with this, the shoulder of a cylinder should be colour coded and an expiry date should be present. On the cylinder itself should be a standardized identification label that includes relevant safety precautions. Larger cylinders do not have the pin identification system: the valves for non-flammable gases are right-hand screw and for flammable gases left-hand screw. Some cylinders come with Schrader sockets already *in situ.*

Maintenance

Every 5 years an internal examination of a cylinder is carried out with an endoscope to check for cracks and corrosion. The plastic disc around the neck is coded by colour and shape according to the year of manufacture and the year of its last service.

Cylinder size and construction

The cylinders are manufactured from steel, often reinforced with small amounts of other metals such as molybdenum, and are without seams so as to minimize weak points. There is a balancing act as to the thickness of the walls of the cylinder for strength versus the weight. Lightweight cylinders made from aluminum or carbon fibre composite are produced for small transport cylinders but are more costly.

Cylinder size uses an alphabetical labeling system: *A* being the smallest and *J* the largest. Developments in technology and manufacturing have led to increased diversity of demand so that subdivisions of each size are now required such as *AV* and *AZ*. The standard cylinder for anaesthetics is the **D** size, and these are the cylinders that are attached to most anaesthetic machines. For exact data, manufacturers such as BOC produce comprehensive data charts on their websites.

Cylinder storage

Because cylinders store gases at very high pressures, a number of precautions must be observed.
- Gas cylinders should ideally be stored indoors in a dry area at a steady temperature.
- Full and empty cylinders should be stored apart, and the full cylinders should be stored in rotation.
- They should ideally be stored upright and those cylinders for clinical use must be stored separately from non-medical cylinders.
- Oxygen, nitrous oxide, and gas mixtures containing oxygen (including Heliox and Entonox), all support combustion so should not be stored with flammable gases.

Colour coding

Gas cylinders are colour coded for quick identification. *Table 13.1* summarizes the colour coding system as well as other data for medical gas cylinders. Note that between 2010 and 2025, cylinders will be brought into line with European standards, having white-only bodies (the shoulder colours will remain largely unchanged from the current scheme).

Table 13.1. *Medical gas cylinder data.*

Gas	Body colour	Shoulder colour	Critical temp. / pressure	Pressure kept in cylinder (room temp.)	State in cylinder
Oxygen	Black (US – green)	White	−118°C / 50 bar*	137 bar	Gas
Carbon dioxide	Grey	Grey	31°C / 73.8 bar	50 bar	Liquid & vapour
Nitrous oxide	Blue	Blue	36.5°C / 71.7 bar	44 bar	Liquid & vapour
Medical air	Grey (US – yellow)	White/black quarters	N/A	137 bar	Gas
Entonox (oxygen + nitrous oxide)	Blue	White/blue quarters	N/A	137 bar	Gas
Heliox (oxygen + helium)	Brown	White/brown quarters	N/A	137 bar	Gas

*[Note] 1 bar = 100 kPa.

13.2 Gas that liquefies in a cylinder

The concept of an ideal gas (see *Chapter 9*) was developed to simplify our understanding of the behaviour of gases under various conditions. Real gases show ideal behaviour at pressures near atmospheric pressure, however, at higher pressures, deviation from ideal gas behaviour occurs. Compressed gases in a cylinder can either stay as a gas, or change state to form a liquid due to the higher pressure (both carbon dioxide and nitrous oxide do this).

Nitrous oxide

A graph of pressure against time for nitrous oxide is shown in *Figure 13.2* (the graph may be compared with the one in *Figure 9.5*, which shows a similar graph for an ideal gas); the isothermal lines are shown for 40°C, 36.6°C and 20°C. At 40°C nitrous oxide is above its critical temperature and so it is a gas no matter what the pressure. When it is compressed (moving from right to left along the isotherm) the pressure increases smoothly (as it does in *Figure 9.5*). At 36.6°C (the critical temperature), as soon as the pressure reaches the critical pressure (72 bar), the gas becomes a liquid.

Note the steepness of the isotherm at higher pressures; this is because liquids are much less compressible, so a very high pressure is needed to reduce its volume further. At 20°C, once the pressure reaches 52 bar (the saturated vapour pressure of nitrous oxide at 20°C), some of the gas condenses so that liquid and vapour are both present. Further decreases in volume cause more vapour to condense, with no associated rise in pressure. When all the vapour has condensed to a liquid, any further reduction in volume causes a rapid rise in pressure.

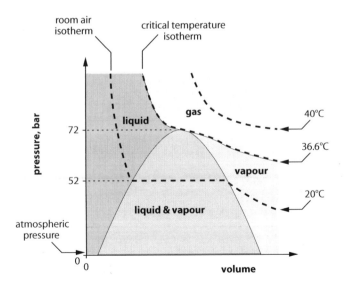

Figure 13.2. *Isotherms on a phase diagram for nitrous oxide.*

Filling ratios

If a gas cylinder was filled completely, so that it contained 100% liquid, it would be extremely dangerous. A small increase in temperature would cause the liquid to expand, greatly increasing the pressure, causing the cylinder to rupture and/or explode. For this reason, cylinders are partially filled so that a volume of vapour is present above the liquid. Any rise in temperature causes expansion of the liquid, which compresses the vapour, causing some of it to condense, which prevents a dramatic rise in pressure. Cylinders are filled by weight and to counter the danger of over-filling, a **filling ratio** is used:

$$\text{filling ratio} = \frac{\text{mass of contents (of cylinder)}}{\text{mass of water to fill cylinder}}$$

 13.1 Learn

In the UK a maximum filling ratio of 0.75 is used, while in hotter climates, 0.67 is recommended. The **tare weight** is stamped onto the cylinder and is simply the weight of cylinder when empty.

Units. The filling ratio has no units (being a ratio). It can be expressed as a fraction (two-thirds), a decimal (0.67) or a percentage (67%).

Pressure in a gas cylinder containing liquid

For a gas that, once compressed, has become a liquid in a cylinder, not only is there a liquid in the

cylinder but also a vapour (gas) above the surface of the liquid; it is this vapour gas that is drawn off when the valve of the cylinder is opened. The vapour is replenished by molecules from the liquid evaporating.

If a gas is stored in the liquid phase in a cylinder, the pressure gauge for the cylinder does not act as a guide as to how full the cylinder is. While liquefied gas is present, no matter how full the cylinder is the pressure will be simply that of the saturated vapour pressure as shown in *Figure 13.3*. Therefore, as gas is released from the cylinder, the pressure remains steady until all the liquid

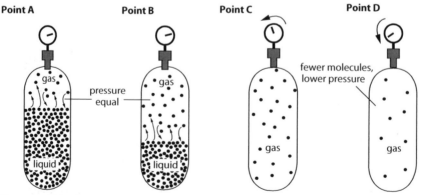

Figure 13.3. *The drop in pressure as a nitrous oxide cylinder empties. While any liquid is present in the cylinder, the pressure above the liquid (saturated vapour pressure) is independent of the volume of liquid in the cylinder. As the cylinder empties, all the nitrous oxide becomes gas and the pressure starts to drop (exponentially) as the number of gas molecules in the cylinder drops.*

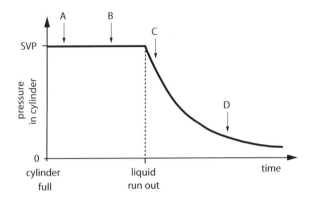

Figure 13.4. *Graph of pressure against time within a discharging cylinder of nitrous oxide. Points A–D relate to the states of the cylinders shown in* Figure 13.3.

has evaporated. The pressure then falls as the remaining gas molecules escape. *Figure 13.4* shows a graph of pressure against time of a cylinder discharging nitrous oxide.

Entonox

Entonox is a mixture of 50% oxygen and 50% nitrous oxide. An Entonox cylinder is prepared by adding nitrous oxide to the cylinder first and the cylinder is then inverted and oxygen is bubbled through it. It is stored in a cylinder at 13 700 kPa (137 bar) in a liquid state. It should be kept warmer than –5.5°C, its **pseudo-critical temperature**; below this temperature nitrous oxide is liquefied and the mixture partially separates, a process known as lamination (the Poynting effect) or liquefaction. At temperatures below –5.5°C, the result is a liquid in the cylinder containing nitrous oxide with some oxygen (about 20%) dissolved in it and a gas of high concentration oxygen above it. As the level of liquid in the cylinder drops the high concentration oxygen gas is gradually replaced by a vapour that contains only a small amount of oxygen. Initially therefore, the patient would receive less analgesic effect, gradually followed by hypoxia.

In large Entonox cylinders a 'dip-tube' delays this hypoxic inhalation by sampling from the liquid at the bottom of the cylinder as shown in *Figure 13.5*, although eventually a hypoxic mixture will be delivered when the liquid has emptied. To reverse the lamination, the cylinder must be rewarmed and the contents mixed by repeatedly inverting the cylinder.

Worked example

Question
The nitrous oxide has been flowing from a cylinder for one hour at a high flow rate. Why might a frost be seen on the outside of the cylinder?

Answer
A full nitrous oxide cylinder contains both liquid and gas as long as the ambient temperature is below its critical temperature of 36.5°C. When gas is withdrawn it is the vapour above the liquid that is being released. Higher energy molecules that have escaped the liquid replenish the vapour above the surface of the liquid. Bonds need to be broken to convert liquid to gas, which requires energy which is taken from the contents of the cylinder. Therefore the cylinder cools considerably. Water vapour in the air condenses on the cool cylinder, and freezes when the cylinder temperature falls below 0°C.

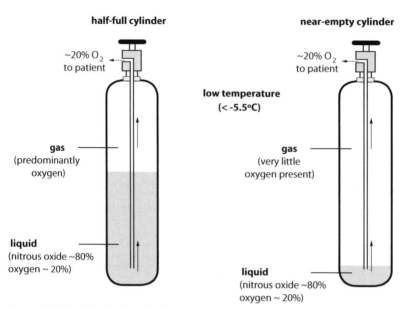

half-full cylinder

~20% O$_2$
to patient

gas
(predominantly
oxygen)

liquid
(nitrous oxide ~80%
oxygen ~ 20%)

**low temperature
(< -5.5°C)**

near-empty cylinder

~20% O$_2$
to patient

gas
(very little
oxygen present)

liquid
(nitrous oxide ~80%
oxygen ~ 20%)

Figure 13.5. *The 'dip-tube' in a cylinder containing Entonox is designed to minimize the clinical dangers of lamination.*

13.3 Piped medical gas

Gases used in high volumes are usually supplied through a piped system. Piped gases include oxygen, nitrous oxide, medical air (used to blend with oxygen) and compressed air (used to power pneumatic instruments). The sockets that link piped gas to the hoses leading to the equipment are called Schrader sockets. The sockets and the probes which fit into them are colour coded and the fit for each socket is specific to the gas, preventing the hose being plugged into the incorrect gas supply. A 'tug test' is recommended to ensure that the Schrader socket has clicked in securely. The system of piping gas along with the centralized vacuum system is called the **piped medical gas and vacuum** (PMGV). Other gases such as carbon dioxide and xenon are not supplied through piped systems and are instead supplied in individual cylinders.

Producing oxygen

Oxygen is manufactured by fractional distillation of liquefied air and this yields oxygen that is 99.6% pure. A chemical oxygen generator, a zeolite molecular sieve that absorbs nitrogen, can also produce oxygen and this is used in home oxygen concentrators. The electrolysis of water is another source of generating oxygen and this is the process by which oxygen is generated in submarines. Oxygen has a critical temperature of –118°C and a critical pressure of 50 bar; at atmospheric pressure it has a boiling point of –182.5°C.

Piped oxygen gas

A central supply of oxygen is organized in two ways. In smaller hospitals cylinder manifolds might be used, where multiple oxygen cylinders are connected together. In a larger hospital a vacuum insulated evaporation set-up is used to store liquid oxygen, though a cylinder manifold system is retained as back up.

Cylinder manifold. An oxygen cylinder manifold (*Figure 13.6*) allows multiple gas cylinders to centrally supply the needs of a small hospital. Two banks of oxygen cylinders are employed such that when the pressures on one side drop it indicates that the cylinders are emptying and there is automated changeover to the other bank of cylinders. The number of cylinders in each bank is dictated by the estimated needs of the hospital, and ideally each bank of cylinders should last for at least 2 days. The pressure of oxygen in the cylinders is 137 bar and a pressure-reducing valve drops this to the 4 bar value of the piped supply. Oxygen is stored as a gas in cylinders at room temperature no matter how much pressure builds up within the cylinder. For it to become a liquid in the cylinder it would first have to drop below its critical temperature of –118°C.

Vacuum insulated evaporator. For larger hospitals with a high usage of oxygen, oxygen cylinders are inadequate, and instead oxygen is stored as a liquid (LOX) at high pressure and a low temperature, namely about 700 kPa (7 bar) at a temperature between –150 and –180°C. It is held in a thermally insulated vessel which is essentially a very large vacuum flask known as a vacuum insulated evaporator (VIE), as shown in *Figure 13.7*. The VIE has an inner shell of stainless steel and an outer of carbon steel. The liquid state delivers a large amount of gas per unit volume: one litre of liquid oxygen gives 842 litres of gaseous oxygen at STP. An electrical warmer is needed to bring the oxygen up to room temperature.

Compressed air supplies

Medical air has been compressed by a pump into a cylinder or piped from a central supply with a central compression pump. Portable pumps can also be used in the clinical setting to give increased flow rates of air. Medical air must be produced such that it is free of oil mist generated from the pump used to compress it and a filter removes this; oil mist can be harmful to the patient when inhaled and can also increase the risk of explosion. Medical air must also have an accurate percentage of oxygen.

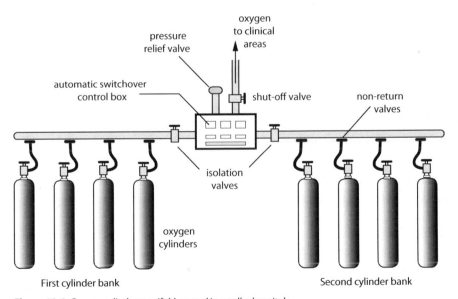

Figure 13.6. *Oxygen cylinder manifold as used in smaller hospitals.*

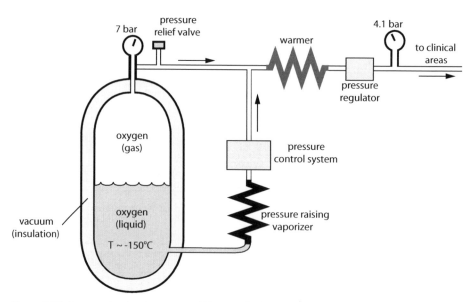

Figure 13.7. *A vacuum insulated evaporator (VIE) as used in hospitals with a high oxygen demand.*

Air is delivered at two pressure levels with dedicated Schrader sockets for each. For ventilation the lower pressure of 400 kPa (4 bar) is used and for driving power tools the higher pressure of 700 kPa (7 bar) is needed.

13.4 Vacuum and suction

A true vacuum is devoid of any matter and the nearest that nature comes to this is in space where there are but a few gas molecules per cubic metre. Aristotle's famous words that 'nature abhors a vacuum' holds true because a true vacuum is difficult to create or maintain. The pressure in a vessel containing a true vacuum is zero because there are no gas molecules present to collide with the vessel wall.

The word vacuum in the clinical setting is often used to refer to pressures lower than atmospheric pressure. So a vacuum source to deliver suction is not a true vacuum in the sense that physicists think of it. Instead it is a pressure notably lower than the ambient pressure: enough to create a pressure gradient.

Suction is the removal of fluids or solids by generating a negative pressure gradient; that is, there must be a negative pressure relative to the ambient pressure. There are three main ways of delivering a negative pressure in the clinical setting: a mechanical pump, a centralized piped vacuum source, and a venturi effect driven by gas from cylinders. A suction system must be capable of generating negative pressure of at least 400 mmHg. A surgical suction source should be capable of reaching −500 mmHg within ten seconds and be capable of removing 25 L·min⁻¹.

The suction apparatus (*Figure 13.8*) must have a reservoir to collect the suctioned material and a bacterial filter to disperse suctioned gas to the atmosphere. There must also be a filter in line to protect the suction source. A pressure gauge is needed to indicate the level of suction and the established practice is to have negative pressure as anti-clockwise (and positive clockwise). Centralized suction (often referred to as wall suction) has a yellow coloured Schrader valve. The suction tubing needs to

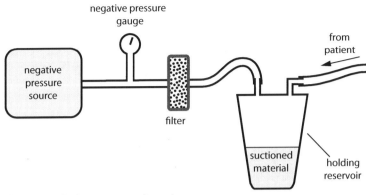

Figure 13.8. *Basic components of a suction system.*

be relatively stiff, having a low compliance so it does not collapse on itself, and to be wide bored so that the resistance to flow is low.

13.5 Combustion risk

Operating theatres and anaesthetic rooms present an increased risk of fires and explosions due to the presence of oxygen and nitrous oxide. Although neither of these gases is flammable, they both support combustion by acting as oxidizing agents. The fire triangle or combustion triangle (*Figure 13.9*) is a model to aid understanding of the ingredients necessary for fires to occur: there must be a flammable substance (fuel), oxygen and also a source of ignition that could be heat, a flame or a spark.

All episodes of combustion, including explosions, are in essence exothermic oxidation, a chemical reaction between a substance and oxygen. New compounds are formed, along with the production of energy predominantly in the form of heat, but often accompanied with light, sound and pressure. Combustibles are substances capable of reacting with oxygen to produce heat at high temperatures.

A measure of the extent of oxidation is the **stoichiometric composition**. It is defined as the composition where the amounts of fuel and oxygen present are such that there is no excess of fuel or oxygen after the chemical reaction has occurred. The stoichiometric composition or ratio can be regarded as the composition giving the most explosive mixture. It is the chemically correct air–fuel ratio necessary to achieve complete combustion of the fuel. The ratio is always in a whole numbers of moles, as determined by the chemical equation of combustion. As an example, the stoichiometric air–fuel ratio of ethanol (by mass) is 9:1.

Definition
Stoichiometric composition: in air the stoichiometric composition of a fuel is the concentration range that will allow oxidation of all the fuel and the consumption of all oxygen.

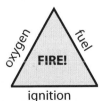

ignition

Figure 13.9. *The triangle of combustion.*

Zone of risk

The zone of risk of fire or explosion is defined as an area extending 25 cm around any part of the anaesthetic apparatus. Leaks from the circuit can produce a high percentage of oxygen gas. Avoiding problems means reducing the amount of oxygen that enters the atmosphere. So closed circuits are preferable to open ones, scavenging is helpful and open-mask anaesthesia intubation is better. Optimum ventilation in the theatre complex reduces oxygen build up. Particular caution is needed around diathermy and ether, though rarely used now.

Ignition sources

Obvious sources of ignition include naked flames (which should never be used in clinical areas), and any hot object. Hot wires including ordinary light bulbs, halogen lamps and cautery apparatus are potential ignition sources, as are hot plates and toasters. Electrical appliances can cause sparks and arcing whenever faults are present. Simply switching on a light switch or ripping a plug from a socket has been known to ignite flammable gases and vapours in the air causing explosions. Finally, static electricity can cause sparks, and is discussed in *Section 20.6.*

Flammable substances in the operating theatre

Diethyl ether (an anaesthetic agent that has now largely been phased out), when mixed solely with air, does not readily ignite when a spark is present. However, when in the presence of either oxygen or nitrous oxide (or both) the danger of explosion is much greater. Relatively cool heat sources such as hot wires and plates can result in ignition, and it burns with an invisible flame. An even greater risk was presented by the anaesthetic agent ethyl chloride, which burns easily and an explosion can happen in the presence of oxygen or nitrous oxide or simply in the presence of air.

Alcohol, used for cleansing skin or surfaces is a volatile flammable liquid. It also burns with an invisible flame, and vapour can collect in confined areas causing an explosion risk. Gaseous hydrocarbons such as methane (a major constituent of the gas generated in the gut), propane and butane are explosive when mixed with air.

Modern volatile gases such as isoflurane and desflurane are non-flammable.

Summary
- Medical gas cylinders are available in a range of sizes, and use colour coding to aid identification.
- Pin-index systems prevent connection of the wrong gas to a piece of equipment.
- Some gases, including nitrous oxide and carbon dioxide, condense into a mixture of liquid and vapour when pressurized at room temperature.
- If liquid gas is present in a cylinder, such as in the case of nitrous oxide, the pressure gauge on a gas cylinder gives no indication of the amount of remaining gas.
- Cylinders are never completely filled with liquefied gas, otherwise any thermal expansion of the liquid would rupture the cylinder.
- Piped oxygen is supplied either from pressurized cylinder manifolds at normal temperature or from vacuum insulated evaporators which store liquid oxygen at low temperatures.
- Nitrous oxide and gas mixtures containing oxygen support combustion. Special care must be taken in clinical areas where these gases are used, to prevent fire and explosion.

Single best answer questions

For these questions, choose the single best answer.

1. The stoichiometric composition is best described as:
   (a) the effective concentration of a cleaning fluid
   (b) the formula used by the fire brigade for extinguishing fires
   (c) a form of anti-static floor
   (d) an indicator as to the ratios of fuel present that might lead to a fire or explosion
   (e) a vaporizer design used for flammable anaesthetic agents

2. The filling ration can be best described as the ratio of:
   (a) the mass of a gas in a cylinder to the mass of air which would fill the cylinder
   (b) the mass of the cylinder to the mass of water which would fill the cylinder
   (c) the pressure of a gas in a cylinder to the pressure of water which would fill the cylinder
   (d) the density of a gas in a cylinder to the density of water which would fill the cylinder
   (e) the mass of a gas in a cylinder to the mass of water which would fill the cylinder

3. The definition of a true vacuum in physics is best stated as:
   (a) a vacuum is low negative pressure in a chamber
   (b) a vacuum is devoid of any matter
   (c) a vacuum contains only noble gases
   (d) a vacuum has high pressure but minimal atoms present
   (e) a vacuum is where one zone has significantly lower pressure than another

Multiple choice questions

For each of these questions, mark every answer either true or false.

1. Which of the following statements regarding the storage of gas in a cylinder are true?
   (a) Modern pressure gauges show how full a cylinder is regardless of the state in which the gas is stored.
   (b) It is stored at a pressure significantly lower than atmospheric pressure.
   (c) A phase diagram shows what state a substance will be in at a known pressure and temperature.
   (d) All gases (once compressed) are stored as liquids in a cylinder unless at high altitude.
   (e) A pressure regulator controls the temperature of gas leaving a cylinder.

2. The triangle of combustion:
   (a) highlights the key components that are needed for a fire
   (b) is a simplified model of the combustion process
   (c) involves oxygen, ignition and fuel
   (d) involves oxygen, electricity and fuel
   (e) has pressure as a central component of the model

3. Which of the following gases are stored as liquids in medical cylinders?
   (a) Oxygen.
   (b) Entonox.
   (c) Carbon dioxide.
   (d) Oxygen.
   (e) Nitrous oxide.

4. Which of the following substances can be considered flammable?
   (a) Isoflurane.
   (b) Diethyl ether.
   (c) Oils and grease.
   (d) Oxygen.
   (e) Desflurane.

Chapter 14
Breathing systems and ventilation

Having read this chapter you will be able to:
- Understand the Mapleson classification of breathing systems.
- Explain the key components of the circle system.
- Understand how carbon dioxide is removed with soda lime.
- Appreciate the need for scavenging of exhaled gases.
- Understand the principles behind active and passive scavenging.
- Appreciate the history and development of mechanical ventilation.
- Understand the differences between anaesthetic and ICU ventilators.
- Explain pressure and flow gas delivery mechanisms.
- Appreciate the different modes of ventilation available.

The flow of gas in a breathing system is sometimes difficult to envisage from a simple line diagram and text alone; the website www.equipmentexplained.com has some excellent moving images that will complement the content of this chapter.

14.1 Key components in breathing systems

Definition
Breathing system efficiency: the efficiency of a breathing system can be quantified by the fresh gas flow rate required to prevent rebreathing of alveolar gases.

A breathing system is the collection of components that connect the patient's airway to the ventilator/anaesthetic machine through which the patient breathes. The cost of clinical gases such as oxygen and air, as well as anaesthetic vapours, is considerable and a desire to conserve both gas supplies and anaesthetic agents has led to ultra-low flow systems.

Adjustable pressure-limiting valve

The adjustable pressure-limiting (APL) valve is also known as the expiratory valve (see *Section 6.3*). It prevents the build up of pressure within the system, and allows exhaled gas to leave a circuit. It also allows excess fresh gas to leave the breathing circuit. Hooke's law for the extension of a spring (Equation 2.1) means that as pressure increases relative to atmospheric pressure the spring is depressed proportionally. At a set point the spring is depressed enough to allow the valve to release gas from the breathing system. The level of pressure to trigger opening is adjusted by altering the height of the spring. It is simple and reliable but there is a risk of the disc of the valve sticking, either in the 'hold' or 'release' position.

Reservoir bag

As its name suggests the reservoir bag acts as a collapsible reservoir for fresh gas, ready to be drawn upon during inspiration. It can also be used to deliver ventilation either partially or fully. It serves as a useful visual indicator of the presence and pattern of a patient's spontaneous breathing.

A crucial property of the ellipsoidal bag is its capability to expand to a surprisingly large size; if it were not for this the pressure in the circuit could rise alarmingly fast. The compliance of the bag allows it to distend. Laplace's law for a sphere (Equation 2.5) states that a large pressure rise is needed for a given increase in radius when the bag is almost empty. A distended bag, however, 'absorbs' a greater pressure rise (ΔP) without greatly increasing its radius (r):

$$\Delta P = \frac{2 \cdot T}{r}$$

14.1

So as the radius of the bag increases, the pressure should rise to no more than 40–60 cmH$_2$O. It is similar to blowing up a party balloon: the initial inflation requires the most effort and it then gets easier to inflate, although eventually the balloon will pop! In the same way, the grossly distended reservoir bag will eventually burst.

Fresh gas flow

Fresh gas flow is the delivery of fresh gas that is yet to be inhaled. It should be noted that fresh gas flow is supplied at a pressure far greater than atmospheric pressure, but considerably lower than pipe-line pressure.

Tubing

The tubing for breathing systems must not kink and to prevent this corrugated tubing is used. A large internal diameter to the tubing will produce a lower resistance to gas flow.

14.2 The circle system

The circle system is an almost ideal anaesthetic system and is widely used. The idea behind the circle system is both elegant and simple; a schematic diagram is shown in *Figure 14.1*. Air flows around a circuit (the 'circle') in one direction only, and the circuit may be thought of as comprising two 'limbs'.

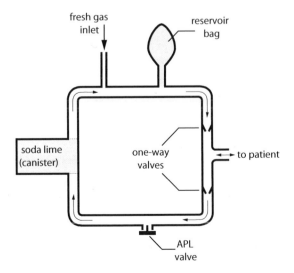

Figure 14.1. *A circle breathing system.*

A breathing bag is positioned in the inspiratory limb between the fresh gas inlet and the patient. The key components are:

- two unidirectional valves, one in each limb of the circuit
- fresh gas flow positioned proximal to the inspiratory valve
- exhaust (APL) valve positioned on the expiratory limb
- carbon dioxide absorbing material
- soda-lime canister used to absorb carbon dioxide
- reservoir bag

Assuming the soda lime is functioning at 100% efficiency and there are no leaks in the circuit, the fresh gas flow need only match the basal oxygen consumption – typically 250–500 mL per minute. Gas enters the inspiratory limb having passed through the soda lime with a contribution from the fresh gas flow outlet. The gas then passes through the one-way inspiratory valve due either to drive from a distal ventilator or via the negative pressure created by a spontaneously breathing patient. An initial flushing of the circuit is needed with fresh gas flow to de-nitrogenate the circuit prior to attaching the circuit to the patient.

On a normal anaesthetic machine the vaporizer is situated out of circle and so a volatile agent enters with the fresh gas flow. It is possible to have a circle system with a 'vaporizer in circle' (VIC) although this is rarely encountered in modern practice (see *Section 12.2*). During expiration, pressure down the inspiratory limb closes the one-way valve, forcing the expired gas down the expiratory limb. This then collects in the reservoir bag which vents via the APL exhaust valve at the set pressure limit.

There is a danger at low fresh gas flow that there will be insufficient oxygen to match the patient's oxygen consumption. Because vaporizers out-of-circle (VOCs) deliver considerably lower concentrations at low internal flows, it used to be the case that a detailed knowledge of uptake and distribution of the various volatile agents, together with reference tables, were required to estimate the concentrations of volatile agent delivered to the patient. This concentration would therefore be an estimate and the attendant clinician would have to pay close attention to ensure awareness did not occur. However, inspiratory and expiratory gas monitoring has considerably reduced the risk of hypoxia and awareness.

For a VOC there is a delay between an alteration to the concentration dialed on the vaporizer and the time it will take to have an effect in the breathing system. This is because the fresh gas flow with this altered concentration will represent only a very small portion of the total gas being delivered to the patient.

Table 14.1. *Typical constituents of soda lime.*

Soda lime	%
Calcium hydroxide	94
Sodium hydroxide	5
Potassium hydroxide (optional)	<0.1
Silica (binding in granules)	0.2
Dye (changes colour when pH <10)	trace

Carbon dioxide removal by absorption

To remove the expired carbon dioxide the exhaled gas is passed through soda lime. There are three reactions that take place, which produce water as a by-product aiding humidification of inhaled gas. One reaction is also exothermic, so produces heat that replaces heat lost in the breathing circuit. Heat and humidification are therefore welcome by-products of the process.

The typical components of commercially available soda lime are listed in *Table 14.1*. Soda lime is also used outside of the clinical environment; it makes up the carbon dioxide scrubbers used to remove carbon dioxide from the atmosphere of submarines and space vehicles.

The overall reaction is:

$$CO_2 + Ca(OH)_2 \rightarrow CaCO_3 + H_2O \ (+ \ heat)$$

14.2 Learn

This reaction is in fact broken down into three stages:

1. $H_2O + CO_2 \rightarrow H_2CO_3$ (slow and rate limiting)
2. $H_2CO_3 + NaOH \rightarrow NaHCO_3$
3. $NaHCO_3 + Ca(OH)_2 \rightarrow CaCO_3 + H_2O + NaOH$ (the NaOH is regenerated and acts as a catalyst)

The pH of soda lime is greater than 10 due to the sodium hydroxide present. As can be deduced from the third stage, because the calcium hydroxide is used up the sodium hydroxide regeneration starts to fail. As the level of sodium hydroxide in the soda lime declines the pH decreases, sodium hydroxide being the strongest alkaline component of soda lime. The lower pH of soda lime slows the formation of carbonic acid from carbon dioxide and water thereby making the soda lime less efficient. The dye added to soda lime (of which there are several varieties/colours) is a pH indicator mixture that begins to change colour as pH reduces to below 10.

Soda lime is the generic compound that has historically been used for carbon dioxide absorption. Potassium hydroxide is sometimes added as an alternative pathway to mop up the carbonic acid. Over time manufacturers have developed their own compounds in an attempt to try and combat some of the concerns generated by soda lime use in very low flow systems.

- Compound A: this is produced by sevoflurane in the presence of soda lime, especially at higher temperatures and also when the soda lime has dried out. Compound A has been shown to be lethal in rats at high concentrations (not achievable in a circle system) and nephrotoxic at lower concentrations (20–50 p.p.m.) that are possible under low flow conditions. Although these findings have failed to be substantively translated into humans, it is not recommended to use sevoflurane at flows less than 1 litre/min.

- Carbon monoxide: many anaesthetic machines have a default low flow of 250 mL·min^{-1} of oxygen even when the oxygen knob is turned off. These low flows of dry gas circulating in closed circuits overnight dry out the soda lime granules. When desiccated soda lime is exposed to the CHF_2 group it can cause carbon monoxide to be produced. Desflurane is the worst offender; carboxyhaemoglobin levels can become significant in infants.

14.3 The Mapleson classification

In a landmark paper in the *BJA*, William Mapleson, a medical physicist, ingeniously classified five breathing systems using the alphabet. Mapleson was tasked with working out what conditions were necessary in each circuit to eliminate re-breathing whilst maintaining economy of gas flow. Given the

Definition
Mapleson classification: an alphabetical categorization of five semi-closed breathing systems (A, B, C, D and E).

five components of the breathing system (fresh gas flow, mask, adjustable pressure limiting or spill valve, tube and bag) there are only five conceivable and functional configurations in which these can be arranged.

The calculations used in the paper were based on a small sample group and made four assumptions.

1. A regular pattern of respiration.
2. A tidal volume not so large as to drive it back into the bag where it would mix with fresh gas.
3. A sharp division between dead space and alveolar gas.
4. The sharp division remains sharp as the gas moves in the tubing.

14.4 Mapleson A, B and C systems

In all of these circuits the bag stems from the afferent or inward flowing limb of the circuit and they are often primarily classified as afferent systems. Another way of identifying one of these systems is that the APL valve is the most proximal component to the patient's mask.

Mapleson A

System A is known as the Magill circuit (*Figure 14.2*). This configuration was often used when gas induction was common.

In this system (in fact, in any of Mapleson's A–C circuits) there are three resistances that determine the direction and the flow of fresh gas at any time during the respiratory cycle, namely the bag, the APL valve and the patient. The flow and/or direction of gas flow differs for inspiration, expiration and during the expiratory pause as follows.

- Inspiration – the APL valve closes under the negative pressure generated by the lungs. Gas flows into the lungs from the circuit primed by the fresh gas flow and from the bag acting as a reservoir.
- Expiration – as inspiration stops, fresh gas will begin to refill the now partially collapsed bag. The first 150 mL of dead space gas (containing no carbon dioxide) will be simultaneously expired back down the circuit as the resistance offered by the bag increases as it fills. At a point, roughly equal to the demarcation between dead space and alveolar gas, the resistance offered by the bag plus the patient will be sufficient to overcome the APL valve and the carbon dioxide-containing alveolar gas is vented.
- Expiratory pause – at this point the patient still offers a high resistance to flow from the fresh gas outlet that becomes the overwhelming direction of force. Gas from the circuit proximal to the APL valve that may contain carbon dioxide is vented.

For this pattern of gas flow to occur, a regular respiration and specific ratio of tidal volume to breathing system volume is required. Mapleson calculated that given these parameters, no

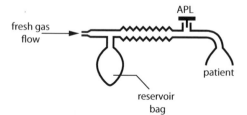

Figure 14.2. *The Mapleson A breathing system.*

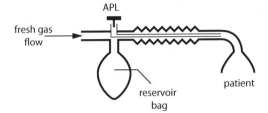

Figure 14.3. *The Lack breathing system.*

re-breathing would occur if fresh gas flow is equal to minute ventilation. If re-breathing of dead space is allowed (non-carbon dioxide containing, warm and humidified gas) then 70% minute ventilation, or alveolar ventilation is achievable as fresh gas flow. This has been backed up by experimental evidence. Mapleson A is therefore efficient for spontaneous ventilation.

During controlled ventilation, fresh gas is moved within the circuit by positive pressure from the ventilator rather than negative pressure from spontaneous respiration. Due to this positive pressure, the APL valve is opened during the inspiratory phase and fresh gas is vented before reaching the lungs. Similarly in expiration, alveolar gas is re-breathed before venting from the APL valve, unless high fresh gas flows are used to increase the overall pressure in the circuit more rapidly. This value is around 20 L/min, which suggests that Mapleson A is therefore very inefficient during controlled ventilation.

Lack circuit. The eponymously named Lack circuit (*Figure 14.3*) is a coaxial configuration of the Magill circuit. In terms of function, it is identical to the Magill. The advantage of coaxial circuits is that they place the APL valve at the bag (and therefore machine) end, meaning that you can remain seated whilst making adjustments.

Mapleson B

The Mapleson B circuit still positions the fresh gas inlet distal to the APL valve, but now the circuit tubing and the bag become the reservoir. This arrangement was not often used in clinical practice because it is inconveniently bulky at the patient end and requires twice the patient's minute volume for both spontaneous and controlled ventilation.

Mapleson C

The Mapleson C arrangement is commonly encountered in the intensive care unit and is more commonly known as the Water's circuit. Very high flow rates are normally used through this circuit and, as such, it is rarely if ever used to administer anaesthetic gas. The bag valve mask commonly found on resuscitation trolleys is another variety of the Mapleson C circuit.

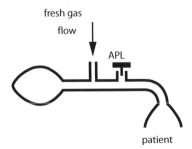

Figure 14.4. *The Mapleson C breathing system.*

14.5 Mapleson D, E and F systems

Mapleson D

The Mapleson D arrangement is the first of the efferent systems, i.e. the bag stems from the expiratory limb of the circuit. This is the only semi-closed circuit still in common use to deliver anaesthetic gases today.

The D system has the fresh gas entering the circuit at the patient end. During spontaneous ventilation the following pattern of gas flow occurs.

- Inspiration – assuming the circuit is filled with fresh gas, negative pressure created by the patient draws gas in from the circuit, collapsing the reservoir bag.
- Expiration – during expiration exhaled gas travels down the circuit, re-filling the reservoir bag. At the same time fresh gas is still filling the circuit, mixing with the exhaled alveolar gas. The distal end of the circuit will contain a mixture of dead space gas, alveolar and fresh gas until such a point where the pressure in the system exceeds that of the APL valve and excess mixed gas is vented.
- Expiratory pause – fresh gas entering the circuit will flow down the corrugated tubing forcing the mixed gas out of the APL valve. However, a fresh gas flow of between 100 and 150 mL/kg/min is required to prevent re-breathing of alveolar gas making Mapleson D **inefficient for spontaneous ventilation**.

During controlled ventilation there are two important differences that occur that make system D more efficient. First, during controlled ventilation the **I:E** ratio tends to be lengthened to 1:2 or 1:3, giving more time for the fresh gas to travel along the tubing towards the APL valve during the expiratory pause. Secondly, there is a tendency toward larger tidal volumes during controlled ventilation. This has the effect of driving more gas into the lungs and, whilst a larger proportion of alveolar gas is re-breathed, it is in turn mixed with a larger proportion of fresh gas reducing the overall percentage and therefore the amount of re-breathing. It is possible to use a fresh gas flow of 70 mL/kg/min making Mapleson D **an efficient system for controlled ventilation**.

The Bain breathing system, introduced by Bain and Spoerel in 1972, is a coaxial Mapleson D system in which the fresh gas flows down the inner tube and the expired gas down the outer corrugated tubing. As with the Lack circuit, this reduces circuit bulk and makes it easier to make adjustments from a seated position. The circuit is particularly useful for anaesthesia where the anaesthetic machine is remote from the patient such as in an MRI scanner.

Note that both Mapleson A and D systems, regardless of the type of breathing, require a fresh gas flow that is substantially greater than that required for a circle system (which can employ very low flows). Confusingly, these systems could lead to dangerous levels of re-breathing.

A danger with coaxial circuits is a covert disconnection that can occur internally. At the machine end where the fresh gas flow/APL valve part of the circuit is constructed, it is vital that the inner tube

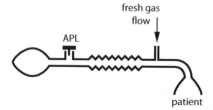

fresh gas
flow

APL

patient   **Figure 14.5.** *Mapleson D breathing system.*

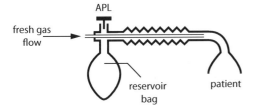

Figure 14.6. *Bain breathing system (coaxial Mapleson D).*

does not become disconnected to allow mixing of fresh gas with expired gas in the distal part of the circuit. This creates an enormous dead space volume that cannot be compensated for, even by torrential gas flows. Two ways exist to check this in the Bain circuit. The first is rather inelegant and requires the destruction of a perfectly good 2 mL syringe. The plunger of the syringe is removed and thrust into the inner tube whereby it causes a blockage and so a build up of pressure that is evident from the dipping of the flowmeter bobbin. A superior method of testing the integrity of the circuit is to first get a modest gas flow through it (about 5 litre/min) and to then press the oxygen flush. The accelerated flow through the narrow inner tube causes gas to be vented from the outer exhaust portion via the venturi effect, visible as a collapse of the reservoir bag.

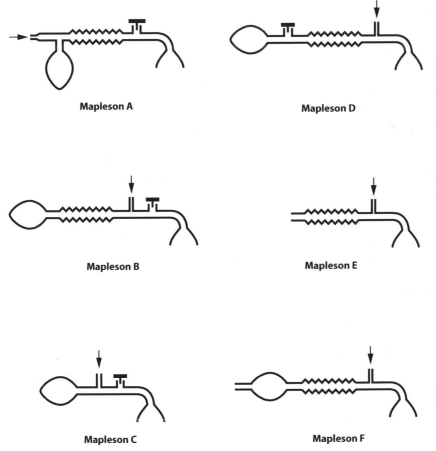

Figure 14.7. *Mapleson's systems.*

Mapleson E

System E is otherwise known as the **Ayre's T-piece** and was developed in 1937 for infants undergoing cleft lip and palate surgery. This circuit has the advantage of providing very little resistance to spontaneous ventilation whilst venting the expired volatile away from the surgeon! However, the system is inefficient for both controlled and spontaneous ventilation, requiring fresh gas flows of around 2–3 times minute volume to prevent re-breathing.

Mapleson only originally classified five breathing systems, A to E. However, the Ayre's T-piece was modified by Gordon Jackson-Rees to include a reservoir bag with a hole cut in the end. This has two main benefits over the conventional T-piece. Whilst still providing a low resistance system, the bag can be observed moving during spontaneous ventilation and the hole pinched to provide controlled ventilation when required. Although not in the original classification this has become known as the Mapleson F. *Figure 14.6* shows all the Mapleson circuits for easy comparison.

14.6 Minimizing pollutants in the theatre environment

Regulations

Volatile anaesthetic agents are potentially harmful to staff and as such come under Control of Substances Hazardous to Health (COSHH) Regulations. There must be an assessment of the risks involved, a plan to minimize these risks, and also monitoring of the exposure to the identified substance. The employer has a legal duty and a legal requirement to control and monitor levels according to the Health and Safety Commission (1996). Concentration of agents is measured in parts per million (p.p.m.) and this is usually as an eight hour, time weighted average (see *Table 14.2*).

Strategy to minimize pollutants

The strategy to reduce pollutants in the theatre environment is three-fold.
- **Minimize** the use of anaesthetic agents. Employing low flow anaesthetic techniques will mean less volatile agent is used. Careful attention to detail when refilling vaporizers.
- **Contain:** use of a circle breathing system. The system should be free of leaks and low fresh gas flow techniques used as appropriate.
- **Remove** gases from both the general environment (**ventilation/air conditioning**) and from the breathing system (**scavenging**).

Ventilation/air-conditioning

Ventilation in theatres should ideally be a non-recirculating ventilation system that changes the circulating air 15–20 times per hour and this should be positive pressure ventilation. Where

Table 14.2. *Maximum concentrations of volatile agents (figures for the UK).*

Pollutant	Maximum level (parts per million)
Halothane	10
Enflurane	50
Isoflurane	50
Nitrous oxide	100

Entonox is used, such as in a maternity unit, the minimum change of circulating volume is five times per hour.

Anaesthetic gas scavenging systems (AGSS)

Scavenging systems can be classed as either passive or active.

Passive scavenging. Passive scavenging is the removal of waste gases by passive means. The technique relies on a residual positive pressure from the breathing circuit to drive the gases down a pipe to outside of the theatre environment. Its advantages are its simplicity and minimal costs. Although it has its limitations: being vulnerable to changes in airflow in the breathing circuit and this can render the scavenging ineffective.

The **Cardiff Aldasorber** is a passive scavenger, removing and filtering waste gases, with activated charcoal absorbing the volatile agents. They weigh 1 kg before use and gain weight on absorption; an estimate of their lifespan can be obtained from the canister's increased weight. It is simple and cheap, however, its weakness is that it does not absorb nitrous oxide

> **Definition**
>
> **Passive scavenging:** the removal of exhaust gases from the breathing system without mechanical assistance.

Active scavenging. Active scavenging employs a negative pressure to generate a flow of gas from the exhaust, through tubing and pipes out of the clinical area, to a vent situated outside (see *Figure 14.8*). The low negative pressure is generated by a fan/pump or a venturi system. In the reservoir there are vents that act as a safety valve and a bacterial filter separates the breathing circuit from the external vent exhaust. The tubing used is 19 mm in diameter to avoid accidental connection to the breathing system.

> **Definition**
>
> **Active scavenging:** the removal of exhaust gases with the aid of mechanically generated negative pressure.

14.7 Ventilators

Mechanical ventilation is the process by which gas is artificially moved in and out of the lungs to facilitate oxygen delivery and carbon dioxide removal. Mechanical ventilation can be undertaken by hand, or more commonly by machine where prolonged periods of ventilation are expected.

Until the worldwide polio epidemic in the 1950s, the most common method of mechanical ventilation was negative pressure ventilation via the iron lung. During the 1952 epidemic in Copenhagen, Bjorn Aage Ibsen, a Danish anaesthetist and one of the pioneers of intensive care medicine, was one of the first clinicians to institute long-term airway protection and mechanical ventilation by intubating polio patients. He enlisted 200 medical students working in shifts to provide around the clock positive pressure ventilation. The enormous reduction in mortality sparked the subsequent rapid development in positive pressure ventilation technology.

At present, the overwhelming majority of mechanical ventilation is performed by positive pressure.

When considering mechanical ventilation it is useful to look at simple anaesthetic machine ventilators and ventilators suitable for intensive care separately. Although they share many features in common, anaesthetic machine ventilators are considerably simpler, being designed for short to medium term ventilation in a patient with relatively normal lung mechanics. Anaesthetic

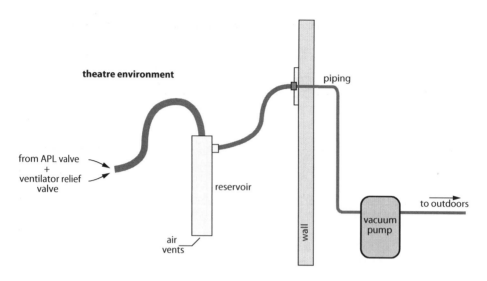

Figure 14.8. *An active scavenging system.*

machine ventilators are also designed to work with an anaesthetic breathing circuit, optimized for economical anaesthetic gas delivery. In contrast, ventilators suitable for intensive care are considerably more complex, encompassing a vast array of different and confusingly named modes. They are capable of coping with extremely deranged lung compliances for extended periods of time. These ventilators incorporate sophisticated feedback mechanisms to enable assisted spontaneous ventilation. Microprocessing units control nearly all currently manufactured ventilators. That said, efficient and reliable gas-powered minute volume dividers are still in use in some anaesthetic rooms and are relied upon for millions of anaesthetics a year in the developing world.

Anaesthetic ventilators

The traditional way of classifying ventilators is by their mechanism of gas delivery. Ventilators are either **pressure generators** or **flow generators**.

- A pressure generator moves gas into the lungs by generating a constant and pre-determined pressure, greater than the intrapulmonary pressure. This results in forward flow of gas. A pressure generator cannot compensate for changes in lung compliance but can compensate for a leak in the circuit.
- A flow generator moves gas into the lungs by generating a constant and pre-determined flow that will move gas into the lungs if the resulting pressure is greater than the intrapulmonary pressure. A flow generator can compensate for changes in lung compliance but not for a leak in the circuit. Most anaesthetic machine ventilators are flow generators of the bag-in-bottle variety.

During mechanical ventilation, expiration is a passive function of the elastic recoil of the lungs as they drop back to atmospheric pressure. The method by which the inspiratory and expiratory phases are changed over is another method of classification. *Table 14.3* summarizes the classification of anaesthetic ventilators.

Table 14.3. *Classification of anaesthetic ventilators by the method through which the inspiratory and expiratory phases are changed.*

Volume cycling	• The ventilator will change respiratory phases at a pre-set volume. • This will be dependent on the flow generated and the lung compliance.
Time cycling	• The ventilator will change respiratory phase after a pre-set time. • This will be independent of lung compliance but could lead to the generation of small minute volumes.
Pressure cycling	• The ventilator will change respiratory phase at a pre-set pressure. • The volume delivered and the time taken to achieve this will depend on the compliance of the lungs.
Flow cycling	• The ventilator will change respiratory phase when a pre-set flow has been reached.

14.8 Ventilator designs

Minute volume dividers

The classic example of this is the Manley MP3 ventilator. This is an entirely mechanical pressure generator, powered by the fresh gas flow. The desired minute volume is delivered to the ventilator and then, through a series of bellows, valves and weights, it is divided into inspiratory and expiratory phases. The anaesthetist then sets the desired tidal volume and inspiratory time.

Penlon Nuffield 200

This is a small, gas-driven flow generator. It is versatile and suitable for use in paediatrics. The Penlon differs from the Manley in that it generates flow from a high pressure gas source that is independent of the fresh gas flow. The anaesthetist sets the inspiratory and expiratory times (time cycled) and then determines the correct inspiratory flow rate to deliver the desired tidal volume.

Bag-in-the-bottle

Most current anaesthetic machine ventilators are of the 'bag-in-bottle' variety. The bellows are filled internally with gas from the fresh gas outlet. Externally, the bellows are surrounded by a bottle that contains gas supplied from an independent high pressure source. The pressure within the bottle can be increased rapidly to collapse the bellows and drive fresh anaesthetic gas into the patient's lungs. This bottle pressure is then released, returning it to atmospheric pressure. The bellows then re-inflate driven by the elastic recoil of the lungs and further fresh gas from the fresh gas outlet.

Ventilators of this design can deliver either a pre-set volume or a pre-set pressure. The tidal volume, inspiratory pressure, the respiratory rate and I:E ratio can all be altered.

Intensive care ventilators

All modern intensive care ventilators are electrically powered, microprocessor-controlled flow generators. There are a myriad different flow patterns that these ventilators are capable of producing thanks to complex and rapid servo-controlled feedback mechanisms. Commonly encountered flow patterns are:

- **constant** (or square wave) where the gas flow is constant until a desired tidal volume or pressure is achieved
- **decelerating** where the speed of gas flow decreases throughout the respiratory cycle
- **sinusoidal** which is more akin to that seen in a spontaneously breathing patient

The different flow patterns create different distribution characteristics within the alveoli of the lung, depending upon the overall compliance and differing time constants.

14.9 Modes of ventilation

Thanks to microprocessor technology and improved manufacturing and safety standards, there is now little to choose between most standard ventilators. There are, however, a large number of confusingly named modes, each with customisable settings, but with a complete lack of any standardized nomenclature. The modes in common usage today are all variations on a theme and can be worked out in terms of pressure or volume delivery, mandatory or spontaneous, invasive or non-invasive.

The majority of ventilated patients on ICU will have a degree of positive end expiratory pressure (PEEP) applied as a baseline pressure delivered by the ventilator. If this is 5 cmH$_2$O, then the pressure in the circuit and lungs will never fall below 5 cmH$_2$O, provided there are no leaks (in the airway device or lungs). A baseline level of PEEP is generally a good idea as a recumbent patient inevitably collapses the basal segments of their lungs, resulting in a reduced functional residual capacity and reduced compliance. PEEP helps to counteract this phenomenon by holding the dependent alveoli open throughout the respiratory cycle. With baseline positive pressure in place, the ventilator then has to create a higher level of pressure to create forward flow of gas into the lungs. As discussed above, there are a number of variable flow patterns by which this can be achieved.

The PEEP/CPAP 'problem'

Definitions

Mandatory breaths: delivered to the patient independent of any trigger.
Spontaneous breaths: delivered in response to a trigger from the patient.

Continuous positive airway pressure (CPAP) is frequently used interchangeably with positive end expiratory pressure (PEEP). In reality they refer to the same phenomenon of raising the total intrapulmonary pressure above atmospheric pressure for the entirety of the respiratory cycle. CPAP is commonly used to refer to the non-invasive ventilation version of PEEP.

Synchronized intermittent mandatory ventilation (SIMV)

This ventilatory mode is the successor to intermittent mandatory ventilation (IMV). IMV was used in patients able to take spontaneous breaths, but unable to facilitate adequate gas exchange without extra support. IMV used a simple demand valve to disconnect the patient from the ventilator circuit and allow a true negative pressure breath. Problems would occur when the ventilator, being unaware of the spontaneous breath, would stack another breath straight on top. Similarly, by inspiring through the valve, any applied PEEP would be lost.

These problems were overcome by SIMV. In an SIMV mode the ventilator senses the patient's attempt at a spontaneous breath (this sensitivity is set by the trigger threshold) and the patient is then allowed to breathe spontaneously through the ventilator circuit, with the ventilator assisting inspiration to a pre-set degree known as the pressure support. The number of mandatory breaths selected by the operator will therefore become the minimum number the patient will receive, but the patient is free to breathe over that number as much as they like.

Once a patient is sufficiently awake to spontaneously ventilate, they can be switched to a spontaneous mode commonly known as pressure support. In terms of the level of support the patient receives from the ventilator, this is identical to the equivalent on SIMV, there is just no delivery of mandatory breaths. On a ventilator without a pure spontaneous mode and only SIMV, the same effect could theoretically be achieved by turning the mandatory respiratory rate to 0.

Pressure control, pressure support or ASB?

There are two ways of regulating a patient's tidal volumes: by delivering a specific volume or a specific pressure. There is no standardized terminology for describing the pressure over PEEP delivered to the patient.

On the majority of ventilators **pressure control** refers to the pressure given over PEEP on a **mandatory breath** and this setting will therefore only be seen on modes with some form of mandatory breath frequency.

Pressure support refers to the inspiratory pressure or assist given by the ventilator by a patient's triggered, or spontaneous breath. Pressure support can also be known as **assisted spontaneous breathing** (ASB).

Advanced control modes

Nearly every setting on a modern ICU ventilator can be customized by the user. A discussion of ramp times, Ti and Te (inspiratory and expiratory times or I:E ratio) and patient trigger settings are beyond the scope of this book, but all can be tweaked to fine-tune oxygenation and ventilation. Optimum settings tend to be very specific to a particular patient's respiratory mechanics and rely, in part, on the clinician's experience with that particular model of ventilator).

Popular and recently introduced modes include **pressure regulated volume guarantee** (PRVG) and **bilevel ventilation**. Since the ARDSnet paper demonstrated a reduction in mortality using 6 mL/kg tidal volumes as opposed to 12 mL/kg, this lower target is becoming a standard of care amongst ventilated patients on the ICU, not just for those with acute respiratory distress syndrome. However, many of the acute complications of mechanical ventilation come not only from the inspired volume but also from the pressure required to deliver that volume. As such, many ventilators will now allow an ideal volume target to be set for a particular patient, but will limit attempts to deliver this volume based on a pre-set pressure limit. The physician (or ventilator) can then attempt to alter PEEP, ramp times and peak flows to find the optimal settings for that patient to achieve the desired volume delivery.

Patients requiring high levels of respiratory support fail to 'sync' well with a ventilator. The traditional remedies are to either heavily sedate the patient (often at the expense of hypotension) or paralyse them (increasing the risk of critical illness polyneuropathy and myopathy). Ventilator dysynchrony is often due to inadequate gas flow resulting in patients attempting to compensate by creating their own negative pressure against the ventilator. One of the solutions to this problem is the bilevel mode. Ventilators capable of providing this mode of ventilation incorporate a sophisticated valve that allows the patient to take an assisted breath at any point of the respiratory cycle during a mandatory breath.

Bilevel ventilation is in essence the next stage in the evolution of SIMV in which a physician-set minimum respiratory rate is delivered, while the patient is able to contribute additional breaths as required. As the patient can breathe and receive a uniform level of assistance whenever they choose to take a breath, many of the uncomfortable aspects of 'fighting the ventilator' are negated and patients typically do not require heavy sedation.

High frequency oscillatory ventilation

In the intensive care setting high frequency jet ventilation has largely been superseded by **high frequency oscillatory ventilation** (HFOV), a novel method of positive pressure ventilation. Many of the consequences of long-term mechanical ventilation, such as pulmonary scarring and fibrosis, are thought to be caused by inflammatory mediators provoked by the repeated inflation of alveoli. This is termed volutrauma. HFOV avoids this repeated inflation by inflating the alveoli once with a relatively high pressure and then delivering fast (up to 900 a minute) breaths with small tidal volumes (typically less than the dead space). Despite tidal volumes being insufficient to achieve dead space ventilation, patients by and large achieve adequate carbon dioxide clearance and superior oxygenation due to the increased and sustained mean airway pressure.

The exact mechanism of gas exchange is not fully understood but is thought to be a combination of phenomena such as the Pendelluft effect, direct bulk flow and cardiogenic mixing. This mode is commonly used for patients with resistant hypoxia secondary to acute respiratory distress syndrome.

Lack of evidence relating to modes of ventilation

Whilst so many modes of ventilation exist, other than the use of smaller tidal volumes in patients with acute respiratory distress syndrome, there is currently no convincing evidence for using one ventilatory mode over another. As is often the case with anaesthetics and intensive care medicine, physician preference and familiarity with a specific piece of equipment is as important as the specific pathology of the individual patient.

14.10 Non-invasive ventilation

Non-invasive ventilation is a method of ventilating patients without intubation: a mask is used instead. The modes and principles of non-invasive ventilation available are almost identical to the invasive modes already discussed.

For patients with obstructive sleep apnoea, airway obstruction rather than oxygenation is the issue. Their condition is improved by the application of positive pressure (CPAP) at night. As a supplementary oxygen supply is often not required, the positive pressure is created by an air compressor that can be applied by a nasal mask and keeps the oropharynx patent in spite of reduced muscle tone.

The management of a hypercapnoeic patient may involve non-invasive 'BiPAP' to help control their carbon dioxide. This mode of ventilation, strictly speaking, should be called bilevel positive airway pressure (BPAP). Non-invasive BPAP ventilation is conceptually exactly the same as invasive pressure support ventilation. However, on many machines designed to deliver just non-invasive ventilation the term PEEP has been replaced with EPAP (expiratory positive airway pressure) and pressure support with IPAP (inspiratory positive airway pressure). Although the terms differ, the effect is the same, the goal being to deliver a larger tidal volume thereby improving minute ventilation and reducing carbon dioxide.

14.11 Negative pressure ventilation

Before the advent of positive pressure ventilation in the middle of the twentieth century, negative pressure ventilation (NPV) via an iron lung was the only means of long-term ventilation available. From a physiological standpoint, positive pressure ventilation has many problems, mainly affecting cardiac haemodynamics. In health, the filling and emptying of the heart has evolved around spontaneous negative pressure ventilation and a sudden switch to positive pressure, especially with the application of PEEP, inhibits right ventricular filling by obstructing venous return and biventricular ejection by an increase in afterload. This reduction in cardiac output is compounded by the cardiovascular depressant effects of anaesthetic agents given to facilitate invasive ventilation. However, these disadvantages are clearly outweighed by the ease and convenience with which positive pressure ventilation can be deployed.

One of the major drawbacks of negative pressure ventilation systems such as an iron lung, is that in order to create sufficient negative pressure to move the chest and create a tidal volume, the whole of the patient's body except the head needs to be enclosed, making monitoring and access extremely difficult. More recent attempts have used a cuirass (breast plate) to make an airtight seal over the anterior chest wall. This has been effective to some degree and has the advantage of not requiring an airway through which to ventilate the patient (unless it is required for airway protection). These ventilators also incorporate a (external) high frequency oscillation mode that has shown some promise, mainly in the paediatric population. Although the ventilator is available for adults, the speed of innovation in positive pressure ventilators (particularly form and functionality) has left NPV with few enthusiasts and little research demonstrating any tangible clinical benefit. However, there is a resurging interest in NPV and with better engineering and microprocessor technology and scaling down of the equipment, negative pressure ventilation may once again regain its popularity.

Summary

- The circle system is the most widely used breathing circuit and minimizes consumption of medical gases and volatile agents, whilst retaining warmth and moisture.
- Mapleson categorized breathing systems built from the core components of an APL valve, a reservoir bag, tubing and a fresh gas supply.
- Scavenging can either be active or passive: it is necessary for the safe removal of volatile agents.
- Ventilators generate a positive pressure gradient causing gas to flow into the lungs.
- Intensive care ventilators are generally more complex than anaesthetic machine ventilators and are able to ventilate spontaneously breathing patients with deranged lung mechanics.
- Traditionally ventilators were classified either as pressure or flow generators, although this is now a largely historic classification.
- Due to a lack of standardized nomenclature and cross-specialty interest, many terms exist to describe similar principles and ventilator modes.
- High frequency oscillatory ventilation (HFOV) is a novel method of positive pressure ventilation although its mechanism is not fully understood.

Single best answer questions

For these questions, choose the single best answer.

1. The best description of breathing circuit efficiency is:
   (a) the oxygen/air mix required to prevent rebreathing of alveolar gases
   (b) the fresh gas flow rate required to prevent rebreathing of alveolar gases
   (c) the gas flow rate required to acheive 100% oxygen saturation
   (d) the oxygen flow rate required to maintain a partial pressure of 12 kPa in arterial blood
   (e) the fresh gas flow rate required to prevent re-breathing of circuit gases

2. The action of soda lime granules can be best described by which one of the following descriptions?
   (a) They chemically remove the carbon dioxide contained in exhaled gas.
   (b) They physically remove the carbon dioxide contained in exhaled gas.
   (c) They chemically remove the carbon monoxide contained in exhaled gas.
   (d) They chemically remove the carbon dioxide and water vapour contained in exhaled gas.
   (e) They physically remove the carbon dioxide and water vapour contained in exhaled gas.

3. Active scavenging is best described as:
   (a) the removal of inhaled gases without the aid of mechanically generated negative pressure
   (b) the removal of exhaust gases with the aid of mechanically generated positive pressure
   (c) the filtering of exhaust gases with the aid of mechanically generated negative pressure
   (d) the removal of exhaust gases
   (e) the removal of exhaust gases with the aid of mechanically generated negative pressure

Multiple choice questions

For each of these questions, mark every answer either true or false.

1. The circle system consists of a number of key components: which of the following accurately describe a component?
   (a) Six unidirectional valves, three in each limb of the circuit.
   (b) Fresh gas flow positioned distal to the inspiratory valve.
   (c) Exhaust valve positioned on the inspiratory limb.
   (d) Carbon dioxide absorbing material.
   (e) Reservoir bag.

2. Regarding scavenging, which of the following statements are true?
   (a) Passive scavenging is the removal of exhaust gases from the breathing system without mechanical assistance.
   (b) Passive scavenging involves a low negative pressure to aid gas removal.
   (c) The Cardiff Aldasorber is an example of an active scavenging system.
   (d) Volatile anaesthetic agents come under the Control of Substances Hazardous to Health (COSHH) Regulations.
   (e) Active scavenging systems are more vulnerable than passive systems to changes in air flow in the breathing system.

3. With regards to breathing systems, which of the following statements are true?
   (a) A danger with coaxial circuits is a covert disconnection that can occur internally.

   (b) Mapleson only originally classified five breathing systems A to E.
   (c) System A is known as the Magill circuit.
   (d) System E is otherwise known as the Ayre's T-piece.
   (e) Mapleson A is efficient for spontaneous ventilation.

4. Regarding HFOV, which of the following statements are true?
   (a) It stands for high force oscillatory ventilation.
   (b) The mechanism of action is not fully understood.
   (c) It is most commonly used during routine surgery.
   (d) Anaesthetic ventilators can deliver this mode.
   (e) This mode involves high airway pressures.

5. Regarding negative pressure ventilation, which of the following statements are true?
   (a) An iron lung provides this form of ventilation.
   (b) Airway protection is a weakness with this form of ventilation.
   (c) The negative pressure is applied to the external thoracic region.
   (d) Negative pressure ventilation is better known as BiPAP.
   (e) Intubation is not needed.

Chapter 15
Optics

Having read this chapter you will be able to:
- Explain refraction of light and Snell's law.
- Understand the principle of optical fibres.
- Understand the principles behind a fibreoptic pressure transducer.
- Appreciate how fibreoptic bundles are used in endoscopes.
- Understand how Beer's law describes absorption of light.
- Explain how pulse oximeters work.
- Understand the principle of transcranial near-infrared spectroscopy.

15.1 Refraction

Looking into a fish tank the fish appear to shift their position depending on the angle you look at the tank. Swimming pools appear shallower than they really are, and a straw seems to be bent at the point where it enters a glass of water. These are all consequences of the law of refraction, summarized by Snell's law (Equation 15.2). Snell's law allows us to predict the path of a beam of light traveling from one medium (through the air for example) to another (e.g. water).

> **Definition**
>
> **Critical angle:** when light is incident on a boundary between two materials at an angle greater than the critical angle, it is internally reflected from the boundary rather than refracted out of the material.

Transparent materials are characterized by their **refractive index**, which is the ratio of the speed of light in a vacuum to the speed of light in the material in question. In glass, the speed of light is about two-thirds the speed in a vacuum, so glass has a refractive index of approximately 1.5. In air, the speed of light is only very slightly less than in a vacuum, so the refractive index is close to 1.

$$n = \frac{\text{speed of light in a vacuum}}{\text{speed of light in the material}}$$

15.1

Figure 15.1 shows a ray of light entering a glass slab. All angles are measured relative to the **normal** line, a line at right angles to the boundary between the two materials. It can be seen that the **angle of refraction** (the angle at which the ray exits) is less than the **angle of incidence** (the angle at which the ray enters); in other words, the ray is refracted towards the normal line.

Snell's law

If we know the refractive index of the air and the glass we can use Snell's law to calculate the angle of refraction from the angle of incidence:

$$n_1 \sin\theta_1 = n_2 \sin\theta_2$$

15.2

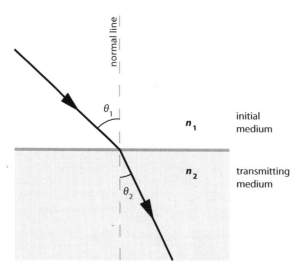

Figure 15.1. *A ray of light passing from air (initial medium) to glass (transmitting medium). The ray is refracted towards the normal line.*

where n_1 is the refractive index of the initial medium
    θ_1 is the angle of incidence
    n_2 is the refractive index for the transmitting medium
    θ_2 is the angle of refraction

Now consider a ray travelling upwards underwater, towards the water's surface. This time the ray leaves the surface at a larger angle than the incident angle, i.e. the ray is refracted away from the normal. If the ray has a small incident angle, i.e. it is traveling upwards at a steep angle; it will escape into the air. If the incident angle is large, however, the ray will be reflected back off the lower surface of the water, a phenomenon known as **total internal reflection.** This effect can be observed underwater whilst diving with a mask or goggles. If you look at the surface of the water straight up,

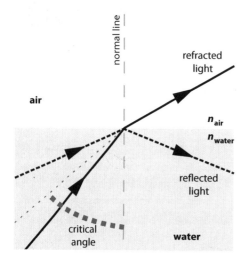

Figure 15.2. *A ray of light passing from water to air is only refracted if the incident angle is less than the critical angle, otherwise total internal reflection occurs.*

you will see the sky, but in the distance, the water's surface looks like a mirror reflecting objects such as the seabed below.

Total internal reflection can be understood by considering that there is an angle of incidence where the angle of refraction is 90° (i.e. the ray will try to leave along the surface of the water) as shown in *Figure 15.2*. This angle of incidence is known as the **critical angle.** Total internal reflection can occur in glass, or indeed any medium whose refractive index is greater than air. Total internal reflection is how light stays inside an optical fibre allowing fibres to transmit light over great distances (see next section and *Figure 15.3*).

The critical angle for any medium can be calculated from Snell's law by setting the angle of refraction to 90°:

$$n_1 \sin\theta_c = n_2 \sin 90°$$

sin 90° = 1, so:

$$\sin\theta_c = \frac{n_1}{n_2}$$

(15.3)

15.2 Optical fibres

Optical fibres have revolutionized telecommunications by enabling transmission of telephone calls and other digital information encoded in optical signals over vast distances. Optical fibres traverse the oceans of the world, and can carry thousands of times more information than copper wires. Optical fibres are made from extremely high purity silica glass, which is highly transparent. To transmit information, a data link converts data from an analogue electronic signal, such as a telephone conversation, into digital pulses of infrared laser light. These travel through the optical fibre to another data link where a light detector converts them back into an electronic signal. As the signal travels along the fibre it becomes weaker and needs to be boosted, or 'repeated'. To do this, laser signal repeaters are placed every 200 km or so throughout the length of a long-distance cable.

Optical fibres have numerous medical applications, the best known being as a light transmitter in an endoscope. Optical fibres can also be coupled to lasers for delivering infrared light for surgical applications. Fibre optics are also used for photodynamic therapy, while dedicated fibreoptic sensors can be used for physiological measurement.

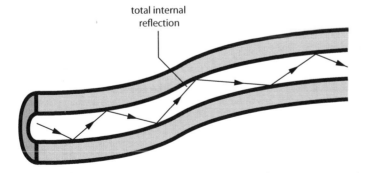

total internal reflection

Figure 15.3. *Transmission of light within a fibre by total internal reflection.*

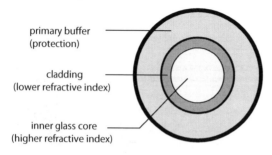

primary buffer
(protection)

cladding
(lower refractive index)

inner glass core
(higher refractive index)

Figure 15.4. *Cross-section of an optical fibre.*

Light must enter the fibre at a small angle relative to the fibre's axis. This ensures that total internal reflection occurs within the core as shown in *Figure 15.3*. A bare core would function as a basic optical fibre, however, contamination such as dirt or grease on the outside of the fibre would increase the external refractive index, lowering the critical angle and causing light to escape. To prevent this, the core is surrounded by a layer of **cladding**, made from glass of lower refractive index than the core, ensuring the core refractive index is always greatest, the condition required for total internal reflection. The cladding layer, being made from glass is brittle, so a third plastic layer is added to protect the cladding, known as the **primary buffer** as shown in *Figure 15.4*.

Fibreoptic catheter tip pressure transducer

Optical fibres can be engineered with special properties enabling measurements of physical quantities. One example is the fibreoptic pressure sensor, a specialized sensor constructed from a bundle of optical fibres and a reflective metal membrane (*Figure 15.5*). The membrane is distorted by external pressure causing the reflected light intensity to vary, so that measuring the reflected intensity allows the pressure to be calculated by the monitor.

Fibreoptic pressure transducers are used for measurement of intracranial pressure. They can also be placed directly in a vessel, with no need for a saline-filled catheter to transmit the pressure to an external transducer (see *Section 6.8*). This device has a rapid response time and no resonance and damping problems, allowing for accurate reproduction of the arterial pressure wave on the monitor screen. The limitations of this sensor are that it is expensive, delicate and difficult to calibrate, so external transducers are used more commonly for blood pressure measurement.

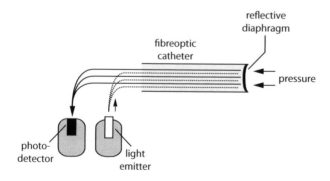

reflective
diaphragm

fibreoptic
catheter

pressure

photo-
detector

light
emitter

Figure 15.5. *Fibreoptic pressure transducer.*

15.3 Fibreoptic endoscopes

The flexibility afforded by optical fibre endoscopes, introduced in the mid-1950s have enabled previously inaccessible sites to be viewed in both awake and sedated patients. Previous generation rigid endoscopes can only be used in certain sites, and insertion of the endoscope can cause undue trauma to the patient.

A typical fibreoptic bronchoscope contains an **ordered (coherent) bundle** of optical fibres whereby 5000–40 000 fibres are aligned so that the position of the fibres is preserved (*Figure 15.6*). The image is focused onto the distal end of the bundle where it is transmitted to the observer. Thus each fibre represents an element of the image (analogous to a pixel on a computer screen). A non-ordered (incoherent) bundle is used to transmit light from an external source such as a halogen lamp to illuminate the visual field. Non-ordered bundles are used for this purpose because they are considerable cheaper to manufacture than ordered bundles.

The shaft of the endoscope connects the distal end to the proximal end and holds the light guide, imaging bundle and the ancillary tubes together. They are often constructed of steel mesh to stiffen the endoscope and protect the delicate components inside. Some endoscopes have a more flexible distal end that can be bent by mechanical control. Usually there are thin wires that run inside the shaft. By turning a control wheel on a hand piece, the physician can move the end in either one or two perpendicular directions. This allows the view to be changed or the endoscope steered along the desired path within the body (e.g. along selected branches of the bronchial tree). The shaft of the endoscope is sheathed in a plastic jacket that is biologically inert and forms a hermetic seal. This protects the internal components from damage from body fluids and allows the scope to be cleaned and sterilized after use.

Fibreoptic endoscopes are expensive to manufacture due to the technical challenges arising during production of ordered bundles. The fibres are delicate and degrade gradually as tiny cracks appear during repeated use and sterilization. Improvements in small digital photodetector arrays may soon render fibreoptic scopes largely obsolete.

Fibreoptic bronchoscope

A bronchoscope is a type of endoscope with special features dedicated to viewing the airways. A mouthguard is used to protect the delicate shaft of the scope. An ordered bundle of optical fibres for viewing and an unordered bundle for illumination are bound within a flexible watertight shell of outside diameter typically 4–5 mm. There is also a channel for suction of mucus and other debris from within the airway. The suction channel can also carry dedicated surgical tools such as biopsy forceps. The distal tip of a bronchoscope is shown in *Figure 15.7*.

The bronchoscope allows viewing using an eyepiece or by connecting it to a video system allowing images to be viewed on a screen and also be recorded. The limitations of bronchoscopes

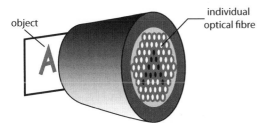

Figure 15.6. *An ordered optical fibre bundle: the view of a letter A.*

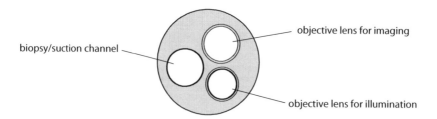

biopsy/suction channel

objective lens for imaging

objective lens for illumination

Figure 15.7. *The distal tip of a bronchoscope.*

are primarily from obstructions from saliva, mucus and other debris and for this reason suction and flush are required to improve the view. Cleaning and sterilizing the bronchoscope between patients is time consuming and requires dedicated equipment.

15.4 Absorption of light: Beer's law

If a light is shone through a glass of red wine, clearly not all the light passes through. The liquid appears dark as the tannins and other coloured compounds in the wine absorb visible light quite strongly. The wine appears red because the absorption is wavelength dependent: red light is absorbed less than other colours, which are strongly absorbed, leaving just red light reaching the eye.

Beer's law, also known as the Beer–Lambert law, describes the absorption of light travelling through any medium containing an absorbing substance. If monochromatic light of intensity I_0 enters the medium, a part of this light is transmitted through the medium while another part is absorbed. The intensity I_1 of light travelling through the medium decreases exponentially with distance:

$$I_1 = I_0 \cdot e^{-\varepsilon \cdot c \cdot d}$$

15.4

where ε is the **molar extinction coefficient** ($L \cdot mol^{-1} \cdot cm^{-1}$)
c the concentration ($mol \cdot L^{-1}$)
d the **optical path length** through the medium (cm)

Figure 15.8 shows light passing through a dye solution. A fraction of the light is absorbed, and is converted into thermal energy. The remaining light is transmitted through the solution. As we might expect, and as confirmed by Equation 15.4, the intensity of the transmitted light decreases if the concentration of the dye increases or the distance the light has to travel through the dye increases. The molar extinction coefficient is a measure of how strongly absorbing the dye is for a given wavelength: green dye absorbs red light much more strongly than it absorbs green light. Note that by convention, units of cm are used for optical path length.

Definition
Beer's law (Beer–Lambert's law): for light passing through a solution there is a linear relationship between absorbance and the concentration of that solution.

The Beer's law equation above (15.4) is useful if we are interested in how much light is transmitted by a substance. If we wanted to describe how strongly absorbing a substance is we can use a variable known as the **absorbance**. The absorbance is given by the following equation:

$$A = \varepsilon \cdot c \cdot d$$

15.5

Remember that the extinction coefficient varies for different wavelengths, therefore so does absorbance. Dark compounds such as melanin or haemoglobin have a higher absorbance of visible light than say water or fat. For light passing through a solution, there is a linear relationship between

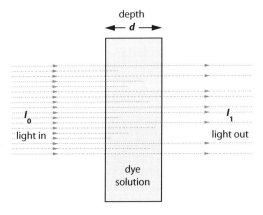

Figure 15.8. *Light passing through a dye solution.*

absorbance and the concentration of that solution. Equation 15.5 is simply an alternative way to express Beer's law.

15.5 Haemoglobin absorption spectra

All coloured compounds have an absorbance which varies across the visible spectrum. This forms the basis of the science of spectroscopy, whereby a compound can be identified and its concentration determined by studying its absorption spectrum. The absorption spectrum is simply a plot of absorbance (or extinction coefficient) against wavelength. Extending these spectra into the ultraviolet or infrared regions can reveal even more information about the compound. Pulse oximeters and CO-oximeters both work by measuring the relative absorbance of haemoglobin.

Figure 15.9 shows the absorption spectrum of oxyhaemoglobin and deoxyhaemoglobin from the red part of the visible spectrum to the near-infrared. It can be seen that the spectrum of oxyhaemoglobin differs considerably from that of deoxyhaemoglobin, although there is one point

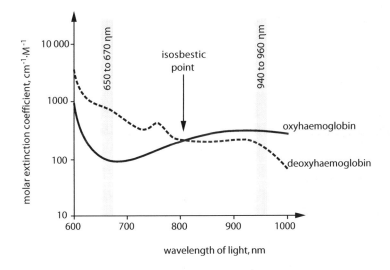

Figure 15.9. *Absorption spectra of oxyhaemoglobin and deoxyhaemoglobin in the visible (red) and near-infrared range showing two wavelengths commonly used in pulse oximetry.*

where the two curves cross, so the absorbances are equal at one wavelength. This wavelength is known as the **isosbestic** wavelength, and occurs at 805 nm for these two haemoglobin species. The molar extinction coefficient is much higher for deoxyhaemoglobin than for oxyhaemoglobin in the red region of the spectrum (around 670 nm). Deoxyhaemoglobin is more transparent to radiation in the wavelength range 805 to 1000 nm. The difference in the absorption spectra accounts for the difference in colour between arterial and venous blood, because the former has a much higher oxygen saturation and thus much more oxyhaemoglobin than deoxyhaemoglobin.

15.6 Pulse oximetry

Pulse oximetry is a noninvasive method for the continuous measurement of arterial oxygen saturation. A probe is placed on an extremity, such as the finger or earlobe, and an instrument unit displays an estimate of oxygen saturation along with other information such as heart rate. Since its invention in 1971, the pulse oximeter has become standard equipment in anaesthetic rooms, operating theatres, intensive care units, and ambulances.

Pulse oximeters determine the oxygen saturation of arterial blood by measuring the light absorbance of the blood at two different wavelengths. A probe (*Figure 15.10*) transilluminates the finger with two wavelengths of light. The arterial oxygen saturation (SpO_2) is determined from the ratio of the absorption of radiation at the two wavelengths. The choice of light wavelength is important: the two wavelengths chosen are typically 650–670 nm (in the red part of the visible spectrum) and 940–960 nm (in the infrared part of the spectrum). At these wavelengths there are significant differences in the extinction coefficients of deoxyhaemoglobin and oxyhaemoglobin.

Pulse oximeters take advantage of the arterial pulsation to discriminate between the arterial blood and other absorbers in the tissue. The arteries and arterioles within the tissue contain more blood during systole than during diastole. The absorbance of light in tissue containing arteries increases during the systolic phase of the cardiac cycle due to the increased optical path length of the blood-filled arteries. The absorbance thus varies periodically during the cardiac cycle. The time varying component of the transmitted intensity is referred to as the **photoplethysmograph** or **pleth waveform**.

Pulse oximeters have certain limitations which should be considered when interpreting oxygen saturation readings. The presence of dysfunctional haemoglobins causes the pulse oximeter to read inaccurately. Patients suffering from smoke inhalation, for example, often have elevated levels of carboxyhaemoglobin, which if high enough can cause the pulse oximeter to over-read and report normal saturation, even though the actual value may be critically low. Pulse oximeters are also sensitive to excessive limb movement or poor peripheral perfusion during states of hypervolemia or hypothermia, or low cardiac output. Newer pulse oximeters address these limitations by using

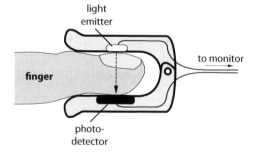

Figure 15.10. *A pulse oximeter finger probe.*

several wavelengths of light, thereby separating the absorbance of carboxyhaemoglobin and the other haemoglobin types. They also utilize advanced algorithms to correct for movement and low perfusion.

15.7 Trans-cranial near-infrared spectroscopy

The head is simply too big to pass infrared light through one side and detect on the other side like the oxygen saturation finger probe does. Visible light is largely unable to penetrate biological tissue to a thickness greater than approximately 1 cm because it is attenuated by absorption and scattering within the tissue: bone is particularly poor at transmitting light. The most abundant component of tissue is water, which has a strong absorption at wavelengths greater than 1000 nm. This leaves an effective window of wavelengths in the visible to the near-infrared region between 650 and 1000 nm in which photons are able to penetrate far enough to illuminate deeper structures such as the cerebral cortex. **Near-infrared spectroscopy** (NIRS) is a technique that can be used for the measurement of oxygen saturation of blood within brain or muscle tissue (*Figure 15.11*).

A near-infrared light source placed on the forehead (*Figure 15.11*) illuminates the tissue of the cerebral cortex and dual detectors placed on the skin surface several centimetres away detect the light back-scattered from the brain tissue. From the relative detected intensity of light of each wavelength, the instrument calculates the oxygen saturation of the blood in the brain tissue beneath the probe. As the measured oxygen saturation contains contributions from the arterial and the venous compartments, the value lies somewhere between the arterial and venous oxygen saturation of the blood within the cerebral tissue.

The technique has found most utility in monitoring cerebral oxygen saturation, but the technique may also be used to estimate changes in blood volume, brain blood flow and oxygen consumption. NIRS is fairly well established for monitoring neurosurgical and head injury patients, and the technique has proved itself a useful indicator of cerebral hypoxia in premature neonates. NIRS has been used in intensive care for several years both with adults and infants and is likely to become a standard monitoring technique. NIRS has also been demonstrated as a useful monitoring tool for patients undergoing major surgery.

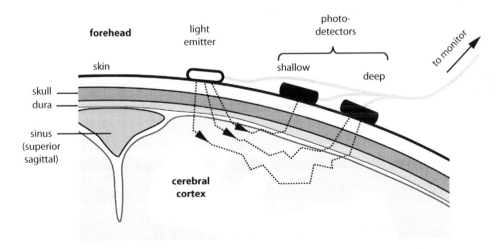

Figure 15.11. *Transcranial near-infrared spectroscopy.*

15.8 CO-oximetry

The **CO-oximeter**, also known as the **haemoximeter**, may be found either as a standalone instrument or incorporated within some blood gas analysers; it is considered the 'gold standard' measurement of oxygen saturation. This is due to its high level of accuracy and ability to distinguish between different types of haemoglobin. The CO-oximeter is indicated for patients with carboxyhaemoglobinaemia or other conditions where pulse oximeters may give erroneous readings. The CO-oximeter uses many more wavelengths of light than a pulse oximeter, so it is able to differentiate several haemoglobin types, because each type has a different absorption spectrum. CO-oximeters, unlike pulse oximeters require a blood sample, so they do not provide a continuous monitoring of oxygen saturation and other measurements.

A small (100 µl) heparinized blood sample is introduced into the input port of the haemoximeter and is transferred to the cuvette. The sample undergoes ultrasonically induced haemolysis in the cuvette in order to rupture the walls of the red blood cells so that their content is mixed with the blood plasma, giving an optically clear solution. Light from a halogen lamp is sent to the cuvette and the light transmitted through the cuvette is guided to the spectrometer via an optical fibre. A diffraction grating separates the light into several wavelengths within the visible and near-infrared region of the spectrum, and the intensity of the light is measured at each wavelength using a photo-detector array. These data are sent to the analyser's computer where the concentrations of all the haemoglobin types present in the blood are calculated. The CO-oximeter produces a report showing the total haemoglobin concentration, oxygen saturation, as well as individual concentrations of deoxyhaemoglobin, oxyhaemoglobin, carboxyhaemoglobin, methaemoglobin and other dysfunctional haemoglobins. Some instruments can also measure bilirubin concentration.

Summary
- Light is refracted when it crosses a boundary between two materials with differing refractive indices.
- Total internal reflection can occur in glass or water, and is a result of light trying to exit the material at too shallow an angle, i.e. an angle greater than the critical angle.
- Light stays in an optical fibre because of total internal reflection.
- Fibreoptic pressure sensors can be used to measure intracranial pressure as well as blood pressure without the need for a saline-filled catheter.
- Endoscopes use ordered fibreoptic bundles for imaging, and non-ordered bundles for illumination.
- Pulse oximeters, NIRS systems and CO-oximeters all rely on the varying absorbance of haemoglobin to measure oxygen saturation and other variables.

Single best answer questions

For these questions, choose the single best answer.

1. Which one of the following statements best describes the critical angle?
    (a) The minimum angle of refraction which produces total internal reflection.
    (b) The maximum angle of refraction which allows total internal reflection.
    (c) The maximum angle of incidence which allows total internal reflection.
    (d) The minimum angle of incidence which allows total internal reflection.
    (e) The only angle of refraction or incidence which allows total internal reflection.

2. Which one of the following statements best describes the isosbestic point?
    (a) The absorbance of two absorbers of equal concentration.
    (b) The wavelength where two absorbers have the same molar extinction coefficient.
    (c) The wavelength where the absorbance has a maximum or minimum.
    (d) The absorbance of two absorbers of equal molar extinction coefficient.
    (e) The wavelength where the molar extinction coefficient is zero.

Multiple choice questions

For each of these questions, mark every answer either true or false.

1. Which of the following statements are true of pulse oximetry?
    (a) Pulse oximetry measures oxygen saturation by measuring the arterial blood flow and relative absorbance of red and infrared radiation.
    (b) Pulse oximeters can fail or mis-read in patients with hypothermia.
    (c) Pulse oximeters can underestimate oxygen saturation in patients with carboxyhaemoglobinaemia.
    (d) Pulse oximeters are not affected by nail varnish.
    (e) Pulse oximeters produce a continuous estimation of oxygen saturation.

2. Beer's law states that:
    (a) absorbance is proportional to absorber concentration
    (b) transmitted intensity is inversely proportional to concentration
    (c) transmitted intensity is proportional to incident intensity
    (d) absorbance is inversely proportional to extinction coefficient
    (e) absorbance is proportional to optical path length

Chapter 16
Blood flow measurement

Having read this chapter you will be able to:
- Understand how washout curves are generated.
- Understand the relationship between the washout curve and the flow rate.
- Explain how cardiac output is measured by dye injection, thermodilution and other techniques.
- Understand the Doppler effect.
- Explain how ultrasound Doppler is used for measurement of cardiac output.
- Explain how a laser Doppler flowmeter works.

16.1 Measurement of liquid flow

In anaesthesia, the measurement of liquid flow is usually concerned with measuring blood flow through vessels, from large vessels such as the aorta to the smallest capillaries. Not surprisingly, measurement of cardiac output requires a different technique than measurement of microcirculatory flow, and a confusing array of techniques are available in clinical practice. There are only a few basic approaches to liquid flow measurement: dilution of dye or other substance, thermodilution and use of a Doppler flowmeter.

Cardiac output is defined as the volume of blood pumped by either side of the heart in one minute, therefore:

$$\text{cardiac output} = \text{stroke volume} \times \text{heart rate} \qquad \textbf{16.1}$$

Injecting a substance, such as a dye, into the circulation and measuring the concentration as it changes over time, at a location downstream of the injection point, allows cardiac output to be measured. Alternatively ultrasound or light are used to sense motion of blood cells using the principle of the Doppler effect.

16.2 Dye dilution and washout curves

Simple flow model

Definition
Washout curve: a graph of concentration of a substance against time if the substance is removed or washed away by a flow of liquid. The most basic washout curve is simple exponential decay, while specific systems produce variations of the basic curve.

Imagine a large container or tank with a tap at the bottom, being filled by another tap, as shown in *Figure 16.1*. The taps are connected by a mechanism that allows the flows to be adjusted, keeping the flow from each tap the same. Clearly the water level in the tank will remain constant, regardless of the flow. Imagine a quantity of dye is added whilst a stirrer at the bottom of the tank keeps everything thoroughly mixed. The colour of the water flowing from the tank would be seen to immediately darken and then gradually lighten as the dye concentration in the tank falls due to dilution from the upper tap.

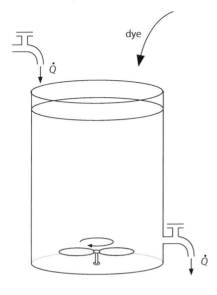

Figure 16.1. *A tank fitted with taps such that the flow into the tank is also equal to the flow out. If dye is added the concentration of dye falls exponentially.*

If we were able to measure the concentration of dye using, for example, an optical sensor, the change in concentration of dye in the water draining from the tap would look like the graph in *Figure 16.2*. This graph is called a washout curve. The dye is removed from the tank at a rate equal to the flow rate $\dot{Q}$ multiplied by the concentration of dye in the water flowing from the tap.

$$\text{rate of dye removal} = \dot{Q} \times \text{dye concentration} \qquad \boxed{16.2}$$

The concentration of dye in the water leaving the tank is equal to the concentration in the tank, and is proportional to the mass of dye left in the tank. This is a feature of exponential decay which is discussed further in *Chapter 28*. Since the flow rate is constant, it follows that

$$\text{rate of dye removal} \propto \text{quantity of dye in tank} \qquad \boxed{16.3}$$

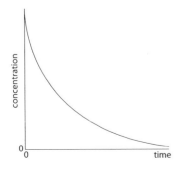

Figure 16.2. *Graph showing the change in dye concentration measured in the tank over time. The concentration is seen to fall exponentially, producing a basic washout curve.*

The concentration reduces more quickly at higher flow rates; in fact the area under the graph is inversely proportional to the flow rate. It follows that the flow rate can be calculated using the following equation:

$$\text{flow rate} = \frac{\text{amount of dye added}}{\text{area under the graph}}$$

16.4

Circulatory flow model

The tank model described above is an oversimplified model of the human circulation because there is no circulation of liquid. A more realistic circulatory model is shown in *Figure 16.3*. Cardiac output may be measured by injection of indocyanine green dye via a large vein (on the left of the diagram). The dye is then washed out of the heart chambers and pulmonary vessels by the cardiac output, and measured somewhere in the peripheral arterial tree (right of the diagram) using an optical-based sensor.

Figure 16.4 shows a graph of concentration measured against time produced using this model. If the dye is injected at time t_0, the dye is not detected until later, t_1, because it takes a finite time for the dye to travel from the injection point to the sensor. There is a rapid rise in concentration, but the maximum concentration does not occur straight away. Instead of a spike, a slightly rounded peak occurs due to the fact that laminar flow is occurring, so the dye travels at a range of velocities from the injection point to the detector. Also, some dye takes a more straightforward path through the system, while some swirls around in eddies within the heart chambers, for example. Exponential decay of concentration is then seen. Before all the dye has gone, a second peak occurs, which is caused by recirculation of the fastest moving dye.

The cardiac output may be calculated as for the simple tank model by dividing the amount of dye injected by the area under the graph. However, the recirculation peak complicates the calculation of cardiac output, so we must somehow ignore its effect. Extending the exponential part of the graph downwards, as shown in *Figure 16.5*, does this. Extrapolation of an exponential graph is mathematically straightforward (if you see how the decay begins, you can predict how it will end!).

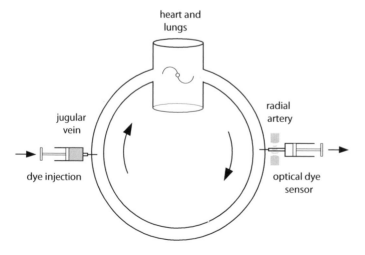

Figure 16.3. *Model of human circulation. Dye is injected into a large vein (e.g. the jugular vein) and detected at a site such as the radial artery.*

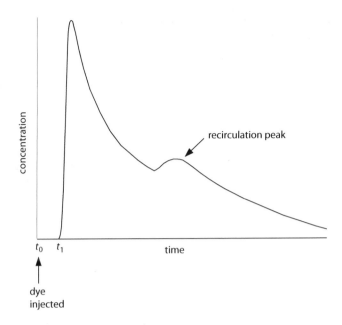

Figure 16.4. *Washout curve from the circulatory system shown in* Figure 16.3. *There is a delay before dye is detected, and a second peak caused by recirculation of dye.*

The area of the extrapolated graph is then used in order to calculate cardiac output. The equation for cardiac output is as follows:

$$\text{cardiac output} = \frac{\text{amount of dye injected}}{\text{mean concentration of dye} \times \text{time interval } t_2 - t_1} \quad \boxed{16.5}$$

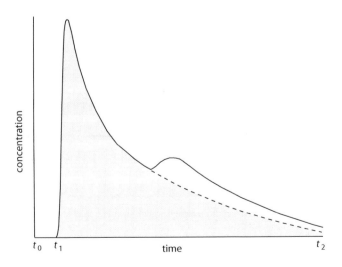

Figure 16.5. *The exponential decay of the washout curve is extrapolated, so that the recirculation peak is ignored. The cardiac output is calculated from the area under the 'reconstructed' curve.*

If t_2 is the time when the dye concentration reaches an insignificant level, the mean concentration of dye equals the amount of dye injected, divided by the volume of fluid flowing past the sampling point during the interval $t_1 - t_2$. This volume is the product of the fluid flow rate and the time interval $t_1 - t_2$. So the equation for calculating cardiac output becomes:

$$\text{cardiac output} = \frac{\text{amount of dye injected}}{\text{area under the graph}} \qquad \text{16.6}$$

Many different indicators have been used for the dye dilution technique. Indocyanine green (ICG) is one of the most popular because it is easy to detect and is 50% metabolized by the liver in 10 minutes, allowing a repeated measurement after a suitable time interval.

16.3 Thermodilution – pulmonary artery catheter

Cold injectate method

Pulmonary artery catheterization is an accurate method of measuring cardiac output and has the added advantage that pulmonary artery pressures may also be recorded by connecting the catheter to a pressure transducer. The pulmonary artery catheter is sometimes referred to as a Swan–Ganz catheter, named after its inventors.

The most common techniques rely on measurement of a temperature change in blood flowing past the catheter. Originally this temperature change was induced by injecting cold saline at approximately 0°C and measuring the thermal washout curve using a similar basic principle as for the dye injection method. The temperature change is measured by a pair of temperature sensors, one upstream and one downstream from the point of injection.

The catheter itself is a tube, made of flexible plastic, with a number of lumens, as shown in *Figure 16.6*. At the distal end, there is a small hole, the distal lumen, through which the intravascular pressure is measured. Just behind the hole there is a balloon that should be inflated with air so that the catheter tip is carried by the blood flow to the correct position. Just behind the balloon is a thermistor and 20–30 cm along from this is the cold saline injection port. At the proximal end there are several lumen hubs, to inject drugs, take blood samples and for inflating the balloon. There is also an electrical connection for the thermistor.

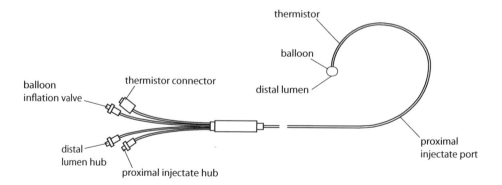

Figure 16.6. *A Swan–Ganz pulmonary artery catheter.*

The catheter is inserted into the jugular or mammary vein and advanced until the tip is in the pulmonary artery and left in this position for monitoring. To make a measurement of cardiac output, a bolus (single injection) of cold saline is injected and the dip in temperature (usually no more than 1–2°C) is recorded downstream with the temperature record corresponding to the dye curve (see Figure 16.7). No blood sampling is required and temperature is measured directly with the thermistor mounted downstream (distally) to the proximal injection port. The cold saline is dispersed in the systemic circulation and therefore there is no recirculation peak and the measurement can be repeated as often as required.

The temperature of the saline must be known. At the time of injection, a button is pressed on the cardiac output computer to indicate the time of injection. The cardiac output is automatically calculated, using the following equation:

$$\text{cardiac output} = \frac{\text{volume of cold saline injected} \times (T_{blood} - T_{injectate})}{T_{mean} \times \text{time interval}\,(t_2 - t_1)} \qquad \boxed{16.7}$$

where T_{mean} is the average temperature measured by the thermistor
T_{blood} is the blood temperature
$T_{injectate}$ is the injectate temperature
t_1 time at which the temperature drop is first observed
t_2 time when the temperature returns to near-normal

Continuous thermodilution method

A method for continuous cardiac output measurement is now widely used because no user intervention is required. The instrument continuously monitors the cardiac output and can display a trend graph and alert clinical staff if the value falls below a certain value. It works by heating the blood using a heating filament incorporated into the catheter, between two thermistors. The heating filament is

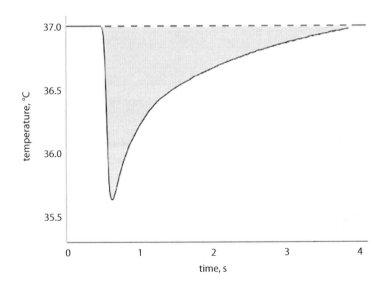

Figure 16.7. Thermodilution washout curve produced by injection of cold saline using a pulmonary artery catheter.

switched on and off by a random signal, so a series of mini washout curves is produced of varying length. The cardiac output monitor switches the heater on and off and uses an algorithm to calculate an equivalent theoretical washout curve from the measured temperature rise, by cross-correlating this value with the input signal. The cardiac output is calculated from the curve using Equation 16.7 as before.

16.4 Lithium chloride dilution

Pulmonary artery catheters are still considered the 'gold standard' for accuracy in the measurement of cardiac output. However, they are highly invasive and their use is decreasing because the benefit of high accuracy is often outweighed by the risk incurred to the patient. Lithium chloride dilution, which uses the same principle as for the dye dilution technique described earlier in the chapter, is now considered comparable in accuracy. An electrochemical lithium-ion detector is used in place of an optical dye detector. The injection point is the jugular vein and sampling point is the radial artery.

A small bolus of lithium chloride is injected via a central or peripheral venous line; the resulting arterial lithium concentration–time curve is recorded by withdrawing blood past a lithium sensor attached to the patient's existing arterial line. The dose of lithium marker needed is very small and has no known pharmacological effects.

Recent developments have enabled continuous measurement of cardiac output by analysing the patient's arterial blood pressure waveform. This measurement is calibrated every few hours by a lithium dilution. The accuracy of the waveform-derived continuous measurement has been shown to be comparable to thermodilution over a wide range of cardiac outputs and when cardiac output varies between calibrations.

16.5 Doppler velocity and flow measurement

Continuous-wave ultrasound Doppler velocity measurement

The Doppler effect may be exploited to estimate blood velocity, providing an indication of blood flow through a vessel. The simplest method in terms of equipment is to use an ultrasound source and measure the Doppler shift of the sound waves reflected from moving red blood cells. Ultrasound is defined as any sound wave with a frequency above the audible range (i.e. > 20 kHz). Continuous-wave ultrasound Doppler is used to insonate large arteries and veins, most commonly in limbs, to check the adequacy of blood flow in the vessel. A higher than normal velocity indicates that a vessel may be narrowed or partially occluded.

The principle of the Doppler effect is explained in *Section 5.7*. When using a stationary source and a moving target (the blood cells), the frequency is changed twice: the red cells 'see' a Doppler-shifted sound wave because they are moving relative to the transmitter. Reflection of the wave occurs so the cells can be thought of as tiny transmitters; a second Doppler shift occurs because they are moving relative to the receiver. If the detector and receiver are incorporated together into the probe, the Doppler shift may easily be calculated. The relative frequency shift Δf caused by a sound wave reflected from a blood cell moving directly towards (or away from) the transmitter/detector is given by the following:

$$\frac{\Delta f}{f} = \frac{2v}{v+c} \approx \frac{2v}{c}$$

16.8

where f is the sound wave frequency (Hz)
        v is the blood cell velocity
        c is the velocity of sound in the tissue (≈ 1500 m·s^{-1})

This agreement is valid because the speed of sound c is much greater than the blood velocity v. The velocities do not all act along the same straight line, so we add an angle factor

$$\frac{\Delta f}{f} = \frac{2 \cdot v \cdot \cos\theta}{c}$$

16.9

where θ is the angle between the beam of sound and the axis of the blood vessel, as shown in the diagram.

The most common implementation of Doppler velocity measurement is a 'pencil' probe connected to a small handheld monitor. *Figure 16.8* shows a Doppler velocimeter probe. The oscillator and detector are low impedance crystal transducers mounted in the tip of the probe. The probe is held against the skin and angled as shown, otherwise the sound would be emitted at right angles to the flow, and no Doppler shift would be seen. An impedance-matching gel ensures efficient transmission of sound between the probe and the tissue. The Doppler effect is insensitive to direction of flow so a positive velocity is recorded, regardless of whether the blood is moving towards or away from the sensor.

The ultrasound carrier frequency is in the ultrasonic range (i.e. several MHz) but the Doppler shifts are in the audio range (i.e. several hundred Hz). The difference between the carrier frequency and reflected frequency is produced as an audible tone that may be listened to using an audio speaker. The pitch of the sound heard is proportional to the blood cell velocity. If the probe is placed over an artery, the pulsatile flow produces a 'whooshing' sound. Some Doppler systems calculate and display the blood velocity and/or show a pulsatile waveform.

Pulsed-ultrasound Doppler

Continuous-wave flowmeters give an 'average' velocity measured in the vessel, but cannot record flow, because the diameter of the vessel must be known. In addition, flow characteristics affect the relationship between flow and velocity; for example, if laminar flow (*Section 8.2*) occurs the velocity profile varies across the diameter of the vessel. Pulsed-ultrasound Doppler flowmeters address these limitations by operating in a radar-like mode. These instruments are used most commonly in the oesophagus for insonating the aorta, producing an accurate estimation of

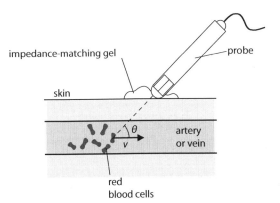

impedance-matching gel

probe

skin

θ

v

artery
or vein

red
blood cells

Figure 16.8. *Continuous-wave Doppler ultrasound probe.*

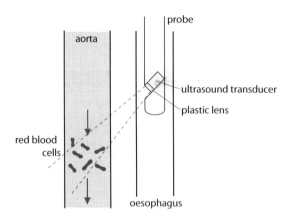

Figure 16.9. *A trans-oesophageal pulsed-ultrasound Doppler probe.*

cardiac output. A schematic diagram of a pulsed-ultrasound Doppler probe *in situ* is shown in *Figure 16.9.*

The transmitter is excited by a brief burst of electrical signal. The transmitted wave travels in a single packet, and the transmitter can also be used as a receiver, because reflections are received at a later time. The delay between transmission and reception is a direct indication of distance, so we can obtain a complete plot of reflections across the blood vessel. By examining the Doppler shift at various delays, the velocity profile across the vessel may be discerned.

To achieve a good range resolution, the transmitted pulse duration should ideally be very short, but to achieve a good velocity discrimination, the transmitted pulse duration should be long. A good compromise is an 8 MHz pulse of 1 microsecond duration, which produces a travelling sound wave 1.5 mm long. Trans-oesophageal pulsed-ultrasound Doppler is a non-invasive method of measuring cardiac output (CO) that is considerably less invasive and therefore potentially much less harmful to the patient than cardiac catheter placement. Continuous-wave and pulsed trans-oesophageal Doppler systems are available, but pulsed systems have become more popular due to their increased accuracy.

The magnitude of the Doppler shift is directly proportional to the velocity of the blood flow. Cardiac output (flow rate) can be calculated by multiplying this average blood velocity during an ejection cycle by the cross-sectional area through which the blood flows (the cross-sectional area of the descending aorta which is obtained from nomograms based on age, weight and height). A correction factor is required to transform the blood flow measured in the descending aorta to a reported cardiac output value. Doppler ultrasound cardiac output measurements are considerably less accurate than those from a cardiac catheter, but the lower risk outweighs the loss of accuracy in many patients, where changes in cardiac output measurement from baseline are usually sufficient for clinical purposes.

Laser Doppler flowmetry

Laser Doppler flowmetry (LDF) is a method for estimating blood flow in the microcirculation: that is the capillaries, arterioles and small venules lying close to the skin surface. This technique may also be used internally for assessing blood flow in the epithelial surface of the gut or the surface of other organs. It works by detecting visible light that has been scattered from the moving blood cells.

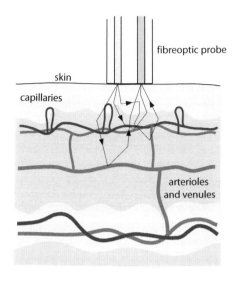

skin

capillaries

fibreoptic probe

arterioles
and venules

Figure 16.10. *Laser Doppler flowmetry probe.*

The He–Ne laser is the light source traditionally used in many LDF systems, although modern systems often use diode lasers. The wavelength of the He–Ne laser is 633 nm or 4.74×10^{14} Hz. LDF probes use optical fibres to transmit the laser light to and from the tissue (see *Figure 16.10*). Assuming a head-on interaction with a red blood cell travelling at 1.5 mm·s^{-1} (a typical value for a capillary), then from Equation 6.8, the fractional shift in light frequency would be only 4.7 kHz. This corresponds to a very small change in the wavelength of the light; however, if the frequency-shifted beam and a portion of unshifted light combine and interfere with each other, the resulting light is modulated at a frequency equal to the difference between the two wave frequencies. This signal (in the kHz range) is readily detected.

Like ultrasound Doppler, the laser Doppler system cannot discriminate between positive or negative frequency shifts (blood cells moving towards or away from the probe) because it only detects absolute differences in frequencies between incoming waves. Flow towards or away from the probe will therefore contribute equally to the signal. In fact, because light is diffusely scattered on entering the tissue, and because of the random orientation of blood vessels, the signal from LDF does not have any significant directional sensitivity. Equation 6.9 may then be rewritten for the average velocity, thereby ignoring any directional bias.

$$v \approx c \frac{\Delta f}{f}$$

16.10

Note: since light from all angles is detected, all angles must be included in the equation. Since the mean cosine for all angles is equal to 0.5, the factor of 2 disappears from the equation.

Laser Doppler flowmeters do not measure actual blood flow because red blood cells are needed to reflect (frequency shifted) light back to the probe. Instead they measure a quantity known as **flux**, which is defined as the product of the blood cell velocity and the **concentration of moving blood cells** (CMBC). The difference between flow and flux can be understood by imagining an attempt to compare blood flowing in a tube with flowing water. Flow is the rate of change of volume, whereas flux is the amount of red cells passing through a volume of tissue in a given time. Because pure water contains no particles, the flux would be zero, regardless of the flow rate.

Summary

- The washout curve of dye concentration in a tank against time with constant flow has the shape of an exponential decay curve.
- The human circulation requires a more sophisticated model incorporating circulatory flow.
- This circulatory flow model allows calculation of flow by extrapolation of the dye washout curve, to eliminate the effects of recirculating dye.
- Dye dilution using indocyanine green in conjunction with a cardiac catheter may be used to calculate cardiac output.
- Thermodilution, either by cold bolus injection or continuous heating using a filament, may also be used to measure cardiac output using a pulmonary artery catheter.
- Analysing the arterial pressure waveform allows continuous cardiac output monitoring. The flow measurement is calibrated by periodically injecting a lithium compound and calculating cardiac output from the washout curve.
- Continuous-wave ultrasound Doppler may be used for measuring blood velocity in large vessels.
- Trans-oesophageal pulsed-ultrasound Doppler allows non-invasive estimation of cardiac output; however, it is not as accurate as dilution methods using a cardiac catheter.
- Laser Doppler flowmetry provides an indication of microcirculatory blood flow.

Single best answer questions

For these questions, choose the single best answer.

1. Which one of the following statements is true of the thermodilution method for measuring cardiac output?
   (a) The recirculation peak must be eliminated by extrapolating the washout curve.
   (b) A temperature rise of 5 degrees is typically measured.
   (c) The measurement can be repeated as many times as needed.
   (d) Knowledge of either temperature or volume of the injectate is needed.
   (e) The exact moment of injection must be recorded.

2. Which one of the following statements is true of ultrasound Doppler?
   (a) Continuous-wave Doppler measures blood flow and velocity.
   (b) Continuous-wave Doppler measures direction of flow.

   (c) Continuous-wave Doppler uses sound waves from 10 to 20 kHz.
   (d) Ultrasound Doppler is unsuitable for assessment of microcirculatory flow.
   (e) Pulsed-ultrasound Doppler does not require knowledge of the aortic diameter to measure flow.

3. Pulmonary artery catheters:
   (a) have a balloon at the distal end which is inflated with saline
   (b) incorporate a thermistor proximal to both injection ports
   (c) measure pulmonary artery pressures and cardiac output
   (d) produce less accurate cardiac output measurement than lithium dilution methods
   (e) cannot be used with dye

Multiple choice questions

For each of these questions, mark every answer either true or false.

1. When dye is washed from a tank at a constant flow rate, the rate of dye removal is
   (a) proportional to flow out
   (b) proportional to the volume of water in the tank
   (c) proportional to the amount of dye in the tank
   (d) constant
   (e) inversely proportional to the volume of water in the tank

2. Regarding the circulatory model of flow, which of the following statements are true of the secondary peak appearing in the washout curve?
   (a) It is caused by dye flowing in the opposite direction to the main flow.
   (b) It is caused by recirculation of dye.
   (c) It does not affect the measurement of cardiac output.

   (d) It does not occur at very slow flow rates.
   (e) It may be eliminated by extrapolating the washout curve.

3. Which of these statements are true of laser Doppler flowmeters?
   (a) They measure blood flux which is equal to the velocity multiplied by the vessel density.
   (b) They require an impedance-matching gel to work most effectively.
   (c) The Doppler shift is directly proportional to the blood velocity.
   (d) They can cause heating of the tissue, so must be used with caution.
   (e) Use light with frequencies in the 10^{14} Hz range.

Chapter 17
Equipment management

Having read this chapter you will be able to:
- Understand safety-critical systems and no single point of failure.
- Appreciate the need for good equipment management practice.
- Understand the importance of safety when using critical medical equipment.
- Appreciate how safety principles in design can reduce the risk of serious incidents.
- Distinguish between cleaning, low and high disinfectant, and sterilization.

17.1 Equipment management principles

Several decades ago, new equipment was often developed by anaesthetists and tested in an *ad hoc* fashion in the anaesthetic room or operating theatre. This led to the routine use of a variety of homespun anaesthetic apparatus, some of which were successful; several familiar pieces of equipment came into being in just such a way, such as breathing systems. In today's more litigious society where we are much more constrained by protocol, this behaviour is not condoned and the vast majority of innovation is carried out in industrial R&D departments.

As medicine continues to progress, we are becoming more and more equipment-orientated, not just in anaesthesia but also in other specialities and allied fields. As such, it now makes considerably more sense for large hospitals to tender contracts to companies to supply a specific type of equipment, for example a syringe driver. This means that, at least in principle, the use of **standardized equipment** means that the process of training staff and equipment maintenance is greatly simplified, with inherent safety and cost benefits.

Many hospitals have local rules regarding equipment management but they must also adhere to national or international protocols. There are also general principles of good equipment practice that should be strictly adhered to, ensuring safe and reliable use of equipment over its entire life cycle.

Preventative maintenance

Equipment needs to be **serviced** at fixed intervals by the hospital clinical engineering department or, in the case of more complex or critical equipment, by the equipment manufacturer. Records of servicing should be kept and the equipment marked with an identification number. Equipment needing a service should be withdrawn from use until servicing is completed. Failure to regularly service equipment heightens the risks of equipment malfunctioning and could cause harm to patients and staff.

Electrical testing

In addition to regular servicing, the clinical engineering department should regularly check all electrical equipment in a hospital, including appliances used in non-clinical departments (e.g. a kettle in a staff room).

Calibration

Certain equipment may need to be calibrated regularly. In many cases it might be sufficient for this to be carried out during normal servicing. Some devices need more frequent calibration, however, and it may be the responsibility of the clinical staff to calibrate the equipment daily, or prior to each use. This is discussed later in the chapter.

Logging and repairs of faults

A system should be in a place to log faults with equipment, so that the circumstances giving rise to a fault are properly communicated to the clinical engineer. Faulty equipment should be removed from service immediately and the fault reported to the clinical engineering department, using the appropriate form to record all the relevant details. Equipment may need to be disposed of or returned to the manufacturer. Equipment may not be used again until it has been repaired and checked by the clinical engineers.

Appropriate use

The manner in which a device should be used should be stated in a **protocol**. This should include who can use the device, and when and how it should be used.

Training, assessment and frequency

Those using a device must be competent, so training is needed. Relevant staff should be taught and then assessed by a competent trainer on how to correctly use a piece of equipment. There must be proof that training has been given. Records should be kept of who has been trained and regular updates to training should be given as appropriate.

Security: access and data integrity

An assessment needs to be made of each device as to how the data it might generate are managed and the security that is in place to secure that data. Patient confidentiality should be strictly adhered to.

Equipment alerts and product recalls

There must be a system in place to receive and act upon notification from manufacturers and relevant organizations such as the MHRA (Medicines and Healthcare Devices Regulatory Authority) and MIMS (Monthly Index of Medical Specialties). These communications can alert clinicians and clinical engineers of potential problems with devices and also of product withdrawals.

Procurement

The process of purchasing clinical equipment is now well structured. Ideally a list of desired specifications should be drawn up and the manufacturers asked to submit equipment for consideration. A shortlist from this should then lead to trials with specified qualities and means of measuring these desired qualities. This should include the frequency and nature of maintenance, calibration and servicing, the cost relative to performance, life span, ongoing running costs and linked disposables and the availability of spare parts, replacement kit and disposables. The aim of the procurement is the best clinical device coupled with the best financial deal for the institution.

Disposal

Equipment that exceeds its design lifetime should be permanently withdrawn from clinical use. Equipment should be disposed of in a responsible way, paying attention to local environmental and decontamination regulations. Some equipment may be recyclable, or re-usable in other countries.

17.2 Safety critical systems

What happens when a pressure sensor on an infusion pump fails? Does the device continue to infuse anaesthetic, causing a potential extravasation injury? Or should the device stop the infusion, thereby putting the patient at risk of awareness if the anaesthetist is not paying attention? Critical systems are those where failure can result in death or harm. Most devices found in hospitals fall into this category, particularly in anaesthesia and intensive care. When designing these systems it is important to engineer fail-safe modes in case of complex-system malfunction as well as systems to minimize the possibility of catastrophic device failure.

Single point of failure is a good example of an engineering principle used in the design of medical devices. To illustrate this concept, consider the oxygen supply to the hospital, which is generally derived from a vacuum-insulated evaporator (VIE). If the scales measuring the amount of oxygen remaining were to fail, causing an empty tank to go unnoticed, the hospital's oxygen supply would be compromised and patients put in mortal danger. This single point of failure can be addressed in multiple ways. First, two independent devices could be installed to monitor the quantity of oxygen remaining in the VIE. This is a system of **multiple redundancy** that safeguards a critical system. However, the VIE itself represents a single point of failure. Most hospitals get around this by maintaining a separate oxygen cylinder manifold at a different physical location.

A system of multiple redundancies to combat a single point of failure is commonly encountered in both anaesthesia and aviation. There should always be two laryngoscopes on the airway trolley just as an aeroplane will not take off without two pilots. Failure in certain medical equipment has far-reaching consequences, possibly resulting in serious injury or even death. This presents engineering challenges to provide fail-safe design solutions for critical medical equipment.

Clinical considerations

When designing or even simply using a piece of medical equipment, it is worth considering the following points.

- What is the result of failure of the equipment?
- If it does fail, can it fail in such a way as to cause minimum morbidity?
- How reliable is it? Consider the functionality and quality of materials, manufacturing and disposables.
- What are the margins of safety?

Examples of non-medical safety-critical systems include aircraft, cars, lifts and traffic lights. Failure of these devices can cause injury or death, so engineering principles such as multiple redundancy are employed in their design. Medical safety-critical systems include defibrillators, infusion pumps, anaesthetic machines, heart valves and ventilators.

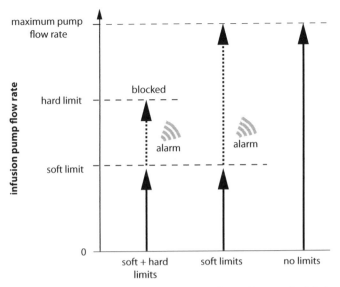

Figure 17.1. *Infusion pumps: restrictions imposed for hard limits and soft limits.*

Clinical example

Infusion pump limits
Infusion pumps in clinical practice attempt to reduce risk by implementing software that guides and can also restrict user choice. An example is shown schematically in *Figure 17.1*. **Hard limits** restrict the maximum flow rate, and this value depends on data in a drug library that have been programmed into the device. A **soft limit** allows the user to override the maximum flow rate, but only after the user overrides a warning alarm.

17.3 Calibration

Precision and accuracy

Although accuracy and precision are often used interchangeably in clinical measurement, they have separate definitions. Repeated measurements are needed to assess accuracy and precision. If the mean value of repeated measurements is close to the 'true' value, i.e. a known value or one determined using a reference method, then the measurement is said to be accurate. The measurement is

Definitions

Precision: an indication of the level of random error.
Accuracy: an indication of the level of systematic error.

accurate even if there is a large spread or deviation in the measurements. Repeated measurements with high precision have much smaller deviation from one another, although the mean may differ considerably from the true value. The difference between accuracy and precision may be summed up by considering the 'target analogy' illustrated in *Figure 17.2*. An archer shooting arrows at a target may miss the centre of the target each time (poor accuracy) although the arrows are grouped together tightly (high precision).

Calibration of any measurement system is essential to ensure accurate and precise reporting of the measured variable. In some cases it is only necessary to calibrate an instrument once at the time of manufacture. This only applies to certain measurements, or certain types of sensor that are not affected by physical changes occurring over their useful lifetime, such as pulse oximeter probes or disposable pressure transducers.

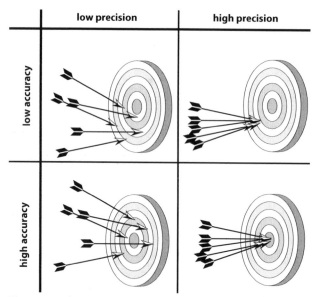

Figure 17.2. *The target analogy for accuracy and precision. An archer would aim to be to both precise and accurate.*

It is much more common for characteristics of the sensor to change over time. Calibration makes changes to the measurement system to adjust for variations in sensitivity (**sensitivity drift**) and also to eliminate other changes in output such as **zero drift**. Usually a measurement is made of a known value; for example, a gas sensor could be calibrated by measuring the concentration of carbon dioxide in a gas mixture containing exactly 5% CO_2.

Most measurement equipment can be put into a calibration mode, so once the calibration measurement has been made, it adjusts its signal processing to take the calibration into account when measuring unknown quantities.

Sensitivity drift

Sensitivity drift causes an error that is proportional to the magnitude of the input. An example cause of sensitivity drift would be a change in supply voltage to a bridge circuit containing a thermistor. Sensitivity drift causes a reduction in accuracy and precision over a measurement range.

Zero drift

This is defined as a constant change in output, independent of input and constant for all input values. Zero-drift can occur, for example, if a photodetector detects ambient light. Zero drift causes a reduction in accuracy only. Often both zero drift and sensitivity drift occur simultaneously.

17.4 Cleaning and disinfection

Spaulding classification

In 1939 Dr Earl Spaulding of Philadelphia put forward a framework for classifying equipment to aid decontamination decisions and he went on to refine his criteria, which are still used by the FDA

Table 17.1. Cleaning and disinfection requirements for Spaulding's classification of reusable equipment.

Spaulding classification	Body contact	Minimum decontamination requirements	Might also need
Non-critical	Intact skin	Cleaning	Low-level disinfectant
Semi-critical	Mucous membrane	Cleaning then high-level disinfectant	Sterilization
Critical	Sterile body cavity	Cleaning then sterilization	- - -

today. Equipment and devices are divided into three categories: non-critical, semi-critical and critical (summarized in *Table 17.1*).

Spaulding's non-critical category

These are items that come in contact with the skin but not mucous membranes. Sterility is not essential because the skin acts as a competent barrier to most microorganisms. This category can be subdivided into patient care items and environmental surfaces. Non-critical patient-care items include blood pressure cuffs, walking aids and patient-controlled analgesia pumps. Non-critical environmental surfaces include bed rails, floors and equipment housing. These can act as a link in the chain of secondary transmission. This category requires cleaning and in some cases use of a low-level disinfectant.

Spaulding's semi-critical category

Semi-critical items contact mucus and this category includes endoscopes. They require a high-level disinfectant as well as cleaning.

Spaulding's critical category

Critical items carry a high risk if they are contaminated with any microorganism and are likely to transmit infection. This category includes objects that would pierce the skin or enter cavities such as surgical instruments or implants. These items require cleaning followed by sterilization between uses.

> **Definitions**
>
> **Cleaning:** the removal of all foreign material.
> **Disinfection:** the process of destroying pathogenic organisms.

Cleaning usually involves water, detergents and mechanical action. It can be mechanized using a medical washing machine, or placed in an ultrasonic bath. Manual cleaning is reserved for delicate instruments or when mechanized cleaning is not available.

Disinfection kills most microorganisms but not all. There are two categories:

- Low-level disinfection – this kills vegetative bacteria apart from TB and endospores, and it also kills some fungi and some viruses. Common low-level disinfectants include chlorhexidine, alcohol (70%) and sodium hypochlorite.
- High-level disinfection – this kills vegetative bacteria but not all endospores, and it also kills fungi and viruses. Note that if the exposure time is long enough this can produce sterilization. Common examples are glutaraldehyde and peroxyacetic acid.

17.5 Sterilization

> **Definition**
>
> **Sterilization:** the process of destruction of all forms of microbial life including bacteria, viruses, spores and fungi.

Sterilization occurs when all microorganisms are destroyed and there are a number of ways of doing this. Boiling and exposure to flames are not considered sterilization processes because they fail to kill all microorganisms.

Dry heat (hot air oven)

The dry heat oven reaches temperatures between 140 and 180°C for up to 3 hours. This technique can be used for powders, oils and glass, and avoids accelerating rusting and corrosion, although it is lengthy and the heat can damage some equipment.

Pressure steam sterilization (autoclaving)

An autoclave uses boiling water in a closed system at a pressure of approximately 35 psi (241 kPa) to produce steam at a temperature of approximately 137°C. This method is a highly effective, cheap and non-toxic method, but it cannot sterilize powders, ointments, oils, or equipment that is heat or moisture sensitive.

Gas (ethylene oxide or hydrogen peroxide gas plasma)

Sterilization by exposure to ethylene oxide (ETO) at 50–60°C is commonly used in industry. It is, however, very toxic and highly explosive so de-gassing must occur post-sterilization to allow the ETO to dissipate. It can be used on rubbers and plastics without damaging them, but it can take days for the process to complete.

Gamma irradiation

Gamma rays are commonly used for sterilization of disposable medical equipment, such as syringes, needles and IV sets. Gamma radiation does not cause irradiated materials to become radioactive, but requires heavy shielding for the safety of the operators. Irradiation also requires storage of a radioisotope (usually Cobalt-60), which continuously emits gamma rays and cannot be switched off.

Clinical example

Prions
Prions are small proteins and they are responsible for transmissible spongiform encephalopathies. Variant CJD (vCJD) is one such disease in this group that has raised particular concerns. The highest concentrations of prions occur in the brain, spinal cord, and posterior eye and it is for this reason that particular attention is given to reusable instruments that have been in contact with these tissues. Post-mortem results from patients who have died from vCJD have shown prion levels to be particularly high in the tonsils, appendix, spleen and gastrointestinal lymph nodes. Prions are resistant to most sterilization processes and their small size allows them to lodge in pits on stainless steel surfaces. However, a large cross-sectional study of 63 007 anonymous tonsil specimens failed to detect any samples containing prions from vCJD, suggesting the population incidence is exceedingly low.

Disposable and reusable devices

The central tenet of infection control is to assume that all patients are an infection risk and so universal precautions should be implemented for all. The aim is to avoid unprotected exposure to blood, other body fluids, non-intact skin and mucous membranes, either between staff and patients or patient to patient. With this has grown an emphasis on single-use (disposable) equipment. Some high-cost equipment such as fibreoptic endoscopes or specialist surgical instruments cannot be single-use and so must be reused; considerable attention must be given to the reprocessing of these reusable devices. All such devices and equipment should have a date as to when it was cleaned, disinfected or sterilized. There also should be an expiry date to indicate for how long sterilization is valid.

Summary

- Good equipment management practice is essential for safe use of critical medical equipment.
- Equipment management includes adherence to protocols covering preventative maintenance, electrical testing, fault reporting, training, procurement and disposal.
- Safety-critical equipment should have no single point of failure, so if a fault develops the equipment defaults to a safe setting.
- Calibration is essential to maintain the accuracy and precision of equipment: manufacturer guidelines and local protocol should dictate how often to calibrate.
- Cleaning, disinfectant use and sterilization offer progressively more aggressive levels of preparation for equipment. The Spaulding classification categorizes the risk.
- Sterilization of medical equipment can be performed by several methods, such as autoclaving, ethylene oxide sterilization or gamma irradiation.

Single best answer questions

For these questions, choose the single best answer.

1. Which one of the following statements is true?
   (a) Precise measurements show small deviation from the mean.
   (b) Accuracy is improved by reducing deviation between measurements.
   (c) Zero drift causes a reduction in precision.
   (d) Sensitivity drift causes a reduction in accuracy and precision.
   (e) Calibration produces improvement in accuracy but not precision.

2. Which one of the following statements is true?
   (a) An oesophageal ultrasound probe falls into Spaulding's semi-critical category.
   (b) Semi-critical items always require high-level disinfection.
   (c) High-level disinfectants include chlorhexidine and glutaraldehyde.
   (d) Semi-critical items never require sterilization.
   (e) High-level disinfection kills all bacteria and viruses.

Multiple choice questions

For each of these questions, mark every answer either true or false.

1. Regarding sterilization, which of the following statements are true?
   (a) Ethylene oxide is the fastest method of sterilization.
   (b) Autoclave sterilization typically takes place at 137°C.
   (c) Surgical equipment may be sterilized by boiling in water for 2 hours.
   (d) Gamma irradiation is unsuitable for disposable equipment.
   (e) Gamma irradiation does not make irradiated items radioactive.

2. Which of the following statements are false?
   (a) The use of multiple redundancy always eliminates single point of failure in a device.
   (b) Single point of failure increases the risk of critical incidents.
   (c) Footbrakes and handbrakes in cars are an example of multiple redundancy.
   (d) A flashing light and an audible alarm on a patient monitor is an example of multiple redundancy.
   (e) A device powered by two 1.5 V batteries contains an example of multiple redundancy.

Chapter 18
Basics of electricity

Having read this chapter you will be able to:
- Know the relationship between electric current, voltage and electrical resistance.
- Understand how current flows around a circuit.
- Appreciate the theory and application of the Wheatstone bridge.
- Be familiar with direct current (DC) and alternating current (AC).

18.1 Electric current

The earliest record of electricity was when the ancient Egyptians observed that certain Nile fish had the ability to shock unsuspecting waders. The Greeks noted that rods of amber rubbed against some materials could then be used to attract other substances (static electricity). The Greek word for amber (*elektron*) was used in the seventeenth century to coin the term electricity.

Electric current is defined as the flow of an electric charge. Charge is one of the fundamental properties of matter. Protons in the nucleus of atoms are positively charged, while negatively charged electrons surround the nucleus, forming a cloud of

> **Definition**
>
> **Electric current:** the flow of an electric charge.

negative charge. The movement of electrons is responsible for current flow though metals and most other conductors. Current can also arise from flow of other charged particles such as ions. Ions can be either positively or negatively charged and are referred to as electrolytes when in solution.

Water flowing from a pipe at the foot of a dam is immediately visible and the flow can be estimated at a glance. The pressure in this pipe depends on the height of the dam: the higher it is, the greater the pressure, the force of the flow and the amount of energy it delivers. For any given driving pressure, the volume of water moving through the pipe will also depend on the resistance it offers: the shorter and wider the pipe, the greater the flow, according to the Hagen–Poiseuille law (Equation 8.4).

The flow of electric charge in a wire is analogous to the flow of a liquid. Each electron carries a tiny negative electric charge, equal to 1.602×10^{-19} coulomb (C). Metals conduct electricity because they contain a 'sea' of electrons that are not bound to a particular atomic nucleus. The electrons are instead free to move throughout the material. Current cannot flow freely, however, because it is restricted by an **electrical resistance**. The resistance of a wire increases with length and decreases as cross-sectional area is reduced. Different metals also conduct electricity with varying ease, and tend to conduct better at lower temperatures.

Electrical current (symbol I or i) is measured in amperes, with 1 ampere defined as 1 coulomb of charge passing a fixed point in 1 second. When current flows from a battery, electrons flow from the negative (−ve) terminal to the positive (+ve) terminal but, by convention, we assume that the current is flowing from the positive to the negative terminal. Circuit diagrams often contain an arrow marked with the symbol I to indicate the direction of the current flow. However, this arrow indicates the direction of conventional current flow, from positive to negative, which is opposite to

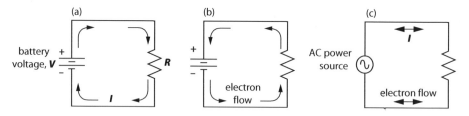

Figure 18.1. *Conventional current flow is in the opposite direction to the flow of electrons, because electrons are negatively charged. (a) Direct current showing conventional current flow I; (b) direct current showing electron flow; (c) alternating current where current and electrons flow in both directions.*

the direction of the flow of electrons (see *Figure 18.1*). The reason for this ambiguity is that when electricity was discovered, it was not known that electrons were the main charge carriers. When J. J. Thompson eventually discovered electrons in 1888 they were found to be electrically negative, by which time the convention had been established.

The current flowing from a power supply may always flow in the same direction, such as in the case of a battery (DC or direct current), or the direction of the current may change periodically, as in the case of the mains electricity supply (AC or alternating current).

18.2 Electric potential

Definition
Voltage: an informal term for electrical potential difference. The potential difference between two points in a circuit is the amount of energy required to move a unit charge between the two points.

Voltage, **potential difference**, or **electromotive force** can be thought of as the pressure or force that pushes charges, normally electrons, through a conductor. Put simply, the greater the voltage, the greater its ability to push the electrons through a circuit. The difference in voltage between any two nodes (or points) in a circuit is known as the potential difference, measured in volts (V).

The definition of a volt is as follows: if a unit charge (1 coulomb) were to move through a potential difference of 1 volt, it would require 1 joule of energy. Alternatively, 1 volt may also be defined as the electrical potential required to drive an electrical current of 1 ampere through a resistance of 1 ohm (see below). Voltages are generally expressed in volts with prefixes used to denote sub-multiples of the voltage, such as

Table 18.1. *A comparison of voltages.*

Example	Typical voltage
EEG	50 μV
ECG	1 mV
Peripheral nerve stimulator	9 V
Car battery	12 V
Mains electricity	240 V
External defibrillator	3–5 kV
Diathermy	200 V–10 kV
Power lines	250–400 kV

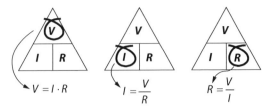

Figure 18.2. *Ohm's law pyramid.*

microvolts ($1\ \mu V = 1 \times 10^{-6}\ V$), millivolts ($1\ mV = 1 \times 10^{-3}\ V$) or kilovolts ($1\ kV = 1 \times 10^{3}\ V$). Voltage can be expressed as either positive or negative, to denote the direction of current flow.

AC voltage sources are supplied to both domestic homes and industry. The domestic mains voltage supply in the UK is 230–240 V AC but is just 110–120 V AC in the USA. Many small electronic devices operate on a low DC voltage of between 1.5 and 24 V, which is supplied by batteries or mains transformers (*Chapter 19*). *Table 18.1* shows some typical voltages of well-known electrical phenomena.

18.3 Electrical resistance

Any material in which current flows will have a **resistance** (except certain materials at very low temperatures known as superconductors). The smaller the resistance, the larger the current for any given potential difference. Ohm's law is crucial to understanding electricity because it defines the relationship between voltage, current and resistance:

> **Definition**
>
> **Ohm's law:** the potential difference between two points is the product of the resistance and the current flowing.

$$I = \frac{V}{R}$$

18.1 **Learn**

where I is the current (A)
             V is the potential difference (V)
             R is the resistance (Ω)

It is important to keep units consistent: if the voltage is measured in volts (V) and the resistance in ohms (Ω), the current will be given in amperes (A). By knowing any two of the values for the voltage, current or resistance, the third missing value can be calculated, as illustrated by the Ohm's law 'pyramid' in *Figure 18.2*.

Worked example

Question
Calculate the current flowing through a 240 Ω resistor connected to a 6 V power supply.

Calculation
Use Ohm's law:

$$I = \frac{V}{R}$$

$$I = \frac{6\ V}{240\ \Omega} = 0.025\ A = 25\ mA$$

Answer
25 mA of current flows through the resistor.

Insulators and conductors

In everyday life we need to be aware of the conductivity of different materials: for example, metals are conductors, so trying to remove bread from a toaster using a fork is highly inadvisable. Solutions containing electrically charged atoms (ions) are also able to conduct electricity, which is why it is also inadvisable to immerse electrical appliances into salt water, such as a hair dryer in a bath (bath water contains many electrolytes). Incidentally, plasma (ionized gas) also conducts electricity, a phenomenon that enables fluorescent lights and energy-saving bulbs to function.

Materials are divided into conductors, semiconductors and insulators, based on their electrical resistance (see *Table 18.2* for examples). The fundamental difference between a conductor and an insulator is the freedom with which charge carriers can move. In metals such as copper (a good conductor), a large number of electrons are relatively unbound to a specific nucleus, forming a 'sea' of charge carriers. In an insulator, by contrast, the electrons are tightly bound so are not able to participate in conduction.

Most of the body can be considered a good conductor because the body largely comprises water containing dissolved ions and so acts as a very capable conductor of current. Skin, however, particularly when dry, acts as a significant resistance to the flow of electricity and so provides some protection from electric shock injury.

Semiconductors

A semiconductor is a material whose resistance is half-way between that of a good conductor and a good insulator. The majority of semiconductors are made from silicon which, much like carbon, is able to form a strong covalently bonded crystalline structure. The 'valence' electrons that form the bonds between adjacent atoms are tightly bound. In this configuration, all of silicon's four outermost electrons are tightly bound to neighbouring silicon atoms. At higher temperatures thermal motion can free some electrons from the lattice, allowing some conduction, but at room temperature pure silicon is an effective insulator.

Table 18.2. *Examples of insulators and conductors.*

Insulators	Conductors
Wood	Metals
Plastic	Saline
Ceramics	Soft tissue
Latex gloves	Blood
Rubber boots	Nerve fibres
Wheels on a hospital bed	ECG electrodes
Insulation on pacing leads	Inner core of pacing leads

In order to make a semiconductor, silicon (Group IV in the periodic table) is 'doped' with small quantities of impurities. These impurities are typically elements such as phosphorus (Group III) or boron (Group V) that have either three or five electrons in their outer shells. These impurities now create either a surplus of electrons, or 'holes' in the crystal lattice. The free electrons can move along the lattice, while the holes can be filled with electrons from an adjacent atom. Either way, electrons can move from atom to atom in the lattice and hence take part in conduction.

The valence electrons and the conduction electrons can be thought of as existing in two separate energy bands, with the valence electrons at a low energy and the conduction electrons at high energy. By absorbing energy, electrons in the valence band can jump up to the conduction band where they are free to move. In a pure (**intrinsic**) semiconductor, the energy bands are far apart, while in a doped semiconductor there are many more conduction bands at lower energies. Electrons can therefore free themselves from the lattice much more readily, allowing conduction through the material.

When different types of semiconductors are sandwiched next to each other they exhibit some very interesting properties. A **diode**, for example, is a device that will only allow current to pass in one direction, while a **transistor** acts as a tiny switch, allowing a small current to control a larger current, forming the basis of an amplifier. These components form the building blocks of electronic circuits and can be miniaturized into so-called **integrated** circuits ('microchips'). Modern electronic devices such as personal computers, patient monitoring systems and smart phones contain **microprocessors**, complicated integrated circuits containing millions, or even billions, of transistors.

Resistance variation with temperature

The resistance of many materials changes with temperature; the resistance of conductors such as metal wire generally increases with increasing temperature. This is because the vibrating atoms in the metal impede the flow of electrons. These materials are said to have a positive **temperature coefficient of resistance**. Semiconducting materials usually exhibit a drop in resistance with increased temperature, i.e. a negative temperature coefficient; in these materials increased thermal energy allows more electrons to jump up from the valence band to the conduction band. Thermistors are made from semiconducting materials and are used for temperature measurement. These devices can have a positive or negative temperature coefficient of resistance, depending upon which material they are made from. Further details on thermistors can be found in *Chapter 4*.

18.4 Rules of electrical circuits

Current in a circuit

When trying to visualize the current flowing around a circuit it must be remembered that the current is actually flow of charge (a quantity). A current obeys **Kirchhoff's first law** (the 'current' law) which simply states that at any junction (or 'node') in a circuit, the sum of currents entering and leaving the node is always zero (see *Figure 18.3*). This is expressed as:

| **Definition** |
| Kirchhoff's laws: firstly, for a junction in a circuit, current going in is equal to current going out; secondly, the sum of the electrical voltages around a closed circuit is zero. |

$$I_1 + I_2 + I_3 + I_4 + I_5 = 0$$ (18.2)

Note that in *Figure 18.3*, I_4 and I_5 have opposite signs to the other currents.

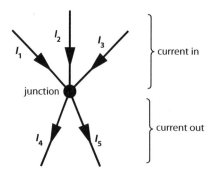

current in

current out

Figure 18.3. *At any junction the current in must equal the current out (Kirchhoff's first law).*

Voltage in a circuit

When we think of current flowing through resistors, the voltage is seen to 'drop' across the resistor (i.e. the voltage is higher on one side of the resistor compared to the other). When there is more than one resistance, there is a larger resistance and consequently a larger voltage drop (in a wire there is only a very small voltage drop because the wire's resistance is very low).

Kirchhoff's second law (the 'voltage' law) states that in any closed loop network (*Figure 18.4*), the total voltage around the loop is equal to the sum of all the voltage drops within the same loop, which is also equal to zero. That is:

$$V_{AB} + V_{BC} + V_{CD} + V_{DA} = 0 \text{ V}$$

18.3

In this example a battery between D and A produces a voltage gain, so all the voltages add up to zero, as demanded by the voltage law.

18.5 Electrical power and energy

Power in electrical circuits

A major advantage in using electrical energy is that it can readily be converted into other forms of energy such as light (light bulb), heat (heating element) or motion (motor). The rate of dissipation of electrical energy is called power. Power is measured in watts, where 1 watt is 1 joule of energy transferred per second, that is:

$$\text{power} = \frac{\text{energy transferred}}{\text{time}}$$

18.4

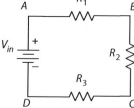

Figure 18.4. *The algebraic sum of all voltages within any closed circuit loop must be equal to zero (Kirchhoff's second law).*

Power transfer in simple circuits is easy to calculate. If a resistor has a voltage V across it and a current I flowing through it, then it will consume power, heating up in the process. The power dissipated (P) is simply the voltage multiplied by the current:

$$P\,(\text{watts}) = V\,(\text{volts}) \times I\,(\text{amps})$$

18.5 Learn

By using Ohm's law and substituting for V, I and R, the formula for electrical power can be found as:

$$P = \frac{V^2}{R}, \text{or}$$

18.6

$$P = I^2 R$$

18.7

Energy in electrical circuits

Electrical energy converted to other forms in an electrical circuit is the product of the electrical power and time (rearranging Equation 18.4):

$$\text{energy} = \text{power} \times \text{time}$$

18.8

Energy is measured in watts and the time in seconds, with the unit of energy given in joules.

For example, a 60 W light bulb connected for 1 hour will consume a total of 60 watts $\times$ 3600 sec = 126 000 J. Prefixes such as kilojoules (kJ = 10^3 J) or megajoules (MJ = 10^6 J) are often used. A **unit of electricity** as shown on your household electricity bill is equal to one kilowatt hour; a 1 kW heater running for exactly one hour would consume one unit.

18.6 Resistor combinations

Resistors in series

In *Figure 18.4* the resistors are connected together in series; therefore the same current passes through each resistor. The total resistance, R_T of the circuit is equal to the sum of all the individual resistors added together:

$$R_T = R_1 + R_2 + R_3$$

18.9

This total resistance is sometimes referred to as the **equivalent resistance**. Remember that when resistors are placed in series, the total resistance (R_T) will always be greater than the value of the largest resistor.

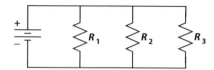

Figure 18.5. *Resistors in parallel.*

Resistors in parallel

Figure 18.5 shows resistors connected in parallel. The equivalent circuit resistance R_T is calculated using the equation:

$$\frac{1}{R_T} = \frac{1}{R_1} + \frac{1}{R_2} + \frac{1}{R_3} + \dots + \frac{1}{R_n}$$

18.10

Here, the reciprocal values of the individual resistances are all added together. Remember that when resistors are placed in parallel, the total resistance (R_T) will always be smaller than the value of the smallest resistor.

Potential divider

Suppose a smaller voltage is required than that of the voltage supplied. One way to reduce the voltage is to use a **potential divider**, a set-up commonly used in electrical circuits. The basic circuit for a potential divider (also known as a voltage divider) is shown in *Figure 18.6*: the circuit is essentially two resistors in series with a voltage output V_{out} 'tapped' between the two resistors.

While the output from a theoretical potential divider can be calculated, in reality the situation is a little different. As soon as any load, R_L (e.g. another resistor or even a measuring device such as a voltmeter) is connected at point B, some current flows through this load and the voltage across R_2 falls. Provided that R_L is of much higher resistance than R_2, then the error is small. Unfortunately, this is not the case when trying to measure biological potentials. Imagine, for example, trying to measure the voltages between nodes of Ranvier. It easy to see consecutive nodes as forming a series of resistors like in the potential divider circuit. Because the currents flowing along the nerves are tiny, as soon as we connect a meter, it will draw some current and give an inaccurate reading. Technical improvement in the meters can help, so that they draw ever less current, but there is a much better solution: the **Wheatstone bridge**.

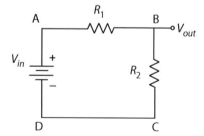

Figure 18.6. *A potential divider circuit.*

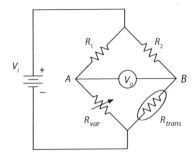

Figure 18.7. *Wheatstone bridge circuit: balancing the variable resistor (R$_{var}$) so that the voltage across A and B is zero allows R$_{trans}$ to be calculated.*

18.7 Measuring small physiological changes: the Wheatstone bridge

Clinical measurement involves the accurate recording of biological quantities, many of which are extremely small. It is usually convenient to convert a physical quantity, usually a form of energy, into an electrical quantity such as a voltage because modern monitoring systems are usually electronics-based. A transducer achieves this process of conversion. An example in anaesthesia is a blood pressure transducer, a type of strain gauge

> **Definition**
>
> **Wheatstone bridge:** a device for measuring small changes in electrical resistance; it consists of four resistors and a power supply and is a key component of many clinical instruments.

(*Section 6.8*) that is constructed from a material that changes its electrical resistance in response to pressure. This change in resistance is very small and so an extremely sensitive circuit is needed to convert this small resistance change into an electrical voltage signal. A circuit known as a Wheatstone bridge fits this requirement exactly. The output of the Wheatstone bridge circuit is then processed by the monitoring system and displayed in units of blood pressure.

The Wheatstone bridge is named after its inventor Charles Wheatstone and allows a component in a circuit with unknown resistance to be measured easily. *Figure 18.7* shows a Wheatstone bridge with an applied DC voltage of V_I. The bridge consists of two fixed resistors R_1 and R_2, a transducer R_{trans} and a variable resistor (or potentiometer) R_{var}. The bridge circuit is essentially two potential dividers in parallel, with their outputs compared by a voltmeter, which reads the difference in output from each divider, i.e. the difference between the voltages at A and B (V_A and V_B, respectively).

The resistance of the potentiometer R_{var} is adjusted until the voltmeter output (V_O) is zero. This happens when the output from each potential divider is equal; the voltmeter shows a zero potential difference, the bridge is said to be 'balanced', and no current flows between A and B so:

$$\frac{R_{trans}}{R_2} = \frac{R_{var}}{R_1}$$

18.11

This allows R_{trans} to be measured without disturbing the current flow through R_2 and R_{trans}, solving the problem described above.

Summary

- An electric current is the flow of charge which is driven by a potential difference: a difference in voltage between two points.
- Potential difference is the product of current and the resistance, as stated by Ohm's law: current is measured in amperes, potential difference in volts and resistance in ohms.
- Semiconductors have an electrical conductivity between that of insulators and conductors.
- Silicon is doped with other elements to produce a surplus of electrons or 'holes' in the crystal lattice. These act as charge carriers, increasing the conductivity.
- Power is dissipated by a resistor and is equal to the voltage multiplied by the current.
- Placing resistors in series produces a resistance equal to the sum of the individual resistances.
- Placing resistors in parallel produces a lower resistance, equal to the reciprocal sum of the individual resistances.
- A potential divider comprises two resistors in series, with a voltage 'tap' at the junction between the two resistors. The output voltage is smaller than the input.
- A Wheatstone bridge circuit allows accurate measurement of small changes in resistance.

Single best answer questions

For these questions, choose the single best answer.

1. Which one of the following is a good conductor of electricity?
   (a) Distilled water.
   (b) Wheels on an ITU bed.
   (c) Theatre clogs.
   (d) Saline spilt on the floor.
   (e) Room air.

2. How much current will flow if 1 volt is applied across a resistance of 100 Ω?
   (a) 100 A.
   (b) 10 A.
   (c) 1 A.
   (d) 100 mA.
   (e) 10 mA.

3. What is the total resistance of a 100 Ω and a 200 Ω resistor in parallel?
   (a) 300 Ω.
   (b) 200 Ω.
   (c) 150 Ω.
   (d) 67 Ω.
   (e) 33 Ω.

Multiple choice questions

For each of these questions, mark every answer either true or false.

1. Which of the following are true of semiconductors?
   (a) Undoped silicon is a very good conductor.
   (b) The conductivity of semiconductors decreases if the temperature is increased.
   (c) Addition of Group V elements introduces unpaired electrons that can take part in conduction.
   (d) Valence electrons are the main charge carriers in a semiconductor.
   (e) Boron is a suitable doping element for semiconductors.

2. Which of the following statements are true of resistor networks?
   (a) The combined resistance of parallel resistors is always smaller than the largest resistor.
   (b) The combined resistance of parallel resistors is always larger than the smallest resistor.

   (c) A potential divider in open circuit has no current flowing through it.
   (d) The voltage drop across resistors in series is equal to the total of the voltage drops across each resistor.
   (e) The current flowing through parallel resistors is equal for all resistors.

3. Which of the following statements are true?
   (a) In a circuit the current entering and leaving any point adds up to zero.
   (b) The voltage drop across a resistor is greater for smaller resistances.
   (c) Power is proportional to the product of voltage and resistance.
   (d) A unit of electricity is equal to 3.6 kJ.
   (e) The voltage drop across a wire is zero volts.

Chapter 19

Electromagnetism and alternating current

Having read this chapter you will be able to:
- Understand the link between electricity and magnetism.
- Know the three types of magnetic materials.
- Appreciate the theory behind a simple electromagnetic dynamo.
- Understand transformers and how they can step-up or step-down a voltage.
- Understand how electricity is generated and distributed to homes and hospitals.

19.1 Magnetic fields

Definition

Magnetic fields: produced by electric currents which can be macroscopic currents in wires, or microscopic currents associated with electrons orbiting an atomic nucleus.

The earth can be thought of as one large magnet and it is the electric currents in the earth's molten core that generate this magnetic field. The magnetic field emerges from the magnetic North Pole, returns into the ground at the magnetic South Pole, and is a result of electric charges moving within the core. In fact a magnetic field is always produced when a charge flows through a conductor. In the case of a **permanent magnet**, it is the movement of charged electrons around the atomic nuclei within the magnet.

Like the earth's magnetic field all magnets have two poles, namely a north (N) and south (S) pole. Opposite magnetic poles attract and like poles repel. This behaviour is similar to electric charge, where the north and south pole are analogous to positive and negative charges. There is a fundamental difference between magnetic poles and electric charges, however, in that magnetic fields are dipolar. In other words, a north pole cannot exist without a coupled south pole whereas an electric charge, either positive or negative, can exist alone. Magnetic fields are analogous to (though distinct from) gravitational or electric fields, but exactly how similar they are to each other causes great excitement amongst physicists.

A familiar example of magnetic attraction is that of a compass needle. Both the needle and the earth have magnetic properties. A compass has a small, lightweight magnet (the needle) balanced on a pivot and the north pole of the needle points in the direction of the North Pole. Paradoxically, because opposite poles attract, the earth's magnetic North Pole is actually a physical magnetic *south* pole and the magnetic South Pole is actually a *north* pole.

While preparing for a lecture in 1820, Hans Christian Ørsted made a surprising observation. As he was setting up his equipment, he noticed a compass needle deflected from magnetic north when the electric current in a nearby circuit was switched on. Ørsted discovered that when current flows through a wire, it generates a cylindrical magnetic field around the wire. The field lines rotate around the wire as shown in *Figure 19.1*. This deflection suggested that a wire carrying an electric current produces a magnetic field. In 1831, Michael Faraday showed that a magnetic field induces an electric

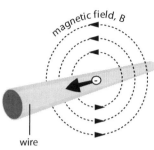

wire

⊖ = electron,
negative charge

Figure 19.1. *Moving charges generate a magnetic field perpendicular to their direction of travel. In the case of a wire, this results in a cylinder-shaped magnetic field.*

current in a wire moving through the field. Both these observations demonstrate that electrical and magnetic fields are inextricably linked.

Figure 19.2 shows a permanent magnet and a coil (solenoid). Both generate a magnetic field because of the movement of electric charges or currents. The permanent magnet has currents flowing at the atomic level, whereas the solenoid has current flowing through the wire. The number of turns of wire in the coil determines the strength of the magnetic field: more turns produce a stronger field. Wrapping the solenoid around an iron core can further enhance the strength of the magnetic field. Electromagnets have many uses because their fields can be switched on and off at the flick of a switch. Fire doors are held open by electromagnets that lose their magnetism when the alarm is triggered and the current is switched off.

A permanent magnet can be induced in certain materials such as iron when exposed to a magnetic field. The strength of a magnetic field is defined by the **magnetic flux**, a measure of the amount of magnetic field passing through a given surface. The magnetic flux (Φ) may be thought of as the 'amount' of magnetic field, and is proportional to the number of magnetic field lines and is measured in **webers** (Wb). The **magnetic flux density** (B) describes the strength of a magnetic field at a single point, for example, at a point on the earth's surface. Magnetic flux density is measured as flux per unit area, so is measured in Wb·m^{-2} (or **tesla**).

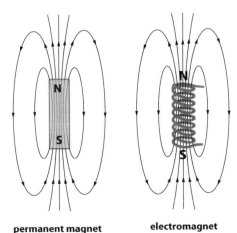

permanent magnet   electromagnet   **Figure 19.2.** *A permanent magnet and an electromagnet.*

The relationship between magnetic flux and magnetic flux density is as follows:

$$\Phi = B \cdot A$$

19.1

where

Φ is the magnetic flux
B is the magnetic flux density
A is the cross-sectional area

Magnetic materials

> **Definitions**
>
> **Ferromagnetic:** ferromagnetic materials are strongly attracted to magnetic fields.
> **Diamagnetic:** diamagnetic materials are repelled by magnetic fields.
> **Paramagnetic:** paramagnetic materials are weakly attracted to magnetic fields.

There are three types of magnetic material: ferromagnetic, paramagnetic or diamagnetic.

- Ferromagnetic materials have a large and positive susceptibility to an external magnetic field. They can retain their magnetism as their unpaired electrons have, a net magnetic moment, which means that the atoms act like tiny magnets and can align themselves to an applied field. The material is strongly attracted to the magnetic field, as can be seen when an iron bar is attracted to a magnet. When the applied field is removed, the atoms retain their alignment to the original field direction, which imparts some magnetism to the material. The length of time the material will retain this induced field depends on several factors including the material, its purity and its temperature. There are only a few materials that exhibit this behaviour and they include iron, nickel and cobalt.
- Diamagnetic materials have a weak and negative susceptibility to magnetic fields (i.e. they are repelled by magnetic fields). They have all paired electrons that prevent a permanent net magnetic moment forming in the atom. Examples include most elements including copper, silver, and gold, but also common substances which display no obvious magnetic properties such as water, most organic compounds, as well as superconductors.
- Paramagnetic materials have a small and positive susceptibility to magnetic fields. An external magnetic field causes the unpaired electrons to realign themselves. Examples include magnesium, molybdenum, lithium, tantalum and oxygen.

19.2 Electromagnetism

The electric motor

The English physicist Michael Faraday decided to confirm or refute a number of speculations surrounding Ørsted's discovery. Faraday devised a simple experiment to demonstrate whether or not a current-carrying wire produced a circular magnetic field around it. Faraday took a dish of mercury and placed a permanent fixed magnet in the middle. Above the magnet, he dangled a freely moving wire, so that the free end of the wire dipped into the mercury. When he connected a battery to form a circuit, the current-carrying wire circled around the magnet. This was the first demonstration of the conversion of electrical energy into mechanical energy, and as a result, Faraday is credited with the invention of the electric motor.

Faraday's motor was not at all powerful so its energy could not be harnessed for useful work. In the decades which followed, more powerful electric motors were designed which contained large coils in place of Faraday's hanging wire. When an electric current is passed through the coils, they move in response to electromagnetic forces, turning the spindle of the motor. The rotational speed can be controlled by varying the current. Nowadays, motors find applications in a wide range of electrical equipment including hairdryers, fans and electric drills.

The dynamo

A dynamo is the opposite of an electric motor; it converts mechanical energy into electrical energy. In fact, dynamos are constructed in exactly the same way as electric motors. An electric motor can be used as a dynamo; if the spindle of the motor is turned, it will produce an electric current in its coils.

Figure 19.3 shows a simple dynamo consisting of a wire coil, which when rotated cuts through the field lines of a fixed magnet, and as a result, a current flows in the coil. An alternative design moves the magnet whilst keeping the coil stationary, while more advanced designs use several magnets and/or coils. A simple generator produces alternating current, with the frequency of the AC equal to the number of rotations per second of the coil. Large generators in power stations are simply large dynamos attached to steam turbines. Wind generators contain dynamos attached to large turbine blades; of course the speed of rotation, and thus the output, is highly variable, depending on the wind speed.

19.3 Alternating current and power

A battery generates a current flow in just one direction and this is known as direct current (DC). However, electricity is often supplied as an alternating current (AC), such as the electricity supplied to hospitals and homes via wall sockets, known as mains electricity. Here the current is regularly reversing direction and mains electricity is transported as alternating current.

> **Definition**
>
> **Alternating current:** has a flow of electric charge that periodically reverses direction.

Mains electricity is transported and delivered as an alternating current for a number of reasons. Electric power station generators naturally produce alternating current and the use of AC allows the voltage to be changed up and down relatively easily using transformers. This is important because electricity is transported along power lines more efficiently at high voltages.

Devices such as electric heaters or light bulbs work just as well whether the current is AC or DC. For most electronic devices a DC current is needed and the current therefore has to be converted

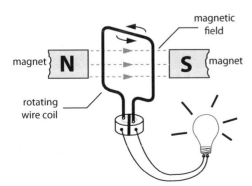

Figure 19.3. *A simple dynamo. The current flows through the circuit powering the light bulb as a result of the wire rotating through the magnetic field.*

from domestic AC to DC, using rectifying circuits in the electronic devices. The conversion is inefficient, and the energy wastage is apparent when feeling the heat produced by a laptop adapter.

Alternating current has no set positive and negative terminals because the current (or the direction of the electron flow) keeps changing direction periodically. The frequency of the AC supply is the rate at which the current switches back and forth and is expressed as hertz or cycles per second. In the UK the frequency of the AC supply is 50 Hz, while in the USA and many other countries the frequency is 60 Hz.

Consider two lumberjacks cutting down a tree with a two-person saw: whilst one pulls, the other pushes. *Figure 19.4* shows a graph of voltage against time for an AC supply – a graph of the saw moving relative to one of the foresters with respect to time would look similar to this graph. For the saw, the negative section of the graph still represents effective sawing. Work is still being done on both the "push" and the "pull".

An alternating current (AC) is often sinusoidal in shape on a graph with the voltage plotted against time. This creates a problem as to what the effective voltage is over a whole cycle. The average is zero because the negative and positive voltages cancel one another out, which does not help when trying to calculate the power in a circuit. The root mean square (RMS) is the value normally quoted for the effective voltage. It is calculated by squaring every point in the signal (this makes everything positive), then calculating the mean over the whole waveform and finally taking the square root. The RMS is equal to 0.707 (the square root of 2 divided by 2) multiplied by the peak amplitude. UK mains electricity has an RMS voltage of 240 volts. The RMS value of the current may also be calculated in the same way.

Worked example

Question
Calculate the peak voltage of the UK mains supply.

Calculation
The RMS voltage is 240 V. The peak voltage must be higher, and is in fact equal to
240 V / 0.707 = 339.4 V

Answer
The peak voltage is 339.4 volts.

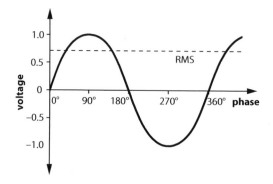

Figure 19.4. *A typical AC electricity supply consists of a sinusoidally varying voltage.*

Impedance and power

Instead of resistance as used in calculations involving DC, an equivalent quantity, **the impedance** (Z), is substituted for resistance in calculations involving AC. When calculating power in AC circuits, the impedance takes into account the inductance and capacitance of the circuit.

Calculating the power in an AC circuit is straightforward if the RMS voltage and current are known. The equation has exactly the same form as for DC circuits (Equation 18.5), but impedance replaces resistance and RMS values of voltage and current are used:

$$P = I_{RMS} V_{RMS}$$

19.2

$$P = \frac{V_{RMS}^2}{Z}, \text{ or } P = I_{RMS}^2 Z$$

19.3

19.4 Transformers

An elegant way to demonstrate electromagnetic induction is to align two coils of wire side by side. If a current is switched on in the first coil, the electric current generates a magnetic field. The magnetic field lines cut through the windings of the second coil inducing a current (by exactly the same principle as the dynamo). This is known as coupled induction, and the device described is a

transformer. Transformers rely on alternating current to work, because the magnetic field must be constantly changing to induce a current in the second coil.

Transformers are familiar everyday objects used to power small electrical devices and for charging batteries. *Figure 19.5* shows a simple 'step-down' transformer. The iron core of the transformer has the effect of maximizing the magnetic flux. The voltage generated in the secondary circuit is dependent on the relative number of turns in the wire for the two coils. In this way voltage in a circuit can be manipulated: it can stepped-up (increased) or stepped-down (decreased). A step-up transformer has a higher output voltage than its input and contains a greater number of turns in its secondary winding than in its first.

The voltage generated in the secondary coil is dependent on the ratio of the number of turns in each coil.

$$V_S = V_P \left(\frac{N_S}{N_P} \right)$$

19.4

where N_S is the number of turns in the primary coil
  N_P is the number of turns in the secondary coil
  V_S is the voltage across the primary coil
  V_P is the voltage across the secondary coil

According to the law of conservation of energy, the amount of power available from the secondary coil cannot be more than that dissipated by the primary coil. Therefore stepping-up the voltage results in the current being stepped-down. Transforming the voltage and current with induction is analogous to gearing with cogs (*Figure 19.6*). The speed of the cogs may be thought of as the current, while their torque (twisting force) is analogous to voltage.

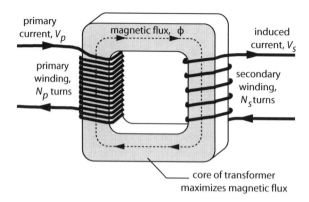

Figure 19.5. *A simple step-down transformer with an iron core to maximize the magnetic flux.*

19.5 High voltage power transmission

Electricity is generated at relatively high currents and low voltages (a few hundred volts). The voltages are raised using step-up transformers to around 400 000 volts before being transmitted over long distances by overhead electrical cables carried by pylons or via underground cables (*Figure 19.7*). The reduced current in the high voltage lines allows thinner, cheaper cables to be used when building the grid and reduces power wastage in the form of heat. The reason for this is that for a given rate of power transmission, a lower current is needed, which results in lower losses in the cables due to electrical resistance. This may be understood by considering that the power lost in the cable, which has fixed resistance R, is equal to I^2R; lowering the current clearly reduces the resistive loss of power. The high voltage is stepped-down to 240 V by transformers located at an electricity substation and distributed to homes and offices. Some industrial premises and hospitals also use 415 V supplies for more powerful appliances. For the National Grid, the ability to use transformers to step-up and step-down AC voltages provides great advantages over using DC.

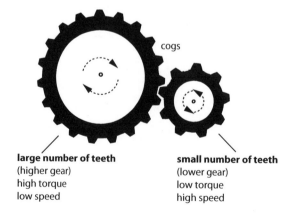

Figure 19.6. *Cog analogy for a step-down transformer.*

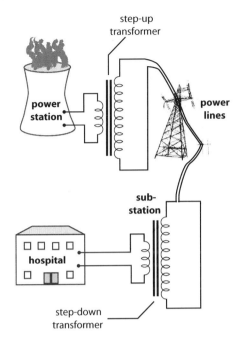

Figure 19.7. *Transformers are used to step-up the voltage at the power station end, to allow energy-efficient high voltage transmission. A second transformer at the electricity substation lowers the voltage for hospitals.*

UK domestic power supply

In the UK electricity is supplied at 240 V at 50 Hz, in contrast to North America's 120 V at 60 Hz supply. Human tissue is most sensitive to frequencies between 40 and 150 Hz, making domestic power supplies particularly hazardous, with 50 Hz being optimal for causing ventricular fibrillation. UK power outlets incorporate shutters on the live and neutral contacts and usually include a separate on/off switch. British Standard (BS) 1363 plugs (*Figure 19.8*) also contain a fuse within the plug,

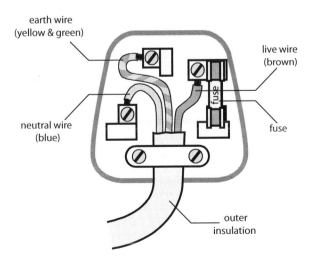

Figure 19.8. *A domestic plug (UK-type: BS1363).*

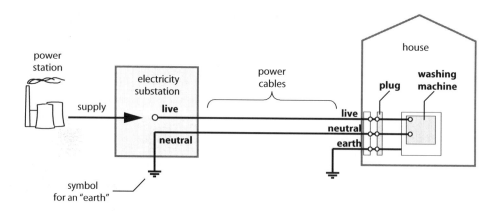

Figure 19.9. *The three wires used in UK domestic supply and their connections.*

making them arguably the safest in the world. Despite this, their design causes controversy, as they are extremely bulky, especially when carried with portable equipment.

Why are there three wires on a UK plug?

UK plugs contain three wires, **live** (brown), **neutral** (blue) and **earth** (yellow with green stripes). These wires connect to the pins in the plug, which correspond to the three terminals on the wall socket (see *Table 19.1*). The earth terminal is connected to a local earth, usually a metal spike buried in the ground just outside the building (see *Section 20.2*). The live terminal is the 'active' connection from the power station generator (or substation), and its voltage goes from +240 V RMS to –240 V RMS during each mains cycle. For this reason, the live wire is the most dangerous because if touched, electrocution can result. The neutral terminal provides the electrical return path for current to flow back from the appliance to the substation. When nothing is connected, the voltage remains at 0 V, so neutral can be thought of as the 'earth connection at the substation' (see *Figure 19.9*). The power station generator's other output is also connected to ground that supplies a reservoir of electrons. It is important that plugs for electrical appliances are wired correctly, although safety regulations now insist that electrical appliances have pre-wired plugs attached. Nevertheless, familiarity with the wiring scheme of a plug can potentially prevent serious injury or death from electric shock.

Table 19.1. *The role of the three wires used in UK domestic plugs.*

	Colour of wiring cover	Function	Description
Live	Brown	Active	Driving force for current
Neutral	Blue	Passive	Completes the circuit Provides return path for current
Earth/ground	Green/yellow	Safety	Path for errant currents to flow safely away

Summary

- A magnetic field is generated by a moving electric charge.
- All magnets must have a north and south pole, and they cannot exist in isolation.
- Materials have one of three types of magnetic properties: diamagnetic, paramagnetic and ferromagnetic.
- Transformers are used to either increase (step-up) voltage or decrease (step-down) voltage. They are employed by the National Grid to ensure electricity arrives at homes and hospitals at the appropriate voltage.
- Direct current (DC) travels in just one direction, whereas alternating current (AC) regularly changes direction: electronic equipment often requires DC and a rectifying circuit converts mains AC to DC.
- Impedance is the equivalent variable to resistance when talking about AC circuits.
- The neutral terminal on a household plug is nominally at zero volts and is connected to the electricity substation.

Single best answer questions

For these questions, choose the single best answer.

1. Which one of the following statements concerning magnetic materials is true?
   (a) Paramagnetic materials are not attracted to magnetic fields.
   (b) Copper is a ferromagnetic material.
   (c) Hydrogen is paramagnetic.
   (d) Cobalt is a diamagnetic material.
   (e) Oxygen is weakly attracted to a magnetic field.

2. The amount of power P produced by an electric heater of impedance Z supplied by voltage V is given by:
   (a) $P = VZ$
   (b) $P = V^2Z$
   (c) $P = V^2/Z$
   (d) $P = Z/V$
   (e) $P = V/Z$

3. Which one of the following statements is true?
   (a) The mean voltage of an AC supply is 0 V.
   (b) Mains electricity is transmitted over long distances at very high currents to minimize losses.
   (c) A step-down transformer increases current.
   (d) The RMS voltage can be positive or negative.
   (e) The peak voltage of the UK mains supply is 240 V.

Multiple choice questions

For each of these questions, mark every answer either true or false.

1. Which of the following statements concerning magnetic flux are true?
   (a) Magnetic flux density is measured in webers.
   (b) Magnetic flux is measured in webers.
   (c) Magnetic flux density is measured in tesla.
   (d) Magnetic flux density is measured in webers per square metre.
   (e) Magnetic flux is dimensionless.

2. Which of the following statements are true?
   (a) Current in a wire produces a cylindrical magnetic field.
   (b) A dynamo converts electrical energy into mechanical energy.
   (c) The coils of a dynamo move through a magnetic field and current is induced in the coils.

   (d) The north pole of a compass needle points to the earth's magnetic South Pole.
   (e) Current will flow in a wire in a steady magnetic field.

3. Concerning transformers, which of the following statements are true?
   (a) Transformers can change voltage but not current.
   (b) A transformer can change the voltage of a DC supply.
   (c) A transformer only works with AC.
   (d) The ratio of output voltage to input voltage is equal to the ratio of the number of turns of wire in the secondary winding to the number of turns in the primary.
   (e) Small electrical devices can run on AC or DC.

Chapter 20
Electrical shocks and safety

Having read this chapter you will be able to:
- Understand the nature of electrical shocks.
- Be able to explain the function of an electrical earth.
- Appreciate the difference between macro-shock and micro-shock.
- Be aware of the principle and dangers of diathermy.

20.1 Electrocution

The old adage, 'it's the current that kills you' is true. However, according to Ohm's law (Equation 18.1) the current that travels through a conducting medium is entirely dependent on the potential difference (volts) driving the electricity and the resistance (ohms) offered by the conducting medium. When you receive an electric shock by touching a live wire with your finger, the current enters through your finger and normally exits to the ground through your feet. As a conducting medium a human has a typical resistance (or impedance for alternating current) of about 1500 ohms between major extremities.

Most of the body's resistance occurs in the outer skin layers, because the internal tissues and blood (largely ionic solutions) that make up the body have very low resistance. Dry skin has much higher resistance than wet or punctured skin, so the figure of 1500 ohms is very approximate. An anaesthetist may reduce the risk of electrocution by wearing insulating footwear and the effective impedance for current flowing through the body would increase to around 240 000 ohms. If we look at this in a simple calculation we can see the difference good insulation makes. Ohm's law (Equation 18.1) states:

$$\text{current} = \frac{\text{voltage}}{\text{impedance}}$$

Applying this to a new-age rocker who is standing barefoot in a puddle at Glastonbury whilst adjusting the feedback on his faulty guitar amplifier:

$$\frac{240\text{ V}}{1500\ \Omega} = 0.16\text{ A} = 160\text{ mA (a probably lethal level of current)}$$

If we examine the same scenario with a piece of similarly faulty medical equipment, operated by an anaesthetist wearing poorly conducting shoes in theatre:

$$\frac{240\text{ V}}{240000\ \Omega} = 0.001\text{ A} = 1\text{ mA (may cause a barely perceptible tingling)}$$

This example highlights the importance of wearing appropriate theatre shoes.

Minimizing risk: isolated systems and low voltages

Definition
Isolated system: a system that does not interact with its surroundings. A patient is said to be isolated if there is no pathway for a current to flow. It is the opposite to being earthed.

As well as Ohm's law dictating that a high resistance reduces current flow, it is also the case that a lower potential difference (voltage) will also reduce current flow. Clearly if an electrical device is likely to come into direct contact with a patient, a low voltage is more desirable than a high voltage: the smaller the voltage, the less harm done in the event of an electrical shock. The voltage supply to a piece of medical equipment can either come from batteries or from a transformer.

Batteries have the obvious advantages of being low voltage and portable. Unfortunately, batteries need regular replacement or recharging. An alternative is to use an isolated (or floating) circuit utilizing a transformer. Because the secondary winding of a transformer is not connected to the primary winding, there is no direct connection between the mains power supply and the equipment attached to the patient. Furthermore, the transformer steps down the voltage supplied to the equipment and so if a fault should occur, and the patient also became earthed, the potential difference driving the current through the patient would be much less than the mains voltage, so minimal injury would occur.

Factors determining the severity of an electric shock

The amount of current flowing through the body provides a rough indication of the likely level of injury caused by electric shock. The severity of the shock is determined by:

1. The voltage of the source.
2. The body's resistance, which can be affected by:
   - the nature of the contact
   - the condition of the skin
   - moisture on or in the skin
   - body mass index
   - the route taken by the current in the body

Table 20.1. *The effects of different currents on the body.*

Electric current (1 sec contact)	Physiological effect	Voltage required to generate current	
		High resistance (10 000 Ω)	Low resistance (1000 Ω)
1 mA	• Threshold of feeling • Tingling sensation	10 V	1 V
5 mA	• Approximately the maximum harmless current	500 V	10 V
10–20 mA	• Current at which person "cannot let go" • Sustained muscular contraction	1000 V	100 V
100–300 mA	• Ventricular fibrillation	10 000 V	1000 V
6 A	• Temporary respiratory paralysis • Burns likely	600 000 V	6000 V

3. Other factors such as:
- clinical risk: some people are more prone to ventricular fibrillation than others
- timing of the shock relative to the cycle of the heart beat

The effects of different currents on the human body are summarized in *Table 20.1*.

20.2 Earthing

If a live power cable falls on top of a car, one might expect the driver to receive a fatal electric shock via the metal frame of their car. In actual fact, the driver stands a chance of surviving the incident. Rubber tyres on a car have a high resistance to the flow of current; in other words they are good insulators. There must be a conduction path for current to flow, and if the car is insulated there is nowhere for the current to flow to. If the driver then decides to exit the car putting one foot on the ground whilst touching the metal car body, then he would inadvertently be

> **Definition**
>
> **Earth (or ground):** a reference point in an electrical circuit from which other voltages are measured. Conventionally, earth also returns to a common return path for electric current, sometimes physically connected to the earth.

acting as an 'earth' or 'ground' and a large current would flow from the cables, through the car body, then the driver and through to the road.

The terms earth and ground are interchangeable: earth is preferred in the UK and ground in the US. In any electrical circuit, a reference voltage is chosen (usually set at zero volts) from which all other voltages are compared. In mains circuits, for safety it is necessary to make a controlled, deliberate path of very low resistance for unwanted current to flow. An effective way to achieve this is to connect the earth point in the circuit to the actual earth itself, which contains a vast reservoir of electrons, through a large metal spike or plate sunk into the ground. In the same way that a bucket of water emptied into the sea would have no measurable effect on the sea level, large currents can flow to earth almost indefinitely.

In the UK, a household plug (*Section 19.5*) usually houses three wires. The live and the neutral are involved with the transmission of current and the third wire, the earth, is there to ensure that there is a safe return path for any wayward currents. The casing of metal appliances is connected to the earth, so that if the casing becomes live through an electrical fault such as a loose wire within the appliance, the current is safely routed to earth, eliminating any shock hazard.

Consider a faulty lamp with a live outer casing. An earthed lamp is much safer because the earth provides a route for harmful currents to be safely conducted away. A patient touching the lamp casing (*Figure 20.1*) would be unharmed even if they were themselves earthed, for example, by touching an earthed bed frame. This is because the resistance of the patient is higher than the earth wire in the lamp, and the current will take the easiest path to earth (i.e. not through the patient). Now consider a lamp which is unearthed, which is often true of old appliances or those with incorrectly wired plugs. Now if an earthed patient touches the lamp casing (*Figure 20.1b*), they will receive a shock, because the current will flow to earth through the body.

An electric shock can only occur under three conditions:
- an accessible object such as the metal casing of an appliance has to be 'live' (connected to a live electricity supply), most likely through a fault
- another accessible object must be earthed
- a person must be sandwiched between the two, with electrical contact between the live and earthed objects

These conditions are sometimes called an electric shock 'sandwich'.

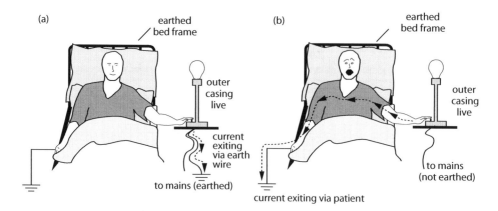

Figure 20.1. *(a) An earthed lamp casing safely conducts current away in the event of a fault. (b) An earthed patient will receive a shock from an unearthed lamp as their body provides a path to earth.*

Lightning conductors

Before a storm, negative charge builds up at the bottom of the cloud and a positive charge builds up at the top of the cloud. The charge in a thundercloud induces positive charge within objects it comes near to. Trees, tall buildings and other structures can be 'hit' by lightning when a positive stream of ions flows from the object up to the cloud and a negative flow of charge flows from the cloud to the object (see *Figure 20.2*). Lightning can generate incredible heat because when a given current flows through an object, the power dissipated is proportional to the resistance R:

$$P = I^2 R$$

Buildings built from brick, stone or glass have a very high electrical resistance and resistive heating can lead to fires and structural damage. A lightning conductor can be used to create a very low resistance path for charge to flow harmlessly to the ground. They are usually connected to a large metal plate buried in the ground to ensure good electrical contact between the conductor and the earth.

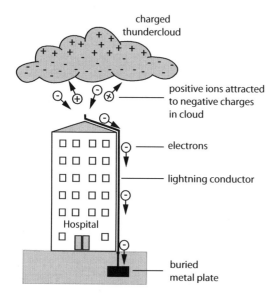

Figure 20.2. *Role of a lightning conductor.*

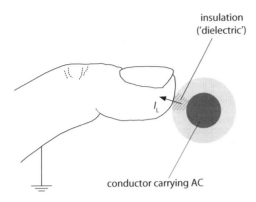

insulation
('dielectric')

I_L

conductor carrying AC

Figure 20.3. *Touching an insulated wire carrying AC can cause a small leakage current I_L to flow to the finger through the process of capacitance coupling.*

Current leakage

Current leakage can occur directly or indirectly. Direct leakage of current can occur, for example, due to faulty wiring. A faulty wire within an electrical appliance may cause the outer casing to become live. If this casing is connected to earth, which can be achieved by simply touching the casing, leaked current may flow.

Alternatively, current can appear to indirectly leak through a phenomenon known as **capacitance coupling**. This phenomenon is the result of charge building up on the casing of AC-powered electrical equipment. As explained in *Section 21.1*, a capacitor appears to conduct electricity if it is connected to an AC source. The equipment acts like a capacitor, with the casing and the wires acting like the opposite plates of the capacitor, and the insulation between them forming the capacitor 'dielectric'. A similar effect may occur by touching an insulated wire carrying AC as shown in *Figure 20.3*. A very small leakage of current can pass to the finger and flow to earth.

A slight tingling feeling on touching the casing of any equipment with a leak might be the only indication of a problem, however, the currents can be large enough to cause injury through micro-shock (see *Section 20.3*). It is for this reason that medical equipment must adhere to strict standards, with the casing being earthed so that any build-up of charge is dissipated and unwanted currents eliminated.

20.3 Electrical safety devices

In order to improve the safety of electrical devices, additional features have been incorporated and these have become more sophisticated over time.

Fuse

A fuse is essentially a thin wire inserted into a circuit. Its length and cross-sectional area (and consequently resistance) are calculated such that when a certain current is reached (the rupture current), the heating effect ($P=I^2R$) is enough to melt the wire, thus breaking the circuit. This simple system provides protection in situations such as described above in which a wire becomes loose and touches an earthed case. A large current flows, 'blowing' the fuse and cutting off the power.

Unfortunately, it is easy to imagine a scenario in which this simple system fails. Imagine that someone tripped over the cable leading from the plug to the lamp described above. As it was tugged, both the live and earth wires became loose, with the live wire coming to rest on the lamp casing, but the earth touching nothing. Even when the patient touches the lamp and receives a shock, the current flow is relatively small and the fuse will not blow, with potentially fatal results. Incidentally, this also explains why the earth wire should always be cut longer than both live and neutral, allowing time for a fault to blow a fuse before the earth can be torn free.

Residual current device

RCDs are electronic devices which measure the currents in the live and neutral wires. From Kirchhoff's first law, the sum of the currents entering and leaving any 'node' must be zero. The node might be a single lamp, or an entire house, but in either case, all the current entering the 'node' via the live wire, should be leaving via the neutral. If there is any difference, then current must be 'leaking' to earth and automatic switches are triggered within the RCD, disconnecting the power. This system is gradually replacing wire fuses in domestic fuseboxes and is common in hospitals, where even small leakage of currents might be very serious. An RCD detects the difference in current between the live and neutral wires and so is able to protect against the example above; it will prevent the patient from being electrocuted even in the event of an earth fault.

Worked examples

Question

What happens when an intravenous infusion of normal saline is spilt over a piece of electrical equipment?

Answer

Due to the electrolytes in saline, namely the ions Na^+ and Cl^-, the spilt fluid acts as temporary wiring within any circuits it seeps into. This can cause serious damage and malfunction and lead to short circuiting, and possible electric shock.

Question

Why are patients, particularly those who are anaesthetized, considered to be so vulnerable to electric shock?

Answer

Usually, when receiving an electric shock while conscious, an unpleasant sensation is experienced and every effort made to avoid further shock. The unconscious patient can neither alert staff nor take evasive action. They are connected to many pieces of electric apparatus that each pose the risk of micro- and macro-shock. The risk of micro-shock is increased by cannula pacing wire and monitoring equipment. Furthermore fluids, including blood, act as good conductors.

20.4 Micro-shock

Definition

Micro-shock: the unintended flow of small but dangerous currents directly, or within close proximity, to the heart.

The consequences of electric shock are dependent upon the path taken by the current. Consider two paths: one path is through the left thumb and exits through the left fore-finger and the other path enters through the central line and out through the left fore-finger. The current entering via the central line probably flows directly through the heart, a much more dangerous scenario, because the shock could trigger the heart into ventricular fibrillation. In practice, a very low current ('**micro-shock**') can lead to death if it enters directly or close to the heart.

In most electric shocks, current travels through the skin and then throughout the body. Because currents take the path of least resistance, micro-shocks take advantage of internal pathways such as pacing wires, central lines and even catheters for the bladder. The barrier of a highly resistant skin is by-passed so that a current that is so low as to be imperceptible to touch could be fatal as a micro-shock.

Not only can the route of a current be critical but also the timing of the shock relative to the cardiac cycle. The most vulnerable time to receive a shock is during the depolarization of the ventricles (the beginning of the T-wave) and the heart is at risk of being thrown into ventricular fibrillation. The minimum current that can cause ventricular fibrillation is 50 μA when in direct contact with the heart. The maximum leak allowed is 10 μA.

20.5 Electrical safety standards

The Electricity at Work Regulations (1989) and Health and Safety at Work Act (1974) aim to minimize the danger from electric shock, electric burns, electrical explosion or arcing, or from fire or explosion initiated by electrical energy. These legislations define different classes of equipment from Class I to Class III.

Class I equipment

The casing of the equipment (or any part accessible to the user) must be earthed. If a fault develops and the casing becomes live, the current will be instantly conducted to earth (via the third prong on a UK plug) and the increased current flow will melt the fuse.

Class II equipment

The equipment is double-insulated. Any part accessible to a user has reinforced insulation rendering shock via a single fault impossible. As a result these do not require earthing.

Class III equipment

Separated (or safety) extra low voltage circuit. This is a low voltage floating circuit, i.e. it is separated from the mains by a transformer with no conducting ground pathway by which to electrocute a user.

Leakage current standards

Devices are again classed according to whether they are for general use (Type B – body) or in contact with the heart (Type C – cardiac). Most leakage current classification also includes an 'F' added to the end to signify that the circuit is floating. *Table 20.2* summarizes the leakage current classification.

Defibrillator-proof equipment

If a defibrillator is discharged through a patient connected to defibrillator-proof equipment, the equipment will not be damaged by the defibrillator's energy. Defibrillator-proof equipment can remain connected to the patient during defibrillation.

Table 20.2. *Leakage current classification standards.*

Leakage classification	Technical information	Comments
Type B	• max leak 100 mA • can be Class I, II or III	• Risk of micro-shock
Type BF	• max leak 100 mA • circuits are isolated from other parts of equipment	• Not suitable for connections to the heart
Type CF	• max leak 10 mA	• Suitable for indirect connection with the heart

20.6 Static electricity

Definition
Static electricity: refers to the build-up of charge on the surface of insulators; it is usually caused by electrons being removed by friction.

Static electricity is normally experienced as nothing worse than a small but annoying shock such as when walking across a nylon carpet and then touching a door handle.

Static electricity is the name given to the potential difference generated between dissimilar surfaces when they are rubbed together, where at least one is an insulator. Electrons are transferred from one surface to the other (depending on which atom is least attached to the electrons in its outer shell), rendering one with an overall negative charge and one that is positive. This charge is dissipated by connecting it to earth. The build-up of static electricity is more problematic in dry conditions. In humid conditions, the higher water content acts to makes the air conductive, gradually dissipating any developing charges.

One of the main dangers of static electricity is the possibility of creating a spark that could ignite flammable gases. In a clinical setting, static can be reduced by:
- theatre shoes having anti-static soles
- theatre floors having an anti-static floor
- ensuring that air does not become too dry, by keeping the humidity levels above 30–40%

Theatre shoes and clogs are designed to have a moderately high impedance (75 kΩ to 10 MΩ), which, while still providing good protection against electric shock, allow static charge to 'leak' to earth.

20.7 Current density and electro-surgery

Definition
Current density: the flow of current per unit of cross-sectional area.

When the new-age rocker from earlier touched his faulty guitar amplifier his finger touched a live wire and he received an electric shock: the current entered through the finger and then exited through the feet. On examination, his finger is a little singed, but not his feet. The degree of damage to a region or organ depends not on the current, but on the **current density**, defined as the current per unit of cross-sectional area. Although the finger and the feet had the same current flowing through them, a finger has a smaller cross-sectional area than a foot, and so a higher current density. The power carried by a flow of electricity is proportional to the square of the current (see *Section 18.5*). Current density, *J*, is given by the following equation:

$$J = \frac{I}{A}$$

20.1

where   *J* is the current density
          I is current
          A is cross-sectional area

Current density is measured in amperes per square meter ($A \cdot m^{-2}$), although amperes per square millimetre ($A \cdot mm^{-2}$) is more practical. A high current density sufficient to cause burns is approximately $5\ mA \cdot mm^{-2}$, while a current density of less than $1\ mA \cdot mm^{-2}$ is harmless in most tissues. Diathermy uses high current densities to heat tissue to very high temperatures in order to destroy it. Diathermy typically produces current densities of $100\ mA \cdot mm^{-2}$ for the purposes of cutting, coagulation and desiccation.

Excitable membranes, e.g. those of nerve and muscle cells, respond to changes in voltage across the cell membranes with changes in voltage-gated ion channels. These proteins have finite response times and while 50 Hz mains frequencies can trigger them easily, they become much less sensitive as the frequencies increase. The use of high frequencies in surgical diathermy ensures that nerve and muscle cells are not stimulated, causing spasms or cardiac arrest.

> **Definition**
>
> **Electro-surgery:** commonly referred to as diathermy, this is the cutting and coagulation of body tissue with a high frequency current.

Unipolar diathermy

Unipolar diathermy (*Figure 20.4*) works on the principle that the body of the patient forms part of the electrical circuit. Electricity passes from an AC voltage source via an electrode through tissue then back to the source via a returning electrode. The cells at the tip of the probe are heated to a high temperature, in excess of 1000°C, so water in the tissue boils, while the tissue itself is cut and blood vessels are cauterized. The frequency of the alternating current is usually 1 MHz, but can range from 0.4 to 3 MHz. This frequency range is called the RF (radiofrequency) range and the effects cannot be felt in nerves and muscles because the frequency is too high.

Placement of the return electrode, the diathermy plate, is crucial for diathermy to work effectively. It must have good contact on the tissue which must have a good blood supply to dissipate heat. The surface area of contact must be large to reduce the current density and not be attached to a bony

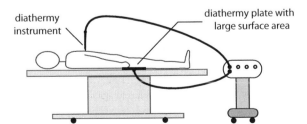

diathermy instrument

diathermy plate with large surface area

Figure 20.4. *Unipolar diathermy.*

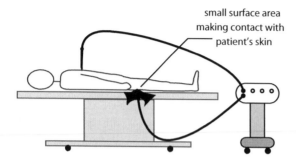

small surface area
making contact with
patient's skin

Figure 20.5. *Reduced contact area between patient skin and diathermy plate creates a high current density, so burns to the skin can result.*

prominence (since bone is a very poor conductor). Finally, the patient should not be touching any metal parts of the surgical table.

Although diathermy is a quick and effective method of halting bleeding and cuts tissue fairly precisely, it generates electromagnetic interference that can disrupt ECG and other patient monitoring and can interrupt the function of pacemakers. If the return plate electrode is not attached properly (*Figure 20.5*) then severe burns can result. Certain implants, particularly those made of metal, can increase local current density and cause thermal injury. Burns have also been observed around ECG electrodes for similar reasons. Capacitance leakage currents can also occur in nearby metal objects, notably the struts in surgical tables.

Minimal access surgery and endoscopic surgery have specific hazards in relation to electro-surgery. Both techniques involve instruments in close proximity and confined spaces. Even if there is no direct contact, capacitance coupling can occur, resulting in current being induced from one instrument to another.

Bipolar diathermy

In bipolar diathermy, the active and return electrodes each make up an arm of the diathermy forceps and the current passes between the two points as shown in *Figure 20.6*. The two arms are separated with an insulating material forming the handle. Bipolar diathermy is perceived to be safer than unipolar diathermy as the current pathway is far shorter, within a small radius of the diathermy forceps. A return plate is not needed.

Bipolar diathermy is used when coagulation is required in peripheral areas of the body or during procedures where pinpoint or micro-coagulation is needed. The technique is also applicable

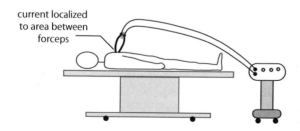

current localized
to area between
forceps

Figure 20.6. *Bipolar diathermy. There is no need for a diathermy pad but it is less powerful than unipolar diathermy.*

Table 20.3. *Types of diathermy.*

Diathermy type	Wave description	Details	Power and current	Effect
COAG	Short bursts of sine waves (pulse-like)	Desiccate	Lower power	Slow drying out of tissues No sparks
		Fulgurate	Higher power	Intermittent heating of cells Cells dry out quickly
Cutting	Continuous sine wave	Higher current but lower voltage than COAG	High current density Delivered quickly	Intense heat Cell explosion due to contents boiling
Blend	Combination of COAG and cutting			Used when both cutting and haemostasis are desired

when a patient is critically dependent upon an implanted pacemaker, as a lower level of electrical interference is generated. Some surgeons consider bipolar diathermy to be less effective than its unipolar counterpart due to a more localized current density.

COAG, cutting and blend

The current delivered during electro-surgery can be manipulated to meet the needs of the task at hand. There are essentially three settings in common use for diathermy: COAG, cutting and blend. COAG consists of short bursts of sine waves and is delivered in either **desiccate** or **fulgurate** forms; these terms are summarized in *Table 20.3*.

Pollutants generated by diathermy – surgical plume

Surgical plume is the name given to the smoke and vapour that is released when an electro-surgery device is used on body tissue (also produced in laser and ultrasonic surgery). This plume can contain toxic chemicals, carbonized tissue, blood particles, viral DNA particles and bacteria. To effectively remove this plume a filter capable of removing such small particulates must be used: general theatre suction is not capable of filtering out the particulate debris so dedicated suction is required.

Summary

- Dry skin has a relatively high resistance, minimizing the risk of serious injury through electrocution in many circumstances.
- Earthing the casing of an appliance can minimize the risk of an electric shock from faulty wiring inside the appliance.
- A lightning conductor minimizes damage to buildings by providing a safe, low-resistance path to earth.

- Micro-shock can occur when very small currents are applied to the heart, in the most serious cases leading to cardiac arrest.
- Theatre shoes are designed to have a small conductance, dissipating static electricity, and reducing the possibility of creating a spark.
- Diathermy produces high current densities at high frequencies, causing thermal effects to tissues; useful for electro-surgery.

Single best answer questions

For these questions, choose the single best answer.

1. Which one of the following is true of theatre shoes?
   (a) They have low resistance to reduce the risk of shock.
   (b) They are insulators.
   (c) They have a small resistance so static electricity is minimized.
   (d) They have a high resistance so static electricity is minimized.
   (e) They are conductors.

2. A correctly applied diathermy plate causes virtually no heating of the underlying tissue because:
   (a) the plate conducts heat away from the tissue
   (b) the current flowing though the plate is very small

   (c) the current density at the plate is much lower than at the probe tip
   (d) the frequency of the alternating current is very high
   (e) the patient is earthed

3. Which one of the following is true of an isolated circuit?
   (a) The circuit is connected directly to the primary winding of a transformer.
   (b) Devices are marked with an 'F'.
   (c) There is no risk of electric shock.
   (d) They are safer than battery-powered devices.
   (e) They eliminate the risk of capacitance coupling.

Multiple choice questions

For each of these questions, mark every answer either true or false.

1. When diathermy is in use it is important to:
   (a) locate the diathermy plate over bony areas
   (b) avoid shaving hairy areas where the plate is to be positioned
   (c) position plate as far away from surgical area
   (d) keep active electrode clear of tissue build-up
   (e) alter the positioning of the plate to avoid prostheses inserted during previous surgery

2. In which circumstances would a patient receive a shock from touching the live casing of a faulty metal appliance?
   (a) Appliance earthed, patient touching an earthed bed.
   (b) Appliance not earthed, patient not touching an earthed bed.
   (c) Appliance not earthed, patient touching an earthed bed.

   (d) Appliance earthed, patient not touching an earthed bed.
   (e) Appliance not earthed, patient standing barefoot on a wet floor.

3. Which of the following statements are true of bipolar diathermy?
   (a) No return plate is needed.
   (b) It is unsuitable for patients with pacemakers.
   (c) It has more powerful thermal effects than unipolar diathermy.
   (d) The risk of burning the skin is much less than with unipolar diathermy.
   (e) Skin burns can result if the patient touches an earthed table.

Chapter 21

Electrocardiography, pacing and defibrillation

Having read this chapter you will be able to:
- Understand the concept of capacitance.
- Know the fundamental principles that underpin the use of a defibrillator.
- Appreciate the difference between monophasic and biphasic defibrillation.
- Understand the nature of cell potentials.
- Have a clear understanding of how pacemakers work.

21.1 Capacitance

A capacitor is an electrical device that stores electric charge. In its basic form a capacitor consists of two or more parallel conductive (metal) plates that are electrically separated either by air or by some form of insulating material, such as paper, wax or porcelain, called the **dielectric**. *Figure 21.1* shows the electrical symbol for a capacitor.

> **Definitions**
>
> **Capacitor:** a device for storing electric charge.
> **Capacitance:** a measure of the charge a device can hold: measured in farads (F).

If a DC voltage is applied to a capacitor's conductive plates, a current flows and charges up the plates (*Figure 21.2*). Electrons collect on one plate, giving it a negative charge, while the other plate becomes deficient in electrons and so has an equal and opposite positive charge. This flow of electrons to the plates is known as the **charging current** and it continues to flow until the voltage across both plates (and hence the capacitor) reaches the applied voltage V_c. At this point the capacitor is fully charged and the charge stored on the capacitor Q is given by:

$$Q = C \times V_c$$

21.1

where C is the capacitance (farads).

The capacitance is dependent on the area of the plates, the separation between them (smaller separation gives larger capacitance) and the properties of the dielectric. *Figure 21.3* shows the voltage between the plates of the capacitor during charging (by connecting to a voltage supply) followed by discharge. Connecting a charged capacitor to a circuit causes electrons to flow away from the negative plate and through the circuit since they are attracted towards the positive plate. During discharge, the charge on the capacitor decreases.

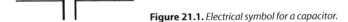

Figure 21.1. *Electrical symbol for a capacitor.*

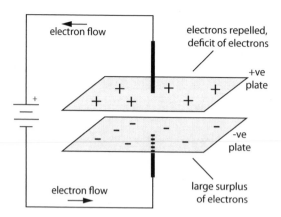

Figure 21.2. *Charging a parallel-plate capacitor.*

As the capacitor's plates charge, an electrostatic field develops across the dielectric, so the electrons building up on the negatively charged plate are attracted to the positive plate. Electrons cannot cross the dielectric 'gap', however, because it is an insulator. In theory a capacitor can hold its charge indefinitely, although in practice the charge leaks very slowly through the casing of the capacitor or through the dielectric.

The capacitance is the charge stored per volt of charging potential:

$$C = \frac{Q}{V}$$

21.2

where C is the capacitance (farads)
Q is the charge stored (coulombs)
V is the potential difference (volts)
The energy stored, E, can be calculated if the capacitance and voltage are known:

$$E = \tfrac{1}{2}C \cdot V^2$$

21.3

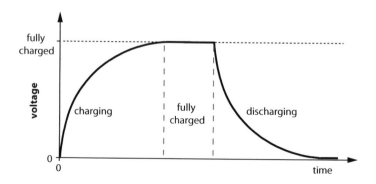

Figure 21.3. *Graph of voltage against time during charge and discharge of a capacitor.*

When used in a direct current (DC) circuit, a capacitor blocks the flow of current through it, but when it is connected to an alternating current (AC) circuit, some current is able to pass straight through. The amount of current passing depends on the frequency of the AC and the capacitance.

Large capacitors are integrated within the power supply of many electronics devices. When there is a disruption to the power supply the capacitors are discharged in a controlled manner to supply power until the main power supply is restored.

21.2 Defibrillators

The defibrillator delivers a charge that travels through the heart as a current to depolarize a critical mass of the heart muscle, with the aim of terminating an aberrant arrhythmia, restoring the function of the sino-atrial node as the natural pacemaker of the heart beat.

Definition
Defibrillator: a defibrillator releases a controlled electric charge that is expressed as units of electric energy.

The resistance of the tissue will determine the magnitude of the current for a given applied voltage. For external defibrillation, the position and degree of contact of the paddles can compromise the success of the defibrillation. There has been a move in recent years to the use of adhesive pads and away from hand-held paddles. This has increased staff safety, the accuracy of positioning and the quality of contact with the skin reducing both burns to the skin and the proportion of energy delivered to the tissue. Internal defibrillators require much smaller voltages to deliver the same energy to the heart because the high resistance of the skin is bypassed.

External defibrillator

The external defibrillator is designed to deliver a controlled shock through a pair of paddles held on the patient's chest, or via self-adhesive contact electrodes. *Figure 21.4* shows a circuit diagram of an external defibrillator. The defibrillator contains a large capacitor that is charged with a prescribed voltage. The capacitor has to be charged with a direct current (DC) that is obtained by passing the AC mains supply through a rectifier. A transformer steps-up the voltage from 240 V to a value in the

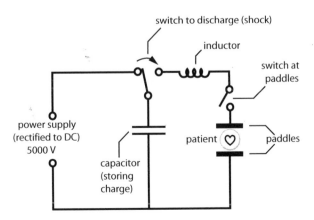

Figure 21.4. *A simplified circuit diagram of an external defibrillator.*

range 3000–5000 V, delivering typically 360 Joules of energy. The capacitor stores energy in the form of electric charge ready to discharge across the defibrillator paddles. An inductor slows down the discharge of the capacitor to around 3 milliseconds, so that during discharge the current flowing through the chest is around 30 amps. For patients at short-term risk of life-threatening arrhythmias, wearable defibrillator vests have been developed.

Automated external defibrillators have the benefit of allowing life-saving interventions in hospitals, ambulances and public places such as airports and shopping malls. They are highly automated, allowing operation by relatively unskilled users. There is, however an appreciable risk of injury from burns arising from incorrectly placed electrodes. There is also significant risk of staff receiving an unwanted shock by touching the patient, a hospital bed or other conducting object in contact with the patient. Finally, misdiagnosis of an arrhythmia can lead to a shock putting the patient into ventricular fibrillation.

Implanted cardioverter defibrillator

The implantable cardioverter defibrillator (ICD) is a small battery-powered electrical impulse generator used to treat patients at high-risk of sudden cardiac death due to ventricular fibrillation (VF) and/or ventricular tachycardia (VT). The impulse generator is usually implanted in the pre-pectoral fascia and is connected to lead(s) that pass through the venous system to the right chambers of the heart. The ICD constantly monitors the rhythm of the heart via these leads. When a dangerous ventricular arrhythmia is sensed by the ICD it may either deliver immediate shocks or attempt to overdrive the heart out of the arrhythmia using anti-tachycardia pacing (ATP). If ATP fails the ICD will deliver shocks. The response of the ICD to ventricular arrhythmias depends upon programmed algorithms usually decided upon at the implantation of the device. These algorithms may be changed at any stage depending upon the patient's clinical condition. The ICD impulse generator usually needs to be changed about every 5 years.

ICDs have the advantage that a life-saving intervention can be given promptly, so these devices are more effective than external defibrillators in patients at high risk of VF. ICDs may occasionally deliver inappropriate shocks causing pain and distress to the patient. These may be caused by damage to the ICD lead, misdiagnosis of atrial arrhythmias by the device, or occasionally due to external interference. Repeated discharges may also cause permanent damage to the myocardium and could cause loss of function due to premature depletion of the battery. Over long periods, electrodes can become coated in tissue or slip out of place, or in extreme cases can cause laceration of the myocardium.

Monophasic and biphasic defibrillation

A **monophasic** defibrillator works by the simple discharge of a capacitor. The **biphasic** defibrillator offers a more sophisticated delivery of electrical energy. It was first developed for implanted defibrillators to prolong battery life and reduce myocardial damage from repeated shocking and is now commonly used for external defibrillators.

In a biphasic defibrillator, the current is delivered through the heart in two directions, or vectors, rather than one. The two-vector method achieves the same effect using a lower peak current and therefore a lower level of energy delivery. *Figure 21.5* shows a typical graph of current against time for a biphasic defibrillator. More sophisticated defibrillators estimate the impedance of the body to be shocked and adjust the shock voltage to be delivered accordingly. This function, in combination with biphasic defibrillation, is less likely to damage myocardial tissue than the traditional monophasic method.

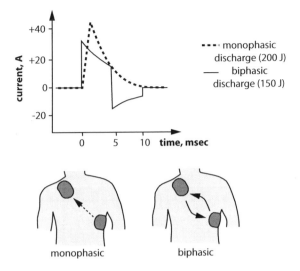

Figure 21.5. *Monophasic and biphasic defibrillators.*

The timing of a shock is unimportant for ventricular fibrillation, but for other arrhythmias a synchronized shock is required. The defibrillator is programmed to deliver a shock synchronized with the ECG R-wave. Incorrect synchronization with the ECG can result not just in a failed defibrillation but can also generate more severe arrhythmias, including ventricular fibrillation. *Table 21.1* summarizes the different types of defibrillators and their features.

Table 21.1. *Types of defibrillators, indications and features.*

Type of defibrillator	Indication	Mode of delivery	Energy (joules)
Emergency defibrillator	Any arrhythmia with associated haemodynamic instability	External pads or paddles	200–360 J
Elective synchronized DC cardioversion	Atrial fibrillation, atrial flutter and ventricular tachycardia	External pads or paddles	50–360 J
Direct to heart	During cardiac surgery	Internal paddles	5–50 J
Implantable cardioverter defibrillators	*Primary prevention:* most commonly patients with poor LV function (LV ejection fraction <30%) due to ischaemic heart disease *Secondary prevention:* most commonly patients who have had VT or VF and were haemodynamically compromised or have poor LV function (for complete indications see NICE guidelines)	Implanted like normal pacemaker	25–40 J

21.3 Biological potentials

The word **cell** refers to a battery as well as a biological cell; this is fitting because biological cells act like batteries generating electrical energy. The cell wall, or membrane, is made from phospholipids and is comparable to a capacitor with the electrical energy stored as a charge on either side of the cell wall, the inside wall being negative with respect to the outside. When cells depolarize collectively they can produce a potential difference that can lie in the microvolts (μV) to millivolts (mV) range depending on the tissue of origin. Like capacitors, cells store electrical energy and after each depolarization energy is required to recharge the cell. This energy is generated by the conversion of chemical energy to electrical energy.

Biological potentials are transmitted through the tissues and so can be detected. Electrodes placed on the skin allow measurement of voltages that are then processed, analysed, recorded and displayed. One technical hurdle to overcome is the reaction between sweat and a metallic electrode, which produces a small voltage that would swamp the small electrical signal from the heart. Also, the salts in sweat degrade many metals, so a non-metallic conductor such as a silver chloride gel is usually placed in contact with the skin as shown in *Figure 21.6*. The gel is backed with a silver/silver chloride disc that forms the connection to the lead while the malleable property of a gel aids contact with the skin.

The skin, and to a much lesser extent the tissue, introduces considerable electrical resistance. This leads to the attenuation of signals so that the signal picked up at the site of the electrode is far smaller in magnitude than the signals emitted by the cells.

Cardiac potentials

An electrical circuit is usually thought of as a collection of wires and components through which a current flows in a controlled fashion. The heart also acts as a circuit, but rather than wires and components there are electrically active cells. Once a myocyte cell is stimulated it in turn prompts depolarization in its neighbouring cell and, like a line of dominos, each one knocks over the one in front of it. In this way the sino-atrial (SA) node initiates the cardiac cycle, creating a wavefront of stimulated myocardial cells allowing this depolarization to sweep through the atria, producing a coordinated ripple of contraction. As *Table 21.2* shows, the heart is a sophisticated circuit where the conduction velocity is not uniform but varies as the wavefront travels.

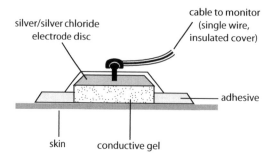

Figure 21.6. *An adhesive skin electrode designed to measure electric potentials.*

Table 21.2. *Conduction velocity in the heart's electrical circuit.*

Myocyte	Typical length (mm)	Conduction velocity (m·s⁻¹)
Atrial	10	1
A-V node	3	0.05
Purkinje fibres	75	4
Ventricle	15	0.3

21.4 Electrocardiography

Other than the skin, most of the tissues and fluids within the body offer excellent electrical conductive properties and for this reason an electrocardiogram (ECG) may be readily obtained. It is the recording of the sum effect of all the individual action potentials of the myocardial cell. The bigger the muscle, the greater the combined numbers of action potentials and hence the greater the deflection seen on the ECG. The size of signal detected by electrodes on the skin surface is far lower than the originating potentials. The current is attenuated as it passes through the intervening tissues, and the skin in particular offers a high resistance to current flow. As a result, an ECG signal of 1 or 2 mV may be all that is detectable.

Generating 'views' with an ECG

The ECG would be very limited if it could not distinguish in which direction the electrical fields exist. Thankfully an electric field is a vector quantity, in other words it has a direction and a magnitude. Strategically placed electrodes on the patient's skin allow a variety of 'views' of the electrical field to be recorded. The ECG reveals the electrical activity of the heart made from 12 different viewpoints in two distinct planes, namely the frontal and transverse planes.

Einthoven's triangle

Willem Einthoven (1860–1927) was a Dutch doctor who constructed apparatus sensitive enough to detect the electrical activity of the heart. Einthoven postulated that the electrical signals he recorded depended on the direction or **vector** of the electrical signal. If the direction of travel of the heart's electrical current is in the same direction as that of the measuring lead, a positive deflection is produced. If the direction of travel of the heart's electrical current is in the opposite direction to that of the measuring lead, a negative deflection is produced. If, however, the direction of travel is perpendicular to that of the measuring lead they cancel each other out and no signal is recorded.

Electrodes placed near the right arm, left arm and left foot make up an arrangement known as Einthoven's triangle. This arrangement, by creating circuits between them, delivers three potential differences that are called **leads I, II** and **III** (see *Figure 21.7*). ECG measurement uses a naming convention largely established by Einthoven, which is historic rather than intuitive.

Bipolar leads

The measurement of potential difference for the electrodes (or leads) that make up Einthoven's triangle are made from one electrode to the other. They are called the standard **bipolar leads** (I, II and III), because the measurement is between two points: the two electrodes. Note that the

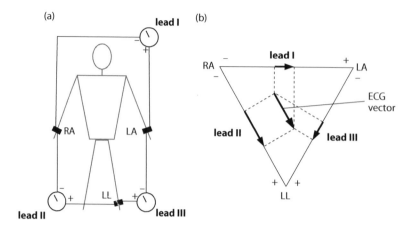

Figure 21.7. *(a) Bipolar leads. (b) Einthoven's triangle.*

word 'lead' originally referred to the physical leads or wires; now the term is used to describe the measurement itself. Lead I measures the potential difference between the right arm (RA) and left arm (LA). By convention, positive deflection is recorded if LA is positive compared to RA. Lead II is between RA and the left leg (LL), while lead III is between LA and LL (LL is taken as positive for leads II and III). Each lead thus gives a different 'view' of the ECG vector. When the three views are all noted together, the direction of the ECG vector may be determined from the relative sizes (**scalars**) of the lead I–III signals as shown in *Figure 21.7*.

Unipolar leads

For diagnostic purposes, **unipolar leads** are sometimes used in addition to bipolar leads. A single electrode placed at different positions on the chest, close to the heart would record higher potentials than at the limbs. Another electrode placed at the centre of the chest would provide a reference (0 V). In practice, this arrangement is impractical, especially during surgery, so combinations of pairs of limb leads are used instead, simulating the exploratory single electrode. The reference voltage is provided by all three limb leads connected together, an arrangement known as **Wilson's central terminal**. *Figure 21.8* shows electrodes RA, LL and LA connected to a circuit with resistors in between each electrode and the circuit itself.

The signal between LA and the reference (Wilson's terminal) is known as **aVL**, that at RA as **aVR** and that at the LL as **aVF**. The small 'a' stands for 'augmented', referring to the way in which the potentials are measured. Each of the three limb electrodes is connected to Wilson's terminal through a resistor of resistance, R, which has the effect of attenuating all the potentials equally. To select a particular electrode, say LL, the resistor connected to LL is substituted for one with a value of $R/2$ (*Figure 21.9*). This boosts or 'augments' the signal from the electrode of interest.

Unipolar precordial leads

The other type of unipolar lead is known as the **precordial lead**. It is similar in concept to the unipolar leads described above, except that six further electrodes are placed on the chest. Because of their close proximity to the heart, they do not require augmentation and also use Wilson's central

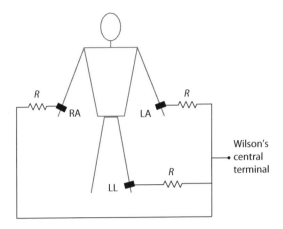

Figure 21.8. *Wilson's central terminal. The electrodes RA, LL and LA are connected together through resistors into a circuit providing a reference potential.*

terminal as a reference potential. These leads are designated by the capital letter 'V' followed by a number, from 1 to 6. These leads provide information about electrical activity in the transverse plane, while the limb leads (bipolar and unipolar) indicate the activity in the frontal plane.

Units. The ECG is measured in mV, millivolts, $1 \text{ mV} = 1 \times 10^{-3} \text{ V}$.

ECG instrumentation

ECG machines are capable of recording all 12 leads simultaneously, although only one or two are displayed for the purposes of anaesthesia. The detected ECG signals are very small so an amplifier is needed to boost the signal. Amplification introduces a problem in that the entire signal is boosted,

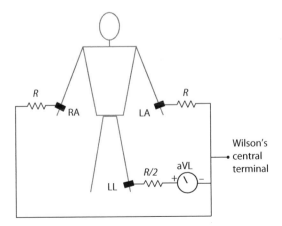

Figure 21.9. *Arrangement for measuring aVL. The resistor R has been substituted with R/2 and the potential is measured between this resistor and the terminal.*

including mains interference induced in the leads and electromyogram (EMG) signals (see *Section 21.5*) from the muscles, so the amplified signal must be filtered to remove this noise. A **low-pass filter** (one which lets through low frequencies and blocks high frequencies) reduces distortions from muscle movement, mains electricity (50–60 Hz) and other equipment, while a **high-pass** filter reduces signals from body movement including breathing. Different levels of filtering can be selected, designated as 'monitoring' and 'diagnostic' modes. A 'monitoring' ECG is heavily filtered, so is less susceptible to interference and artefacts. A 'diagnostic' ECG shows more 'raw' signal information, but is susceptible to interference from electrical equipment and artefacts from patient movement.

The accuracy of ECG is good, despite the attenuation that results from the significant resistance of the skin. It is not without its limitations, however. ECG is reliant on accurate electrode placement and it is susceptible to electrical interference such as from diathermy. Finally, excessive patient movement, especially shivering, can cause considerable artefacts.

Dead myocardium: an electrical window

Infarcted myocardium is electrically inactive and therefore does not generate an electrical field. However, like most tissue in the body, it does **conduct** electricity very well. The view obtained through an infarcted region is essentially that of the myocardium opposite, rather like looking through a window and viewing the opposite wall. This is particularly true of 'old' infarcts, whereas fresh infarcts might have areas where myocytes are undergoing cell death yet still generating some form of a potential.

21.5 Potentials in skeletal muscle: electromyography

The electromyogram (EMG) measures and records the activation signal of skeletal muscle. The potentials range approximately between 50 μV and 30 mV with a frequency of 7–20 Hz. The waveform spikes are shorter than those generated by cardiac muscles and repolarization is faster. The strength of the potential is dependent on the quantity of muscle fibres stimulated, so for a neuron that stimulates a large numbers of muscle fibres there is a bigger potential (or voltage spike).

There are two methods of measurement:

- surface EMG utilizes bio-potential electrodes probes; it is non-invasive, being attached to the skin, but dependent on the temperature and physiology in the area of interest
- intramuscular EMG involves either the insertion of a needle electrode or a needle containing two fine wires into the muscle to be investigated

The EMG records the motor unit action potential that is the sum of electrical activity of a group of motor units. At the same time the nerve conduction down the motor nerve is recorded. By comparing the waveforms produced, the neurophysiologist can delineate where in the circuit the problem lies, either with nerve conduction, at the neuro-muscular junction or at the muscle motor units themselves. Scientists are currently investigating the use of EMG signals to control prosthetic limbs, although attempts are currently hampered by the complexity of EMG signals and the speed at which a considerable amount of post-processing must be achieved to produce a coordinated movement.

21.6 Potentials in the brain: electroencephalogram

The potentials in the brain are very much smaller than those generated in the heart, and as a result are much more difficult to detect. Sixteen electrodes are normally attached to the scalp for an electroencephalogram (EEG) and periodic oscillations are searched for across a range of frequencies. The potentials are the sum of the post-synaptic potentials and are small, in the region of 50 μV (5×10^{-5} V), so considerable amplification is needed. The EEG signals can be plotted directly, like an ECG, although their interpretation is less straightforward. The EEG signals are analysed in terms of the amount of electrical activity in five well-defined frequency bands, known as δ, θ, α, β and γ. *Table 21.3* summarizes the main EEG bands, their properties and examples of how the presence of each band is interpreted.

An evoked potential is the change observed in a continuous EEG recording immediately after a patient has received a stimulus. Auditory evoked potentials have commonly been used when investigating depth of anaesthesia because they are easily applied via clicks close to the ear. Visual evoked potentials require flashing lights. Somatosensory evoked potentials are sometimes used during spinal surgery; for this a peripheral nerve is stimulated and a potential is hopefully recorded on the EEG, demonstrating an intact neural pathway.

A normal EEG shows high frequency activity against a low frequency background. Anaesthetic agents should suppress these high frequency bursts in a dose-dependent manner. At increasing depths of anaesthesia this high amplitude activity can be obliterated, a process known as burst suppression. A burst suppressed EEG indicates a brain at its minimum metabolic rate and this is useful in the treatment of raised intracranial pressure. Note that there is large variation between the characteristic EEG of a neonate and that of an adult.

There are several methods of processing the immense amounts of data gathered from an EEG and new methods are continually being developed by researchers. The **compressed spectral array** is one of the most common. In this technique, the measurement period is broken down into several epochs of fixed duration. A frequency spectrum is produced from the data recorded during each epoch using Fourier analysis (*Section 5.6*) and each spectrum is stacked to form a 3-dimensional representation of how different spectral features evolve with time.

Bispectral analysis (BIS) is used to measure depth of anaesthesia. The EEG signals from the fronto-temporal region are analysed and a dimensionless number is displayed in real time representing the awareness level of the patient (100 = fully awake, 0 = no brain activity). The BIS monitor is a commercial device that uses a proprietary algorithm to analyse the power and phase relationships between the different frequencies in the raw signals. The calculations are based on model data

Table 21.3. *EEG bands, frequencies, location and examples of their interpretation.*

Band designation	Frequency (Hz)	Location	Interpretation
Delta (δ)	0.5–4	Frontally in adults, posteriorly in children; high amplitude waves	'Slow wave' sleep in adults Continuous attention Can indicate subcortical lesions
Theta (θ)	4–8	Away from locations related to task	Drowsiness, idling
Alpha (α)	8–13	Posterior, both sides, higher amplitude on dominant side	Relaxation, eyes closed, coma
Beta (β)	13–22	Both sides symmetrically; low amplitude waves	Alert, active concentration, anxiety
Gamma (γ)	22–30	Somatosensory cortex	Short term memory recall, perception involving two or more senses (e.g. sight and sound).

acquired from a set of anaesthetized patients. The use of BIS has been shown to be more reliable than other methods, including compressed spectral array, for measuring depth of anaesthesia, but it has not been universally adopted. This is probably due to its inconsistency when comparing measurements using different anaesthetic agents and inter-patient variability: some patients, for example, are fully aware with BIS values of 70 while others are unconscious at a value of 75.

Acquiring good quality raw data is full of pitfalls. The potentials that are measured are dominated by signals from the superficial layer of the cortex. Artefacts are plentiful: they can be generated by eye movement, the myocardium, musculoskeletal movement, and from glossokinetics (the potential difference between the tip and base of the tongue).

EEGs can show cerebral hypoxia and with technological advances the sensitivity is improving. There has been much promising research in the applications of EEG monitoring in rehabilitation of patients. Subjects have been able to control prosthetic robotic limbs from a wearable EEG monitor, a role currently restricted to implanted electrodes.

21.7 Cardiac pacemakers

Cardiac pacemakers are most commonly used to treat bradyarrhythmias but are also occasionally used for 'overdrive' pacing of some tachyarrhythmias. Both temporary and permanent pacing systems are used regularly in clinical practice.

Permanent cardiac pacing

Permanent cardiac pacemakers (*Figure 21.10*) are indicated for the chronic treatment of bradycardias, usually second- or third-degree heart block, or prolonged (>3 second) pauses. A permanent pacemaker consists of a pulse generator that usually has a lithium iodide battery and contains the circuits that control the pacemaker timing, sensing and output parameters. The pulse generator is most commonly implanted in the pre-pectoral fascia of the upper chest and is connected via pacing lead(s) that traverse the subclavian vein to the right chambers of the heart.

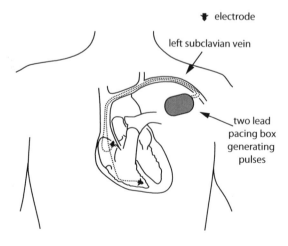

Figure 21.10. *Permanent pacing leads used with an implantable pacemaker.*

A pacemaker is part of a **pacing system**: a pacemaker, a pacing lead, and programmer. Titanium or a titanium alloy makes up the casing and the seal required must be impervious to air and gas (hermetically sealed).

Pacing leads are flexible insulated wires. They have two ends: the connector pin that joins to the pacemaker and the electrode tip, which is placed in direct contact with the heart's surface. The pacing leads transmit impulses from the heart to the pacemaker, allowing the pacemaker to sense the intrinsic electrical rhythm of the heart. In addition, the leads also carry electrical impulses from the pacemaker to the heart, allowing the pacemaker to pace the heart when necessary.

Pacing lead fixation

Pacing leads also have some form of fixation mechanism at the tip, either active or passive. Active fixation has a corkscrew-like tip that is screwed into the heart's surface as shown in *Figure 21.11*. Passive fixation is similar to a ship's anchor, and grips itself onto the heart's surface with the aid of tiny prongs (called 'tines').

Pacemaker principles

The pacemaker senses the intrinsic electrical rhythm of the heart. However, a pacemaker does not record a surface ECG. Rather, it senses the potential difference between two electrodes placed near the tip of the pacing lead. This voltage difference between these electrodes at the lead tip creates an intra-cardiac electrogram (EGM). The EGM represents depolarization of the myocardium at the tip of the pacing lead.

Pacing leads are usually placed in the right ventricle and/or the right atrium. Pacing leads connect to the pacemaker via individual 'channels'. Atrial EGMs and ventricular EGMs will be transmitted via the atrial channel and ventricular channel, respectively. From these EGMs the pacemaker can interpret the electrical rhythm of the heart.

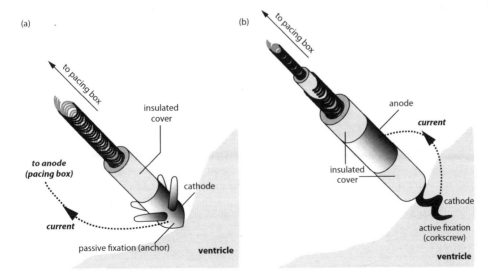

Figure 21.11. *Unipolar lead system uses the pacing box as the anode, completing the circuit. (a) Passive and (b) active fixation can both be used on either a unipolar (a) or a bipolar (b) system.*

The pacemaker generates an electrical pulse at a specific voltage for a defined period of time by a capacitor discharge. This electrical pulse causes the heart's intrinsic electrical system to depolarize and results in the contraction of the desired heart chamber. The **pacing threshold** is the minimum voltage required to cause depolarization of the heart.

Pacing modes

Pacing modes are described by an alphabetic code with up to 5 letters. The **first** letter refers to the chamber that is paced (can be A – atrium, V – ventricle, D – dual (or both A and V)). The **second** letter refers to the chamber that is sensed (can be A – atrium, V – ventricle, D – dual or O – no sensing). The **third** letter refers to the action taken by the pacemaker when an event is sensed (I – pulse inhibition, T – pulse triggered (pacing), D – dual (i.e. I and/or T) or O – no action). The **fourth** letter if present is always R and means rate response. The **fifth** letter, if present, indicates multisite pacing (can be A – atrium, V – ventricle, D – dual, or O – no sensing).

Clinical examples

Common pacemaker modes

VOO: ventricular pacing; no sensing; no response to intrinsic electrical activity
The pacemaker paces the ventricle at a fixed rate, ignoring any underlying intrinsic rhythm. This is the response of many pacemakers to a magnet being placed over the pulse generator.

VVI: ventricular pacing; senses ventricle; pacing inhibited by intrinsic ventricular activation
A minimum ventricular rate is pre-programmed into the pacemaker. The pacemaker will pace the ventricle only if this pre-programmed interval between consecutive ventricular beats is exceeded. If the pacemaker senses intrinsic ventricular electrical activity the pacing is inhibited.
VVI pacing is most commonly used in patients with atrial fibrillation with ventricular pauses.

DDD: dual chamber pacing; dual chamber sensing; dual response (pacing either triggered or inhibited)
If the atrial rate falls below a pre-programmed rate atrial pacing occurs. An AV delay is also programmed into the pacemaker. This represents the time taken for electrical activity to travel from the atrium to the ventricle. Following atrial sensing or atrial pacing, if the time taken for ventricular activation exceeds the AV delay then ventricular pacing will occur. If the intrinsic sinus rate increases, the pacemaker will sense the atrium and, if the ventricle does not respond within the AV delay, then ventricular pacing will occur. DDD is known as physiological pacing – this pacing mode should maintain synchrony between the atrium and ventricles.
DDD pacing is used for pacing when intrinsic atrial activity is present – most commonly second- and third-degree heart block.

Temporary cardiac pacing

Temporary cardiac pacing is indicated when a bradyarrhythmia results in haemodynamic compromise. Temporary cardiac pacing can be established in a number of ways, but the most common technique is temporary trans-venous pacing, where a pacing wire is placed into the right ventricle under X-ray guidance. Usual access sites for this technique include the right femoral vein, right internal jugular vein or right subclavian vein.

External temporary pacing can be achieved via the pads of a defibrillator (with external pacing function) placed on the chest. It is used when trans-venous pacing cannot be established or as a bridge to transvenous pacing in haemodynamically compromised patients. External temporary pacing is uncomfortable because it causes not only the heart but also the muscles of the chest wall to contract rhythmically.

Epicardial pacing involves the pacing leads being attached directly to the epicardium. This is usually only seen in patients immediately after cardiac surgery.

Temporary cardiac pacing for general anaesthesia

The incidence of perioperative complete heart block in patients with asymptomatic bifascicular block or trifascicular block is low, and temporary cardiac pacing is generally not required. Patients with symptomatic bifascicular or trifascicular block should probably receive a permanent pacemaker. This should be undertaken before undergoing general anesthesia.

Summary

- Capacitors store electrical energy in the form of electric charge. They can be used as a short-term back-up during power cuts.
- When a capacitor discharges, it does so in an exponential fashion. A defibrillator is essentially a rapidly discharging capacitor.
- A biphasic defibrillator is a more sophisticated, safer and more efficient defibrillator, discharging in one direction and then in the opposite direction.
- Electrocardiography allows the direction of the cardiac vector to be monitored. Unipolar leads give detailed diagnostic information.
- Electroencephalography measures brain activity by recording very small potentials. Spectral analysis of EEG allows estimation of depth of anaesthesia.
- Pacing may be achieved via several possible conduction paths. Implantable pacemakers use leads fixed to the myocardium.

Single best answer questions

For these questions, choose the single best answer.

1. A capacitor is best described as:
   (a) a specialist resistor that holds charge over short periods of time
   (b) a device for storing electrical energy
   (c) a component for creating an electrical potential
   (d) a short-term battery
   (e) a device for stepping down the voltage in a DC circuit

2. Capacitance is best described as:
   (a) the rate at which a capacitor discharges
   (b) the measure of the rate of current flowing through a capacitor
   (c) a measure of the amount of charge a device can hold
   (d) a base SI unit measuring charge per second
   (e) the energy a capacitor holds on fully charging

3. Concerning defibrillators, which one of the following statements is true?
   (a) An average starting energy for defibrillation is 200 kJ.
   (b) Biphasic defibrillators deliver more voltage than monophasic defibrillators.
   (c) The capacitor in the defibrillator is charged with alternating current.
   (d) Biphasic defibrillators deliver a charge in three directions.
   (e) Poorly attached defibrillator pads can cause burns to the patient following defibrillation.

Multiple choice questions

For each of these questions, mark every answer either true or false.

1. Regarding a capacitor, which of the following statements are true?
   (a) A capacitor is a large resistor.
   (b) A capacitor can have one or two plates depending on intended use.
   (c) The voltage across a capacitor decreases exponentially with respect to time during discharge.
   (d) Capacitors store charge.
   (e) A charged capacitor has a potential difference across it.

2. Regarding capacitance, which of the following statements are true?
   (a) It is the ratio of charge stored to applied voltage.
   (b) It is measured in farads.
   (c) It may be increased in a capacitor if a dielectric material is inserted between the two plates.

   (d) It increases with increasing plate separation.
   (e) The larger the capacitance the greater the ability to store electrical energy.

3. Concerning defibrillator pads, which of the following statements are true?
   (a) Hand-held pads are safer than adhesive pads.
   (b) The better the electrical contact with the patient's skin the less chance of burns to the skin.
   (c) Paddles applied directly to the heart during cardiothoracic surgery must deliver a higher energy to have the same effect as external pads.
   (d) Different types of pads are needed for monophasic and biphasic defibrillator systems.
   (e) Gel applied to hand-held pads that aid contact with the patient must be poor conductors of electricity to aid discharge.

Chapter 22
Processing, storage and display

Having read this chapter you will be able to:
- Appreciate the 'black box' model.
- Understand signal conditioning and signal processing.
- Know the difference between analogue and digital information.
- Understand computer networks.
- Distinguish between software, hardware and operating systems.
- Recognize forms of electronic data storage.

22.1 The 'black box'

Until recently, the home music system for the discerning hi-fi enthusiast came in a number of large components, or 'separates'. Together these separates such as a compact disc player, graphic equalizer, amplifier and speakers combined to convert the raw data, encoded digitally onto the surface of the compact disc, into beautiful sounds emitting from the speakers. The data went through a number of processes, eventually to be heard as music. Advances in miniaturization have resulted in fully integrated systems with little compromise in the quality of sound: everything has been squeezed into one box.

The clinical setting is no different; where once there was a stack of pieces of equipment, all wired to one another, there is now a smaller self-contained unit. Like stereos, the components can now be held within a single box or, at most, a modular system. To simplify matters the components, whether separated or integrated, are often referred to as a '**black box**', so as to acknowledge that a complex process of steps occurs, yet at the same time avoiding an unnecessary description of them. This approach is useful because most complex machinery or instrumentation can be operated perfectly well without specialist knowledge of its mechanism.

Though monitoring equipment is highly complex, there are surprising parallels between equipment used for different types of measurement. Although the method of gathering the raw data is different, the method of processing it is virtually identical in most hospital equipment. There are, in most cases, several readily identifiable steps which are common to almost any physiological measurement application.

Figure 22.1 shows a generalized physiological measurement system. The **measurand** is the quantity we are interested in measuring, for example, blood pressure or skin temperature. A sensor is connected to the patient utilizing a physical or chemical process that responds to the measurand, to produce a signal, often termed a **bio-signal** to indicate that the signal is biological in origin. Many sensors convert one form of energy to another and so are called **transducers**. An example of a transducer is a strain gauge pressure sensor, which converts mechanical strain into an electrical bio-signal. The raw signals from the sensor are often small in amplitude and contain unwanted components (noise and interference). The former problem is corrected by **amplification** to make the signals larger, while the latter problem is addressed by **filtering** to remove unwanted information, 'conditioning' the signal to make it more useable.

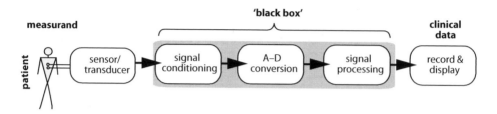

Figure 22.1. *The black box: a convenient description for a multi-stage system for processing raw bio-signals into clinically useful data (A–D stands for analogue to digital).*

The next step is to digitize the signal, in other words to produce numerical data from the signals by an **analogue-to-digital converter** (A–D converter). Most modern medical instrumentation is based on microprocessor-controlled systems that can manipulate digital information to produce clinically relevant information with a high degree of accuracy. This process is termed **signal processing** and relies on an algorithm: a mathematical equation to convert the measured data into a clinical variable, sometimes taking calibration data into account. Once in digital form, the data can be readily stored, displayed and transmitted over local area networks or the internet. The black box model can refer to various configurations, but all of the above processes are usually included in the definition.

22.2 Transducers and signal pick-up

Definition
Transducer: converts energy from one form to another.

The majority of physiological measurements require a transducer of some sort. A transducer is a device that converts one form of energy to another. A typical transducer converts non-electrical phenomena into an electrical signal that is digitized and processed by the monitoring system.

Table 22.1. *Signals from the cardiovascular system.*

Measurand	Typical range	Transducer type
Arterial blood pressure (invasive, e.g. aorta or radial artery)	30–300 mmHg	Bonded semiconductor strain gauge
Venous blood pressure (invasive, e.g. internal jugular vein)	−5 to +20 mmHg	Bonded semiconductor strain gauge
Heart rate	25–200 beats per min	*Derived from ECG, arterial pressure waveform or PPG*
Blood flow (arterial or venous)	0–300 mL·s⁻¹	Electromagnetic flowmeter / Ultrasonic Doppler flowmeter
Cardiac output	0.5–25 L·min⁻¹	Thermal dilution method
Photoplethysmograph (PPG)	–	Transmittance or reflectance probe (two emitters + photodiode)
Oxygen saturation	70–100%	*Derived from PPG*

Table 22.2. *Signals from the respiratory system.*

Measurand	Typical range	Transducer type
Respiration rate	5–50 breaths per minute	Thermistor CO_2 detector Strain gauge transducer
Respiratory flow rate	0–10 $L{\cdot}s^{-1}$	Fleisch pneumotachograph
Tidal volume	250–750 mL	Spirometer *Integrated flow signal from pneoumotachograph*
Expired CO_2 concentration	2.5–9.0%	Infrared sensor
Pulmonary diffusing capacity (using CO)	12–35 mL $CO{\cdot}mmHg^{-1}{\cdot}min^{-1}$	Infrared sensor (CO absorption)
pH	6.8–7.8	Glass electrode
Dissolved CO_2 partial pressure (PCO_2)	2–9 kPa	Severinghouse electrode
Dissolved O_2 partial pressure (PO_2)	6–18 kPa	Clark electrode

Because of the wide range of physiological measurements made, a wide variety of transducer types have been developed, utilizing different principles and physical (or in some cases chemical) processes. Some types produce a current or voltage; others produce a variation in an electrical circuit characteristic such as resistance, according to variations in the quantity being measured. The choice of transducer depends on the nature of the measured quantity, its magnitude, the accuracy required, the measurement site and economic considerations.

Remember that not all forms of measurement need to be converted into an electrical form, for example, the liquid thermometer that is read by a visual inspection. Some bio-signals are already electrical by their nature, such as the electrical activity of the heart and so do not need a transducer. Some signal conditioning is usually still required though to produce high-quality noise-free data. *Tables 22.1–22.3* show some example measurands, their typical ranges and the type of transducer used to measure them.

22.3 Signal conditioning

Signal conditioning can be thought of as 'cleaning up' or improving the overall *quality* of the signal. It is necessary to prepare the signal for digitization and signal processing. In most cases, a signal conditioning circuit will consist simply of an **amplification stage** and a **filtering stage**.

Table 22.3. *Other physiological signals.*

Measurand	Typical range	Transducer type
Central temperature	20–40°C	Pharyngeal probe containing thermocouple or thermistor Intravascular sensor containing thermistor
Skin temperature	12–38°C	Skin-placed thermocouple or thermistor
Galvanic skin resistance	1–500 kΩ	Surface electrodes similar to ECG electrodes

Amplification stage

For musicians and hi-fi enthusiasts an amplifier is a familiar device that makes a small signal into a large signal: in other words changing (usually increasing) the amplitude of the signal. The amount by which the amplitude of the signal increases is known as the **gain** and can be thought of as the 'multiplication factor' of the amplifier. In fact, the gain is the ratio of the voltage at the output of an amplifier to the signal voltage at the input. That is:

$$\text{Gain} = \frac{\text{output voltage}}{\text{input voltage}}$$

22.1

For example, an amplifier that doubles the amplitude of its input signal will have a gain of 2. A hi-fi amplifier has variable gain; the gain is adjusted by turning the volume control up or down. A gain between 0 and 1 would produce an output of smaller amplitude than the input.

Bio-signals require amplification because they are small in amplitude. If they are not amplified, then the signals will deteriorate as noise is added in successive stages of the black box process. Amplification as soon as possible gives the best chance of ensuring that the signal level is boosted above subsequent noise (i.e. the signal to noise ratio remains high). Note that the amplifier does not eliminate noise, or directly increase the signal-to-noise ratio (the noise is amplified along with the signal).

The signal measured by an ECG electrode typically has an amplitude of around 1 mV and is normally amplified by an amplifier with a gain in the order of 1000. An amplifier for a particular biological signal must have sufficient gain to be suitable for the voltage range of the signal. For instance, an amplifier with a very high gain is needed for EEG measurement, because the size of the signal is so small. The types of amplifier used in most medical devices can be fitted onto a small chip and are referred to as **operational amplifiers**, or **op-amps**. They are cheap, reliable and versatile devices whose gain can be adjusted over a very wide range (from 1 to at least 10^6).

Filtering stage

The clinical areas of a modern hospital are awash with a cacophony of electromagnetic noise. They are filled with electrical appliances, both specialist medical devices and everyday 'household' appliances, all of which generate **electromagnetic interference** to some extent. This interference, which is in the form of radiated energy in the radio-frequency range of the electromagnetic spectrum, is normally inconsequential, but it can interfere with sensitive measuring equipment including that used for patient monitoring. Power lines, fluorescent lights, vehicle ignition systems, electric motors, diathermy, computers and displays are all common sources of electrical interference. Some sources of interference originate within the body, for example, the electromyography signal can appear on an ECG trace, especially if the patient is shivering. Interference is often referred to generally as a type of **electrical noise**, or sometimes as **signal artefact**. *Table 22.4* summarizes some commonly encountered sources of signal artefact.

The effect of this interference depends upon the nature of the source, its proximity, as well as the type of measurement being made, but generally the noise shows up as an unwanted high frequency component added to the detected signal. If the signal is small, for example, an ECG recording, the artefact can drown out the desired signal, which makes interpretation of the signal impossible. The

Table 22.4. *Common sources of signal artefact.*

Artefact	Description/explanation
Power line interference	Sinusoidal waves at frequency 50 Hz (or 60 Hz in USA)
Movement artefact	Patient movement causes transducer to momentarily lose contact with the skin
Baseline wander	Low frequency interference appears as waveform baseline drifts in sync with respiratory rate, for example
Muscle depolarization	Muscle contraction generates unwanted potentials and interferes with the ECG
Electrode contact noise	Insufficient electrical contact between skin and electrode leading to distortion
Electrosurgical interference (diathermy)	Interference across the frequency spectrum from intense electrical field at probe tip, causing gross interference to ECG

ECG signal is obliterated when diathermy is used in the operating theatre, a problem familiar to anaesthetists! Amplifying the signal as soon as possible is a partial solution, however, any noise present will be amplified too. To quantify the problem, engineers often refer to a quantity called the signal to noise ratio, which is the ratio of the amplitude of the signal to the amplitude of the noise:

$$\text{Signal to noise ratio} = \frac{\text{signal voltage}}{\text{signal noise}}$$

22.2

If the signal to noise ratio is too low, then the signal is not useable without further signal conditioning in the form of **electrical filtering**. Electrical filters are introduced into the circuit of the ECG to remove some or all of this noise. The household mains electricity supply is a source of interference with a frequency of 50–60 Hz, which is above the highest frequency in the ECG. A **low-pass filter** introduced into the circuit cuts out the high frequency noise but lets through the low frequencies of the ECG.

A **band-pass filter** can cut out high and low frequency interference, letting through only frequencies within a certain range, or **bandwidth**. A filter can be thought of as a frequency selective amplifier with a gain of 1 in the **pass-band** (within the range of frequencies it lets through) and a gain of 0 in the **stop-band** (frequencies which are blocked). As an example, the EMG signal contains frequencies in the range 7–20 Hz (*Table 22.5*) so signals outside of this range can be removed with little loss of integrity to the raw data. *Figure 22.2* shows the response graph (gain against frequency) for a band-pass filter suitable for filtering signals from an EMG electrode.

22.4 Analogue-to-digital conversion

Any waveform, be it sound or an electrical voltage can be recorded as an analogue signal, a representation or replica of the shape of the wave. For example, when sound is recorded by a microphone (a type of transducer) the sound wave is converted to an electrical signal (waveform)

Table 22.5. *Frequency ranges of bio-signals.*

	Frequency	Potentials
EEG	1–20 Hz	10–100 µV
EMG	7–20 Hz	50 µV to 30 mV
ECG	0.5–40 Hz	0.1–5 mV

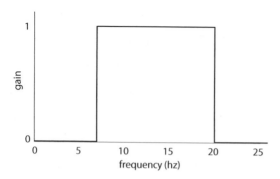

Figure 22.2. *Response of a band-pass filter with a pass-band ranging from 7 to 20 Hz, suitable for EMG measurement.*

that can then be recorded in the form of a groove on a record or the position of tiny magnetic particles on an audio tape.

Alternatively the electrical waveform signal may be transformed into numbers by an analogue-to-digital (A–D) converter, and represented as a binary sequence (0s and 1s). This binary sequence can be manipulated by mathematical transformations and recorded on media able to store binary information such as a computer hard drive or compact disc, and can easily be transmitted as data packets. This is how your favourite band goes from the recording studio, to the online digital music store, and finally through the mobile network to your smartphone. The advantage of a digital signal is that the recording is less susceptible to degradation and distortion, allowing accurate reproduction from stored sources and transmission over long distance networks. Digital information also has the advantage that it can be manipulated by computers, for example, to convert raw bio-signals into clinically useful data. An example of this is in a pulse oximeter, which converts an analogue optical signal (a photoplethysmogram) into a digital signal, which is subsequently used to calculate oxygen saturation by an algorithm stored inside the device. These processes are controlled by a microprocessor running a software program that may be modified and updated over time by the manufacturer to improve the performance of the instrument.

22.5 Hardware, software and operating systems

Hardware

Computer hardware consists of a **processing unit** containing the processor and memory, and **peripheral devices** which are connected to the main unit. Peripherals fall into three main categories: input devices, output devices and external data storage. Peripheral devices such as printers and memory sticks communicate with the microprocessor using an interface known as a data bus, for example, the well-known USB (Universal Serial Bus). In addition, read/write devices such as hard drives are incorporated into the main processing unit.

Input devices. An input device is a hardware device that sends information to the computer. Examples of input devices include a keyboard, mouse, microphone (for speech recognition) or video camera.

Output devices. An output device is any peripheral device that receives output from a computer. An example of an output device is the monitor which receives electronic signals that become images on the screen. A touch-screen monitor combines an input and output device: it both displays an image (output) and receives data when the user touches the screen (input).

Storage devices. Storage devices allow electronic data to be held and accessed at a later date. Magnetic media have been used in the past in the form of floppy disks, and even further back, in the form of magnetic tape. Magnetic hard drives are still used as internal and external storage devices thanks to their low cost and very high capacity. Gradually, however, as their costs fall, solid-state drives are replacing hard disks as the main storage system in personal computers. Optical media such as CD–ROM (read only memory) and DVD–ROM are used for archiving and mass distribution of media such as music and movies.

> **Definitions**
>
> **Hardware:** the physical components that make up a computer system.
> **Software:** a set of instructions or programs, which a computer can interpret and execute; an example of software is an application, which is a program used by the operator for a specific task.
> **Operating system:** software that manages all the applications, handles files and controls the computer's resources.

22.6 Displays

Display technology is one of the fastest-evolving areas of consumer technology. Cathode ray TVs are now almost consigned to museums, while organic light emitting diode (OLED) technology is around the corner, promising stunning image definition combined with very low power consumption. There are currently three main types of displays: LED, LCD and plasma displays. Cathode ray tubes (CRTs) were used for many decades but are now almost completely obsolete, having been replaced by thinner displays.

Display resolution

The **resolution** of a display refers to the number of picture cells, or **pixels**, in the display. The resolution is usually expressed as two numbers (width x height). A computer monitor may have 1600×1200 pixels, which is considerably more than a standard television screen which has a vertical pixel count (number of 'lines') equal to 625. Televisions are designed for viewing at a distance of a few metres, so the smaller number of pixels is not evident. 'High-definition' TV, however, has a vertical pixel count equal to 768 or 1080, which makes a perceptible improvement to the image quality.

Plasma

Plasma screens consist of pockets of gas that emit light when a high enough voltage is applied. Plasma displays can be made very large at a low relative cost, but with lower resolution than LCD or LED, making them suitable for television screens or displays designed for viewing at a greater distance than a computer monitor.

LED displays

LED (**light emitting diode**) displays are an array of red, blue and green diodes that are switched on and off by a complicated electronic circuit. LEDs have high efficiency, while recent advances in manufacturing methods have meant that the individual LEDs making up each pixel on the display can be very small, resulting in a very high quality display.

LCD displays

LCD stands for **liquid crystal display**. When a specific voltage is applied across the crystal they become transparent. With the aid of filters and backlighting this phenomena can be manipulated to produce bright full-colour images. The resolution of LCD displays is unrivalled, making them suitable for viewing high-quality images. The pixel size can be made very small, allowing a high pixel density, so they are suitable for viewing at close-range, for example, in a smartphone.

22.7 Networking

The world is connected together by a network of networks: the internet, which enables seemingly effortless transmission of information. **Local area networks** (LANs) such as hospital intranets are invaluable for conveying patient data from one department to another. For example, real-time physiological data of a patient in theatre can be displayed on a central monitor at a nurses' station in the intensive care unit, or on a handheld device connected to a wireless network. Patient monitors, personal computers, imaging systems and instruments such as blood gas analysers in all parts of a hospital may be connected to a LAN, simplifying the sharing of information. Local area networks can be connected to the internet via a central server, allowing internet access from any computer connected to the LAN. The convenience of hospital networking is undermined by the risk of computer viruses as well as the risk of personal information being used inappropriately, so elaborate security systems are needed.

Wired networks

Computers are often connected by a series of cables, most commonly using a standard of networking called **ethernet**. This method of connecting to the network is often referred to as **hard-wired** and wall sockets are installed in each department enabling connection with an ethernet cable. Wired networking has the advantage of being reliable, secure and can accommodate very high data transfer rates.

Wireless networks

Wireless networking (or **wi-fi**) is very flexible because a single wired hub or base station can serve the networking needs of an entire department. Computers and devices, including mobile devices, exchange data via high frequency radio signals which have a short range (tens of metres). Despite the cost benefits and convenience of not requiring cables, wireless networks are prone to interference and so can be unreliable. They are also potentially less secure and slower than wired networks.

Summary
- The term 'black box' describes a complex electronic system whose function is well understood but knowledge of its mechanism or underlying principles are not needed.
- Patient monitoring systems are a good example of a black box.
- Physiological measurement is performed using a dedicated sensor or transducer. Transducers convert one type of energy into another, usually an electrical quantity such as voltage or current.

- Conditioning of raw signals usually comprises amplification to increase the signal amplitude and filtering to remove noise.
- The gain of an amplifier is the ratio of its output voltage to its input voltage.
- A filter has a gain of zero in its stop-band and a gain of one in its pass-band.
- Digitization of analogue signals allows signal processing using computerized algorithms, and facilitates display and storage.
- Digital information is not susceptible to noise or distortion which affects analogue signals. It can also be transmitted over local area networks or the internet with ease.

Single best answer questions

For these questions, choose the single best answer.

1. Which one of the following statements is true?
   (a) An ECG electrode is an example of a transducer.
   (b) A digital-to-analogue converter is commonly used in physiological measurement systems.
   (c) Digital signals are immune to interference.
   (d) Analogue signals cannot be displayed on a monitor screen.
   (e) A transducer converts one form of energy into another.

2. Which one of the following statements about displays is true?
   (a) Plasma screens have higher resolution than LED screens.
   (b) LCD screens require backlighting.
   (c) The resolution of a screen is the same as the pixel density.
   (d) Cathode-ray screens can now be made as flat screens.
   (e) LED screens have low power efficiency.

3. Which one of the following statements about amplification is true?
   (a) It reduces noise.
   (b) It increases signal to noise ratio.
   (c) The gain of an amplifier is the ratio of output power to input power.
   (d) The gain of an amplifier must be larger than one.
   (e) Amplification boosts the signal to minimize the effect of subsequent noise.

Multiple choice questions

For each of these questions, mark every answer either true or false.

1. Which of the following statements are true?
   (a) Signal processing includes filtering of unwanted signal components such as noise.
   (b) The gain of a filter in its stop-band is 1.
   (c) A low-pass filter removes high frequency noise from a signal.
   (d) An amplifier is a device which increases voltages.
   (e) ECG signals contain frequencies up to 40 Hz.

2. Which of the following measurands always require a transducer?
   (a) Blood pressure.
   (b) ECG.
   (c) Temperature.
   (d) Blood flow.
   (e) Respiratory flow.

3. Which of the following statements are true?
   (a) Wireless networking is faster than ethernet.
   (b) The operating system of a computer comprises both hardware and software.
   (c) A computer mouse is a type of input device.
   (d) USB stands for 'Universal Service Bus'.
   (e) A CD-ROM is an example of external computer storage.

Chapter 23
Ultrasound

Having read this chapter you will be able to:
- Appreciate how reflected ultrasound waves can be used to measure distances within the body.
- Measure flow with ultrasound waves utilizing the Doppler effect.
- Understand the thermal properties of ultrasound and the implications of this.
- Explain the phenomenon of cavitation and its medical applications.

23.1 Ultrasound waves

Definition

Ultrasound waves: sound waves with a frequency greater than 20 kHz, the upper threshold of human hearing.

Ultrasound refers to sound waves whose frequency is too high to be detected by the ear, i.e. the frequency of the waves exceeds 20 000 Hz, the upper threshold of human hearing. Ultrasound is used for diagnostic applications (detection of blood flow, flow measurement, imaging of organs, fetal imaging) and therapeutic applications (fragmenting kidney stones using acoustic energy, a method known as lithotripsy). Ultrasound imaging is one of the key methods of soft tissue medical imaging and at the typically low energies used, ultrasound has no lasting effect on tissue, making it ideal for scanning, even in pregnancy.

The basic properties of sound waves were explained in *Section 5.2*. The basic principle of medical ultrasound is similar to the sonar used in submarines to locate the seabed and other vessels. Unlike medical ultrasound, however, sonar uses frequencies in the audible range. For medical use, the frequency of the ultrasound waves varies according to the application and required range. In general, higher frequencies are more readily absorbed by tissue; so do not penetrate as far as lower frequencies. Typical ultrasound frequencies are in the megahertz (MHz) range, where 1 MHz = 1×10^6 Hz.

The velocity of sound waves in tissue is close to their velocity in water, around 1500 m·s^{-1} although the exact velocity depends on the tissue type. Compare this to the speed of sound in air, which at 330 m·s^{-1} is considerably slower. This is because the speed of sound is dependent upon the medium it passes through; the higher the density of the medium the faster the speed of travel. Diagnostic ultrasound machines typically assume a fixed propagation velocity of 1540 m·s^{-1} for sound waves travelling through 'average' tissue.

The pulse-echo principle

Definition

The pulse-echo principle: measures the presence of, and distance from, an object from which an ultrasound wave has been reflected.

Ultrasound imaging is based on the very simple **pulse-echo** principle. If a person standing in a cave shouts loudly, an echo is heard as the sound bounces off the walls and is reflected back to their ears. The time taken for the sound to travel to the cave wall and back again depends on the distance to the wall: the length of delay being proportional to the length of the cave (see *Figure 23.1*).

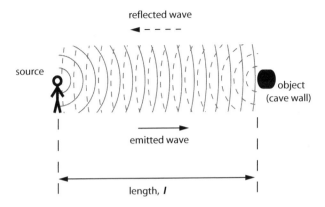

Figure 23.1. *Sound waves reflected from an object.*

An accurate measurement of distance may be obtained using this method if the velocity of sound in the cave is known and the time delay is measured accurately.

Distance is the product of velocity and the time, so:

$$2d = v \cdot t$$

23.1

where v is the velocity of the sound wave

t is the time taken

d is the distance of the object from the source/detector

Car parking sensors are simple ultrasound probes that alert a reversing driver that their car is about to bump into unseen objects. They repeatedly emit and then detect pulses of ultrasound waves: the shorter the time for the wave to be returned to the probe, the closer the object.

Creation of ultrasound waves

Ultrasound must be generated with precision to be of clinical use and the ceramic piezo-electric crystal is a near-perfect source of ultrasound waves. It has the property of expanding when an electric current flows through it in one direction and contracting when the current is reversed. So when an alternating current is applied, the crystal will vibrate at the frequency of the current, if the temperature remains below a certain temperature known as the Curie temperature. This is usually several hundred degrees

> **Definition**
>
> **Piezo-electric crystal:** the piezo-electric crystal contracts and expands when an alternating current is applied allowing sound waves to be generated.

celsius, and is the temperature at which the crystal loses its piezo-electric characteristics. Since the piezo-electric sources emit mechanical rather than electrical energy, ultrasound devices do not interfere greatly with electronic devices and fields.

Detection of ultrasound waves

A piezo-electric crystal also acts in reverse: to detect sound waves. A single probe can act as both an emitter and a receiver of reflected waves, analogous to a loudspeaker and a microphone combined. When the crystal is compressed by a sound wave it produces a small current, while a rarefaction produces a current flowing in the opposite direction. Measurement of the timing, amplitude and frequency of the current reveal all the properties of the arriving sound wave.

Ultrasound waves are emitted only in short bursts so that there are large pauses to allow the probe to carry out its other role as a detector of returning (reflected) ultrasound waves. Crucially it cannot be an emitter and detector at exactly the same time. The size of the gap between bursts must allow for the time taken for all reflected waves to have returned.

Transducer heads

Ultrasound probes are designed with a specific application in mind. The outer surface of the probe is generally shaped to fit the surface anatomy to ensure good acoustic contact between the probe and the tissue. The probe is usually covered in silicone rubber or similar material that matches the acoustic impedance (see *Section 23.2*) of the tissue and therefore transmits sound waves with maximum efficiency. The transducer itself is similarly arranged within the probe to maximize the transmission of sound energy to the tissue. The piezo-electric crystals typically used in ultrasound probes are thin slices of a ceramic crystal that is sized to resonate at the planned frequency of emission. The thickness works out to half a wavelength, in the order of 2 mm, depending on the target frequency.

Phased array

In modern usage, every ultrasound device encountered in the hospital that produces a 2D image on a screen uses a probe known as a **phased array**. A phased array has many small transducer units (emitter/receivers) arranged in a line (array), each unit being capable of transmitting independently. Sending a pulse of current to each unit simultaneously (*Figure 23.2a*) causes a wave to be emitted with its wavefront parallel to the array surface. On the other hand, sending a pulse to each transducer in a sequence (*Figure 23.2b*) causes the wave to exit at an angle. In fact any angle may be chosen, by adjusting the time delay between successive pulses, with a longer time delay producing a steeper angle.

The phased array takes advantage of constructive interference, whereby the spherical wavefronts from each transducer combine to form a straight wavefront that travels through the tissue. A series of waves may be sent out at different angles, effectively 'sweeping' across the tissue to achieve a fan-shaped scan. Phased arrays have greatly increased the capability and flexibility of modern ultrasound imaging systems.

23.2 Imaging modes

Formation of the image

The received pulses are used to form an image on the screen. In the most commonly used method (B-mode imaging), a beam sweeps from side to side, producing a fan-shaped scan. For each scan angle, the time taken for pulses to return to the transducer provides an indication of the depth of the

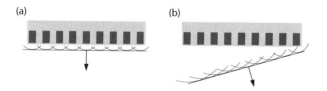

(a)   (b)

Figure 23.2. *A phased transducer array with (a) simultaneous current pulses, and (b) sequential current pulses.*

reflecting structure. The scanner highlights a dot (or pixel) on the screen, the more intense the pulse, the brighter the pixel. The dot is plotted on the screen in a position determined by its depth (and the scan angle). In this way, a linear or fan-shaped (sector) scan is produced which shows the position, shape and density of the structures within the tissue.

A-mode

A-mode is the simplest type of ultrasound. A single transducer scans a line through the body with the echoes plotted on the screen as a function of depth in one dimension. This was the first type of ultrasound but is now virtually obsolete.

B-mode

In B-mode ultrasound, a linear array of transducers scans a plane through the body that can be viewed as a two-dimensional image on screen, so that the position and density of structures is revealed. This is the most common method and is used for most imaging applications.

M-mode

M stands for motion. Ultrasound pulses are emitted in quick succession, and a one-dimensional A-mode image is taken. Each image is represented as a vertical line with brightness representing reflected intensity. Successive images are plotted next to each other (with time along the horizontal axis). This method is useful for finding the boundaries between different regions of the beating heart. The velocity of each structure relative to the probe over the entire cardiac cycle may easily be determined.

Doppler mode

This mode makes use of the Doppler effect (*Chapter 5*) in measuring and visualizing blood flow. The shift in velocity of the reflected pulse provides an indication of the velocity of the reflecting object. The simplest Doppler ultrasound method uses continuous-wave (CW) Doppler (see *Section 16.5*). Doppler information is sampled along a line through the body, and all velocities detected at each time point are plotted against time, in a similar principle to M-mode imaging. A more sophisticated method samples Doppler information from a small tissue volume (defined by the user in a two-dimensional image), and presented on a timeline. This method uses pulsed Doppler to resolve the depth as well as the velocity of the blood.

   Colour Doppler is an intuitive way of representing velocity information as a colour-coded overlay on top of a B-mode image. The velocity is represented as a spectrum of colour: flow away from the probe is usually represented as red, while flow towards the probe is blue. **Duplex imaging** is a commonly used term for the simultaneous presentation of two-dimensional and Doppler information.

Controls

Modern ultrasound scanners allow the user control over the appearance of the image, to maximize the information that can be inferred from the images. *Table 23.1* summarizes some of these controls.

23.3 Attenuation

If the voices of a man and a woman are heard from some distance away, they will often have quite different perceived qualities. The higher pitched female voice will be heard with more clarity than

Table 23.1 *Ultrasound image controls.*

Control	Function
Freeze	Allows image to be held so that measurement and other observations can be made. Images can be stored for diagnostics.
Res/zoom	This magnifies the area of interest (with a reduction in field of view).
Caliper	This allows the distance between two selected points to be measured (often used when the screen has been frozen).
Gain	Similar to a brightness function on a television. A limitation is that artefacts are also amplified.
Time gain compensation	An adjustment in sensitivity that compensates for signal loss when deeper tissue is being viewed.

Definition
Attenuation: the diminution of the energy associated with a sound wave as a result of absorption, spreading, reflection and scattering.

the deeper, lower pitched voice of the man. In contrast a deep male voice may be heard from further away than the higher pitched voice. This is because higher frequency waves are able to carry more detailed information, as more waves are detected in a given time, while the lower frequency waves travel further. A compromise is therefore needed when choosing an optimal frequency of waves for the purposes of medical imaging.

Attenuation is the reduction of amplitude and intensity of a signal and this reduction occurs because of energy loss by absorption, reflection (discussed below), dispersion and scattering (see *Table 23.2*). In ultrasound, attenuation is measured as the reduction in amplitude over distance. The total amount of attenuation is affected by the frequency of the transducer as well as the distance travelled through the tissue. Higher frequencies are attenuated much more strongly than lower frequencies. For example, ultrasound from an 8 MHz transducer will not penetrate very deeply into the body, compared to say a 2 MHz probe. Low frequency ultrasound penetrates deeper because there is less attenuation per unit of distance. The overall resolution produced by low frequencies, however, is poorer.

Table 23.2 *Forms of attenuation for ultrasound waves passing through tissue.*

Form of attenuation	Explanation
Absorption	Energy absorbed by the material the wave is travelling through. The energy is converted into thermal energy, causing a small rise in tissue temperature. The heating effect is too small to cause harm.
Scattering	A fraction of the energy of sound waves is scattered in random directions every time a change in acoustic impedance is encountered. Energy is not lost, but spreads out through the tissue. Higher frequency sound waves are more highly scattered.
Reflection	Reversal of direction propagation at a tissue boundary. This provides a mechanism for imaging using pulse-echo principle (discussed further in *Section 23.3*).
Dispersion	Energy decreases in wavefront as the wave spreads out when it travels from source. Dispersion depends on geometry of the wavefront (e.g. a linear wavefront is minimally dispersed).

Transducer frequencies used in medical ultrasound imaging range from 2 to 19 MHz. High frequencies are suitable for superficial imaging of small structures, e.g. vascular scanning typically uses 10 MHz ultrasound. Low frequencies (e.g. 2–5 MHz) are used in deep abdomen scanning of large structures.

Time gain compensation

Amplification of the signal counters the effect of attenuation by electronic amplification of the ultrasound waves causing a generalized increase in the 'brightness' of the image, allowing fine-tuning of the contrast. This is necessary due to the minor variations in the exact density of an individual's tissue. Time gain compensation (TGC) is an amplification technique used to compensate for increasing attenuation of ultrasound waves when attempting to image through large amounts of tissue. It can be thought of as the ability to increase the gain at specific tissue depths, which would otherwise appear too dark to see, because the waves are weaker. Modern ultrasound machines undertake some degree of automatic TGC, but manual manipulation is still important.

23.4 Reflection and acoustic impedance

Returning to the cave analogy, when a sound wave bounces off the rock face the vast majority of the wave's energy is reflected back while the rock absorbs very little of the energy. This phenomenon occurs as a result of two factors: the properties of the sound wave and the nature of the two materials involved, in this case rock and air. The key is acoustic impedance (Z) and the ratio of the

> **Definition**
>
> **Acoustic impedance:** acoustic energy is reflected at interfaces between tissues with differing acoustic impedances (Z).

impedance of the two structures. For rock and air, the difference in densities is great so nearly all of the sound is reflected. Strength of acoustic reflection increases as difference in Z increases.

Sound waves are changes in pressure propagating through a medium. Acoustic impedance is a measurement of the resistance to oscillation of the molecules in response to these pressure changes. Acoustic impedance is dependent on density in the same way that the speed of sound is dependent on density. In fact, acoustic impedance is directly proportional to tissue density.

Whenever a sound wave meets a material with differing acoustic impedance, a certain proportion of the sound wave is reflected back to the probe, while the remainder of the sound is transmitted across the boundary between the two materials (see *Figure 23.3a*). The fraction of sound intensity reflected is equal to the square of the difference between the impedances divided by the sum of the impedances:

> **Definition**
>
> **Acoustic impedance mismatch:** a large difference in acoustic impedance between two materials is known as an acoustic impedance mismatch, where the vast majority of the sound wave will be reflected back at the interface of the two materials.

$$R = \left(\frac{Z_1 - Z_2}{Z_1 + Z_2} \right)^2$$

23.2

where Z_1 is the impedance of the initial medium
Z_2 is the impedance of the medium beyond the interface

Clearly, if the impedances of the two tissues are very similar, there is minimal reflection. If the impedances are identical, there is no reflectance and the boundary is undetectable. *Table 23.3* lists the acoustic impedances of different body tissues.

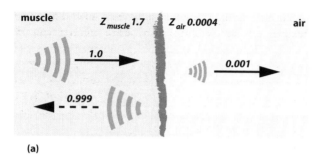

(a)

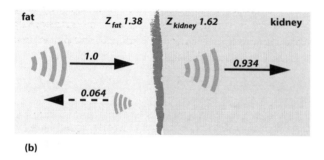

(b)

Figure 23.3. *Impedance and reflection of an ultrasound wave at an interface between materials of differing acoustic impedance.*

Units. The unit of acoustic impedance is the **rayl** (in base units, $Pa \cdot s \cdot m^{-1}$)

Acoustic shadowing

When there is a large disparity in the acoustic impedance between two materials, most of the energy of the sound wave is reflected at the boundary between the two materials. As a result, virtually none of the incident sound wave passes through the boundary to the deeper tissue beyond. Because of this, it is impossible to discern any information about structures lying behind the boundary. The large difference in acoustic impedance between a solid object such as a pacing box

Definition
Acoustic shadowing: occurs when there is near total reflection at an interface obstructing a view beyond the interface.

Table 23.3 *Typical speed of sound and acoustic impedances of different body tissues.*

Material	Speed of sound (m·s⁻¹)	Acoustic impedance, Z (×10⁻⁶ rayls)
Air	330	0.0004
Fat	1450	1.38
Water	1480	1.48
Blood	1570	1.65
Muscle	1580	1.70
Bone	4000	7.80

and tissue means that total reflection effectively occurs and nothing after the solid object can be visualized. Similarly, low impedance structures such as air bubbles can cause near-total reflection of the incoming sound wave.

A large proportion of an ultrasound wave is deflected at the bone/tissue interface making imaging impossible beyond the bone. This is why trans-thoracic echocardiograms (TTEs) are often limited in the views (windows) they can achieve because the probe has to peer through the ribcage. Virtually all of the energy of an ultrasound wave is reflected by an air/tissue interface and because of this imaging of structures near to the lungs is often obscured by air in the lungs.

Micro-bubbles as a contrast agent

Small bubbles are also viewed as distinct white objects and this can be taken advantage of by using micro-bubbles (suspended in agitated saline) as a contrast agent that is injected intravenously during an echocardiographic examination. They are clearly visible by ultrasound, and can be used to help identify septal defects in the heart and liver lesions.

Ultrasound gel

The interface between air and skin (or air and any other tissue) is a very effective reflector of sound waves. Any air between the ultrasound probe and the skin causes virtually all of the sound waves to be reflected before they have even reached the patient. A good acoustic contact is established by the application of **ultrasound gel**. The gel is water-based and has a similar acoustic impedance to skin, greatly increasing the transmission of sound to the tissue.

23.5 Resolution

Depth (or axial) resolution

Depth resolution is the ability to distinguish between two objects lying along the beam axis and is often referred to as axial resolution. When an ultrasound pulse wave is emitted, it is a burst of just two or three cycles, a short length. The length of the pulse determines axial resolution and higher frequency waves give better image resolution.

> **Definition**
>
> **Resolution:** the smallest size of object that can be displayed in the image.

Lateral resolution

Lateral resolution is the ability to distinguish two neighboring objects perpendicular to the beam and parallel to the transducer face. This is determined primarily by the width of the ultrasound beam. It is improved by focusing the beam, i.e. altering the beam width at the depth of interest.

Temporal resolution

The frame rate can be thought of as the number of pictures taken per second. Temporal resolution relates to the number of images captured per second and low temporal resolution might mean a jerky, stuttering image on the monitor screen.

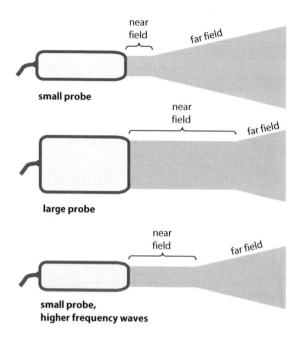

Figure 23.4. *The effect of probe size and frequency on near-field depth.*

Near-field and far-field resolution

In ultrasound imaging, the sonographer is concerned with the performance of the system at different depths within the tissue (or more technically, at different distances from the face of the probe). Two zones are defined, the **Fresnel zone** and the **Fraunhofer zone**, which refer to the near and far depths, respectively. The Fresnel zone is the region of highest image resolution. The size of each zone depends on the frequency (and thus the wavelength) of the ultrasound wave and the width of the ultrasound probe.

The Fresnel zone is the near-depth zone and is the best zone for optimum imaging. The larger the probe diameter the greater the depth of the near field and likewise the greater the frequency of the wave the deeper the near field becomes, as shown in *Figure 23.4*. In the Fraunhofer zone the sound waves start to steadily diverge. This divergence of the ultrasound beam can be corrected using a focusing lens. Modern imaging systems sometimes allow electronic setting of the focal point by the operator.

23.6 Cardiac ultrasound: TOE and TTE

Ultrasound imaging is ideally suited to assessing the heart: it can identify structures, assess function and measure flow. For the **trans-oesophogeal echocardiogram** (TOE), the ultrasound probe is inserted through the mouth down into the oesophagus, usually with local anaesthetic and sedation. The oesophagus is near to the heart, specifically the left atrium, and so this allows superb views of the mitral valve and left atrium, the left atrial appendage and the descending aorta. TOE is an invasive procedure and runs the risk of damaging the structures through which the probe is passed. Contraindications include oesophageal varices, hiatus hernia and previous oesophageal surgery. Complications can include dental damage and oesophageal perforation.

A **trans-thoracic echocardiogram** (TTE) involves placing an ultrasound probe on the external rib cage, but the bones of the rib cage obscure the view. It is well suited for viewing the anterior structures of the heart such as the aortic valve and pulmonary valve, though TTE is poor at looking at the posterior structures of the heart such as the mitral valve and left atrium.

23.7 Therapeutic ultrasound

At a party where there is very loud music being played windows might rattle and a drink on a table can vibrate. Famously, the high-pitched tones of an opera singer can shatter a glass. For these events to happen there has to be a transfer of energy from the sound waves to the objects.

> **Definitions**
>
> **Cavitation** (acoustic): the formation of bubbles in a liquid; the result of extreme negative pressure generated by high energy ultrasound waves.
> **Acoustic power:** a measure of the energy of sound wave per unit of time.

An ultrasound scan usually has waves with energy kept intentionally low so that tissue is not affected, but higher energy ultrasound waves can have dramatic effects on tissue. For each sound wave there is a trough of low pressure and a peak of high pressure, and the peaks and troughs in an ultrasound wave can be increased. This will result in larger fluctuations in pressure in the material the wave is travelling through during each cycle. This can be further exaggerated by manipulating the shape of the wave, making the transition from peak to trough sharper; in other words, there is a greater acceleration between high and low pressures.

Cavitation is the formation and collapse of small bubbles in a liquid. When pressure in a portion of a liquid falls below the vapour pressure for the liquid, then bubbles are created and grow. The bubbles then collapses violently as the pressure changes again. Though ultrasound transfers energy within a medium, it is important to remember that it does not transfer mass.

The beam of ultrasound can be focused on an area the size of a pinhead and this has aided more adept applications of ultrasound. Low-intensity and high-intensity focused ultrasound can be used for tumour ablation and destruction, treating conditions such as prostate cancer. Intensity of a sound wave is the power density measured in $W \cdot m^{-2}$. There are two indices that are used: the thermal index, the ability to raise temperature in tissue, and also the mechanical index, the potential to generate cavitation.

Shock wave lithotripsy

If the collapse of bubbles due to cavitation occurs near a boundary, such as a targeted kidney stone, a high velocity shock wave is formed that impacts the boundary with great force. This force can be sufficient to break up the stone, allowing it to pass naturally out of the body.

Phacoemulsification

Phacoemulsification is used in cataract surgery. Before the cataract is removed a small probe is inserted via a small incision in the cornea. This probe emits ultrasound waves that emulsify the cataract and the resultant fragments are then removed by suction.

Liposuction

An ultrasound 'wand' is positioned amongst fatty deposits and the ultrasound waves causes fat cells to vibrate rapidly, breaking up the cell walls to produce a liquefied fat and this, along with an injected liquid solvent, are then removed by suction.

Ultrasound nebulizers

Water is dropped onto an ultrasound-emitting transducer producing droplets with diameters from 1 to 2 µm. The frequency of the ultrasound is in the range of 1–3 MHz.

Summary

- Ultrasound waves are high frequency sound waves.
- A piezo-electric crystal is used both to generate and detect ultrasound waves.
- The pulse-echo principle simply measures the time a wave takes to hit an object and return and from this time the distance can be estimated.
- The Doppler effect measures flow because sound waves have an altered frequency if they are reflected from a moving object. However, if the flow is perpendicualr to the sound wave the Doppler effect is absent.
- Sound waves carry energy. An ultrasound wave can be used to destroy tissue if it has a high enough energy.

Single best answer questions

For these questions, choose the single best answer.

1. The Doppler effect is best described as:
   (a) an increase in amplitude when the emitting source is moving away from the receiver
   (b) an increase in wavelength when the emitting source is moving away from the receiver
   (c) a decrease in amplitude when the emitting source is moving towards the receiver
   (d) the generation of high positive and negative pressures causing cavitation
   (e) the degree of reflection of waves at a media boundary

2. Cavitation is best described as:
   (a) the solidification in a liquid as a result of extreme negative pressure generated by high energy ultrasound waves
   (b) the forming of bubbles in a liquid as a result of extreme negative pressure generated by low energy ultrasound waves
   (c) the removal of bubbles in a liquid as a result of extreme negative pressure generated by high energy ultrasound waves
   (d) the formation of bubbles in a liquid as a result of extreme negative pressure generated by high energy ultrasound waves
   (e) the generation of images in deep tissue as a result of extreme negative pressure generated by high energy ultrasound waves

3. The Doppler effect is best described as:
   (a) the change in amplification of a wave resulting from motion of the wave's source or the observer
   (b) the delay in reflection of a wave resulting from motion of the wave's source or the observer
   (c) the change in the frequency of a wave resulting from motion of the wave's source or the observer
   (d) the brightness of image resulting from movement of the wave's source or the observer
   (e) the range of frequencies of a wave resulting from reflection from an uneven surface

Multiple choice questions

For each of these questions, mark every answer either true or false.

1. The definition of an ultrasound image is improved with:
   (a) higher frequency of ultrasound wave
   (b) increased wavelength of ultrasound wave
   (c) the closer the object is to the probe
   (d) a decrease in atmospheric pressure
   (e) all media being of similiar densities

2. Regarding the frequency of ultrasound waves travelling trough tissue, which of the following statements are true?
   (a) Higher frequency waves are attenuated less than low frequency waves.
   (b) Higher frequency waves are attenuated more than low frequency waves.
   (c) Higher frequency waves have a higher velocity and are attenuated less than low frequency waves.
   (d) Higher frequency waves have a lower velocity and are attenuated less than low frequency waves.

   (e) Higher frequency waves provide more detailed images than lower frequency waves.

3. Regarding ultrasound imaging, which of the following statements are true?
   (a) The caliper function allows the distance between two selected points to be measured.
   (b) The freeze function allows the image to be held so that measurement and other observations can be made.
   (c) The Fresnel zone is the near-depth zone and is the worst zone for optimum imaging.
   (d) Transducer frequencies used in medical ultrasound imaging range from 20 to 190 MHz.
   (e) Time gain compensation is an amplification technique used to compensate for increasing attenuation of ultrasound waves.

Chapter 24

Lasers

Having read this chapter you will be able to:
- Appreciate the electron energy levels within the atom.
- Understand the principle behind the laser.
- Understand the difference between light from a laser and from other sources.
- Appreciate the risks and precautions needed when using lasers.

24.1 The principle of the laser

> **Definition**
>
> **Laser:** a device that emits a highly controlled continuous beam of coherent monochromatic light; laser is an acronym of **l**ight **a**mplification by **s**timulated **e**mission of **r**adiation.

The American physicist Theodore Maiman invented the laser in 1960. At the time lasers seemed like a novelty with no obvious application, prompting a fellow scientist to describe lasers as a 'solution in search of a problem'. However, within a few years, lasers were well-established scientific and engineering tools. Laser surgery was established by the beginning of the 1970s, and one of the earliest techniques was welding of a detached retina by ophthalmic surgeons. Today lasers have thousands of medical and non-medical uses, and research is still extending their incredible application range.

Lasers are mostly used in surgery for cutting tissue and for thermal coagulation in and around surgical sites. Ophthalmic lasers are used for retinal surgery and for corrective corneal reshaping. Non-surgical uses include photodynamic therapy and tattoo removal.

Energy levels

> **Definition**
>
> **Energy levels:** electrons can only occupy specific energy levels in an atom or molecule, and can jump from one level to another; the lowest level is called the ground state.

Imagine someone climbing a rope while another climbs a ladder. If you wanted to describe how high each one had climbed, it would be much easier to say for the one on the ladder; you would merely need to say which rung of the ladder they had reached. The person on the rope could be in any one of a multitude of positions. One of the revolutionary findings of quantum physics was the discovery that the electrons within the atom act more like the person climbing the ladder than the person climbing up the rope, i.e. they can only exist at certain set energy levels.

As discussed in *Section 1.1*, the Rutherford–Bohr model of the atom replaced the planetary model whereby electrons exist in discrete shells around the atomic nucleus. If the electron drops to a lower level (shell) the energy difference between the two levels is emitted from the atom in the form of a photon (a packet or 'quanta' of electromagnetic energy) as shown in *Figure 24.1*. Conversely, a photon absorbed by an atom can cause an electron to move to a higher energy level.

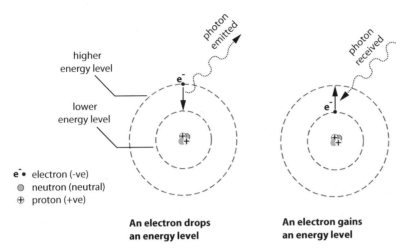

Figure 24.1. *An electron changing energy states.*

A general laser

A laser is essentially a light amplifier, i.e. it produces a high-energy stream of photons, or a laser beam, from a small number of initial photons. A laser comprises a laser tube constructed from an **active lasing medium** that can be a gas, solid or a liquid, with a mirror at each end of the tube (*Figure 24.2*). Injecting energy from an external source causes the lasing medium to become excited. Gas lasers are excited using an electric current applied to either end of the laser tube, while **solid state** and liquid lasers are excited using a high intensity light source. The mirrors cause photons to bounce back and forth within the laser medium, triggering further emission of photons by the process of **stimulated emission**. One mirror is partially reflective which allows some photons to escape in the form of the laser beam. The beam is then focused as required.

Excitation of the lasing medium

As its name implies, a laser is essentially a light amplifier. In order to understand how the laser works we must consider what happens in the medium in which the light amplification takes place. This

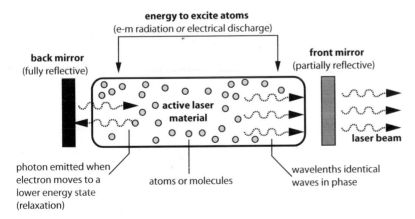

Figure 24.2. *A simplified diagram of a general laser.*

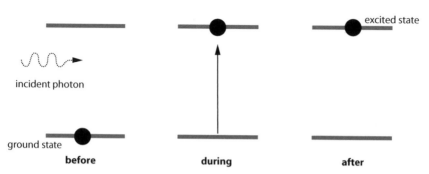

Figure 24.3. *A photon of the correct energy can be absorbed by an electron. After absorption, the electron is in a higher energy state.*

is called the 'lasing' medium and a simplified energy level diagram can represent the atoms in this medium. An electron in the ground state, E_1, can absorb a photon of energy and be excited up to level E_2 as shown in *Figure 24.3*. Alternatively, atoms can be excited by heat or electric charge. In either case, the amount of energy absorbed by the electron ΔE is equal to the difference between the ground state and the excited state, that is:

$$\Delta E = E_2 - E_1$$

24.1

Spontaneous emission

When an electron is excited, it will not stay that way forever. After an indeterminate length of time, somewhere in the order of 10^{-10} seconds, the electron will decay back to the lower energy level (*Figure 24.4*). When such a spontaneous decay occurs, the energy difference between the excited state and the lower energy level is released by the emission of a photon. The wavelength of the photon is inversely proportional to the difference in energy ΔE.

If a bunch of electrons were put into an excited state and allowed to decay by spontaneous emission the resulting radiation would be spectrally limited (i.e. all the photons would have the same wavelength), but the individual photons would all be released at random times and in random directions. This is more or less what happens in a fluorescent light tube.

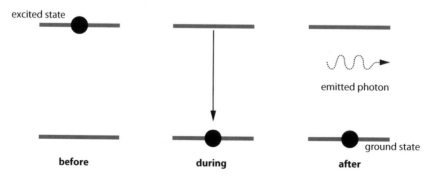

Figure 24.4. *Spontaneous decay results in emission of a photon with the same energy as the difference between the excited and ground states.*

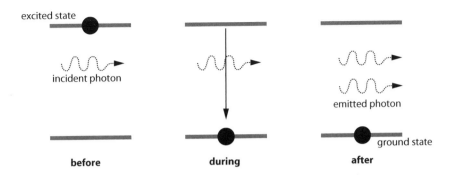

excited state

incident photon

emitted photon

ground state

before　　　　　　　**during**　　　　　　　**after**

Figure 24.5. *During stimulated emission, a photon causes an excited atom to decay to the ground state, causing emission of a second photon with the same wavelength and phase.*

Stimulated emission

Other photons in the vicinity of an atom can affect an atom's state. Specifically, the atom will oscillate slightly as the photon passes, because the electrons are electrically charged and therefore respond to the photon, essentially an oscillating electric field. One of the consequences of this oscillation is that it encourages electrons to decay to the lower energy state, as shown in *Figure 24.5*. When an incident photon causes a **decay**, the emitted photon is emitted at exactly the same time as the passing photon, so the photons are said to be in **phase** with each other, and they travel away in the same direction.

In normal conditions, electrons spend most of their time in the ground state, or at a low energy level. However, a large number of atoms may be excited by a large input of energy in the form of a large injection of photons, heat or electric charge. In this case the electrons are predominantly at higher energy levels as they jump up quicker than they can spontaneously decay back to the ground state, resulting in a so-called 'population inversion'.

Photons of the correct energy passing through a medium exhibiting population inversion can cause stimulated emission. Because we start with one photon and end up with two, we have light amplification. Photons released by stimulated emission can go on to stimulate further emissions, resulting in an avalanche effect. The photons bounce back and forth from the mirrors at each end of the laser tube, and soon a very large number of photons with the same wavelength, direction and timing (phase) are produced. A proportion of the photons emerge from the half-silvered mirror in the form of the laser beam, which is monochromatic, collimated (in a fine beam) and **coherent**. A coherent beam is one that is highly organized so that all its photons are in step with each other, i.e. they have the same phase.

24.2 Types of medical laser

The most commonly encountered medical lasers are summarized in *Table 24.1*. Laser light of any wavelength can cause thermal effects when absorbed by tissue. The exact effects depend on the wavelength and the power of the emitted laser light. Certain wavelengths are absorbed more strongly in tissue, particularly some of the infrared wavelengths. The emitted wavelength depends on the material of the lasing medium, and lasers are constructed with output powers suitable for their intended application, with general surgical lasers exceeding 100 W.

Table 24.1. *Commonly used medical lasers.*

Name	Lasing medium	Wavelength	Uses
Carbon dioxide laser	Gas (carbon dioxide)	Infrared (10.6 µm)	Surgical cutting
Argon ion laser	Gas (argon)	Visible (488–514 nm)	Retinal surgery, e.g. welding detached retina
Nd:YAG laser	Solid (garnet)	Infrared (1.06 µm)	Hyperthermia, coagulation
Dye laser	Liquid (dye solution)	Visible–infrared (380 nm–1.0 µm)	Dermatology, tattoo removal
Ho:YAG	Solid (garnet)	Infrared (2.12 µm)	Surgical cutting via optical fibres
Excimer laser	Gas (noble gas)	Ultraviolet (130–350 nm)	Corrective corneal reshaping

Perhaps the most common medical laser is the **carbon dioxide laser** used for surgical cutting. Its infrared radiation is very strongly absorbed by tissue, producing heat that vaporizes the tissue in the region of the laser spot, so tissue is removed by the process of ablation. The resulting incision is inherently sterile, due to the heat generated in the surrounding tissue, which also cauterizes the surrounding vessels, minimizing surgical bleeding. The **XeF excimer laser** is a UV-emitting gas laser that produces a very precise energetic beam suitable for corrective eye surgery. The **argon ion laser** emits blue–green visible light that is naturally focused onto the retina by the lens of the eye, making it suitable for repair of a detached retina.

Solid state lasers used in medicine include the **Nd:YAG** (neodymium doped yttrium aluminium garnet) laser. Infrared radiation from this laser is weakly absorbed by tissue, which results in dissipation of heat over a large volume, making it suitable for phototherapy and coagulation. Glass optical fibres are transparent to infrared radiation emitted by the Ho:YAG (holmium YAG) laser so it can be used for surgical cutting in conjunction with fibreoptic light guides. Dye lasers are available with a very wide range of emission wavelengths in the visible range, including red, yellow and green. These 'tunable' lasers are used for tattoo removal and other non-surgical applications including treatment of port-wine stains and other dermatological conditions.

Continuous wave lasers produce a constant beam, while **pulsed lasers** switch on and off very rapidly. Pulsed surgical lasers produce much less thermal damage to surrounding tissue than continuous wave lasers of the same power. This is because the pulse delivers a high concentration of energy, causing ablation and removal of tissue. The period between each pulse allows the heat energy to be carried away by the vaporized tissue, and allows cooling of the neighbouring tissues before the arrival of the next pulse.

24.3 Precautions with laser treatment

Lasers are potentially dangerous due to their high energy density (see *Figure 24.6*). The risk is compounded by the invisible nature of infrared laser beams. The power of the laser beam also

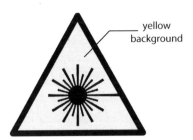

yellow
background

Figure 24.6. *Universal laser warning sign.*

determines the level of risk and this should be assessed and categorized into a class, as outlined in *Table 24.2*. Lasers pose very high risks to the eyes, particularly the cornea, lens and retina; even momentary exposure can cause serious injury including permanent blindness. For this reason, eye protection in the form of goggles is almost always required. The lenses of safety goggles are constructed from different materials depending on the wavelength of the laser. Infrared light from a carbon dioxide laser is completely absorbed by ordinary glass, so glass lenses provide complete protection from eye damage when these lasers are used. This does not apply to all lasers, however, so specific eye goggles should be used. Even very low-powered lasers can cause irreversible eye damage.

Polished instruments can reflect laser beams and for this reason instruments used in conjunction with laser therapy often have a matt surface. The use of high-energy beams of light increases the risks of ignition of flammable substances and of explosion. A patient who is receiving oxygen therapy should be treated with caution as many normally non-flammable materials exposed to a laser beam can combust in the presence of oxygen. Specialist heat-resistant oxygen tubing is manufactured for use when lasers are present.

Table 24.2. *Risk classification for laser beam exposure.*

Class 1	Safe under reasonably foreseeable conditions.
Class 1M	As Class 1 but not safe when viewed with optical aids such as eye loupes or binoculars.
Class 2	The eye is protected by the aversion responses, including the blink reflex and head movement. *Only applies to visible laser beams.*
Class 2M	As Class 2 but not safe when viewed with optical aids such as eye loupes or binoculars.
Class 3R	More likely to cause harm to the eye than lower class lasers but do not need as many control measures as higher class lasers.
Class 3B	Eye damage likely to occur if the beam is viewed directly or reflected.
Class 4	Eye and skin damage likely from the main laser beam and also reflected beams. Heightened risk of fires.

Summary
- Lasers work by stimulated emission of an excited lasing medium.
- Lasers emit monochromatic, coherent and directional light. This allows a focused, high-energy beam to be delivered.
- Infrared lasers are used for surgical cutting, ablation, coagulation and phototherapy.
- Visible light lasers are used for retinal surgery and dermatological treatments.
- Pulsed lasers are used to limit thermal damage to collateral tissue.
- Laser procedures should be categorized by risk and clinicians made aware of the level of risk.
- Care must be taken with lasers: reflected laser beams can cause injury particularly to the eye. Specialist eye protection should be used with all lasers.

Single best answer questions

For these questions, choose the single best answer.

1. A laser beam is best described as:
   (a) monochromatic, in phase and directional
   (b) dichromatic, powerful and directional
   (c) monochromatic, out of phase and powerful
   (d) metachromatic, coherent and directional
   (e) dichromatic, in phase and coherent

2. A laser beam is produced by exploiting:
   (a) the odd numbers of electrons in a nucleus
   (b) the energy levels in neutrons
   (c) certain isotopes with odd electron numbers
   (d) the quantum energy levels of electrons
   (e) paired nucleons at fixed energy levels

3. Which one of the following lasers emits visible light?
   (a) Ho:YAG laser.
   (b) Excimer laser.
   (c) Argon ion laser.
   (d) Carbon dioxide laser.
   (e) Nd:YAG laser.

4. Which one of the following is true regarding laser safety?
   (a) The eye is protected by aversion responses for all lasers.
   (b) Invisible lasers can cause retinal injury.
   (c) Ordinary glass goggles can prevent eye damage from Ho:YAG lasers.
   (d) Class 1 and 2 lasers do not require eye protection.
   (e) Reflected beams from Class 4 lasers only can cause eye damage.

5. Thermal injury to surrounding tissue:
   (a) is minimized by pulsed lasers as the laser is less powerful than a continuous wave laser
   (b) is less likely for a carbon dioxide laser than an Nd:YAG laser
   (c) is less likely for a continuous laser, because ablation removes energy more effectively than with a pulsed laser
   (d) is not possible with visible light lasers
   (e) is less likely for a pulsed laser than a continuous wave laser as the tissue cools between pulses

Multiple choice questions

For each of these questions, mark every answer either true or false.

1. Concerning the production of a laser beam, which of the following are true?
   (a) Changes in energy levels in the nucleus play a significant role.
   (b) Electrons are emitted when the electron is forced to a higher energy level.
   (c) The electromagnetic waves produced are in phase.
   (d) The waves produced are monochromatic.
   (e) All medical lasers use carbon dioxide (gas form) as their 'laser medium'.

2. For laser light to be produced:
   (a) a gas medium must be excited by an injection of energetic photons
   (b) the excitation current must be pulsed rapidly
   (c) a mirror at both ends of the laser tube reflects photons back and forth
   (d) stimulated emission produces monochromatic photons
   (e) light amplification by spontaneous emission must occur

3. Which of the following are true concerning the risks associated with lasers?
   (a) It is only the cornea that is potentially affected when the eye is exposed to lasers.
   (b) All laser beams essentially carry the same risks.
   (c) Standard oxygen tubing is safe for use in the presence of all procedures involving exposure to lasers.
   (d) Polished surgical instruments should be avoided in the presence of lasers.
   (e) Clinicians should be aware of the laser classification associated with the procedure prior to commencing treatment.

4. Which of the following lasers are not normally used for surgery?
   (a) Argon ion laser.
   (b) Carbon dioxide laser.
   (c) Ho:YAG laser.
   (d) Nd:YAG laser.
   (e) Dye laser.

5. Spontaneous emission:
   (a) produces monochromatic, incoherent, directional light
   (b) produces polychromatic, coherent, directional light
   (c) produces polychromatic, incoherent light
   (d) does not require energy input
   (e) takes place in a fluorescent tube

Chapter 25
Magnetic resonance imaging

Having read this chapter you will be able to:
- Understand the principle of magnetic resonance imaging.
- Explain superconductivity and why it helps deliver a powerful magnetic field.
- Understand the importance of proton spin and magnetic dipoles to MRI.
- Know the fundamentals of how images are formed by the scanner.
- Be aware of the safety aspects of MRI scanners.

25.1 Principles of magnetic resonance imaging

<table>
<tr><td>

Definition

Nuclear magnetic resonance: a phenomenon, exploited for medical imaging, whereby the nuclei of molecules placed in a strong magnetic field absorb radio waves supplied by a transmitter at particular frequencies. When the source of the radio waves is turned off nuclei emit electromagnetic waves, which are analysed to produce an image.

</td><td>

Magnetic resonance imaging (MRI) is a medical imaging technique used to visualize detailed internal structures within the body. A powerful magnetic field is used to align the magnetization of atoms (actually the nuclei of atoms) within the tissue. The alignment is manipulated by applying electromagnetic energy, and the response to the applied energy is measured by detecting tiny amounts of electromagnetic energy emitted by the nuclei. These emissions are used to build up a detailed image of internal structures of the tissue. MRI images provide good contrast between different soft tissues, making MRI suitable for imaging the brain, internal organs, muscles and cancerous tissue.

</td></tr>
</table>

The original name for the technique was more descriptive: nuclear magnetic resonance (NMR), but it was thought that the general public would fear the word 'nuclear', associating it with radioactivity, so it was renamed. MRI has the advantage that it does not use ionizing radiation, unlike X-ray or CT imaging.

Superconductivity

<table>
<tr><td>

Definition

Superconductivity: the phenomenon whereby a material conducts an electrical current with virtually no resistance.

</td><td>

Superconductivity is a remarkable phenomenon whereby when certain metals and ceramic materials are cooled to very low temperatures, they completely lose their electrical resistance. The electrons within the material can then move without restraint, so superconductors are able to conduct an incredibly large current

</td></tr>
</table>

without the loss of energy in the form of heat. This phenomenon paved the way for the building of immensely powerful electromagnets (see *Chapter 19*) capable of producing incredibly strong magnetic fields.

At the heart of the MRI machine sits an electromagnet, containing a superconducting coil bathed in liquid helium to maintain the low temperature needed for superconductivity. An electric current transferred to the coil will circulate indefinitely, consuming no energy. The induced magnetic flux density is typically 0.5–3 tesla (the earth's magnetic field is only 0.000006 T), which is so strong that it can propel a metal drip stand through the air. The magnetic fields generated are not only strong but are also remarkably uniform; a quality crucial for high definition imaging. The wire coils are constructed from superconductive material such as niobium–titanium alloy and must be kept at a temperature below –250°C (23 K) to maintain their superconducting properties.

Units. The magnetic flux density is measured in tesla and is between 0.5 and 3 tesla (1 T = 10 000 gauss) in an MRI scanner.

Nuclear spin

The study of the atom over the last hundred years has revealed surprising complexity. Atoms were once thought to be indivisible, but it was shown that each one contains a tiny nucleus surrounded by orbiting electrons. It was then found that the nucleus is made up of nucleons, namely protons and neutrons. Now it is understood that these protons and neutrons are made up of even smaller particles called quarks.

> **Definition**
>
> **Spin:** a property of certain subatomic particles and nuclei; charged particles with spin possess a magnetic dipole.

Atoms with an odd number of protons and neutrons exhibit a property that physicists call **spin**. A hydrogen nuclei (a single proton) has a positive charge, and as all moving charges create a magnetic field, then spinning protons produce a small field known as a **magnetic dipole**. Normally, the directions of the magnetic dipoles of all the hydrogen atoms are randomly aligned, but when they are exposed to an external magnetic field, the dipoles line up with the direction of the applied field. The dipoles align in one of two ways: either *with* the magnetic field or *against* it (parallel or anti-parallel), as shown in *Figure 25.1*. A small but consistent majority align *with* the magnetic field. Because the body is composed largely of water (H_2O), hydrogen is the most abundant element in the human body. The hydrogen nuclei are thus magnetically active and their presence is revealed in MRI images.

The spin of the proton is akin to a spinning top spinning on its axis. In the presence of an applied magnetic field, the proton **precesses** (i.e. rotates) around an axis, tilted with respect to its axis of rotation, as shown in *Figure 25.1*. The frequency of precession is proportional to the strength of the applied field, and is known as the **Larmour frequency**. At the magnetic field strengths used in clinical MRI systems (0.5–3 T), the Larmour frequency of hydrogen ranges from 21.3 to 128 MHz.

Excitation and relaxation of protons

Once the nuclei are aligned with the magnetic field (either parallel or anti-parallel, see *Figure 25.2*), another coil in the scanner emits a pulse of electromagnetic radiation in the radio frequency (RF)

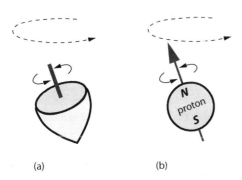

(a)   (b)

Figure 25.1. *Like a spinning top (a) the proton (b) spins or 'precesses'.*

(a)

(b)

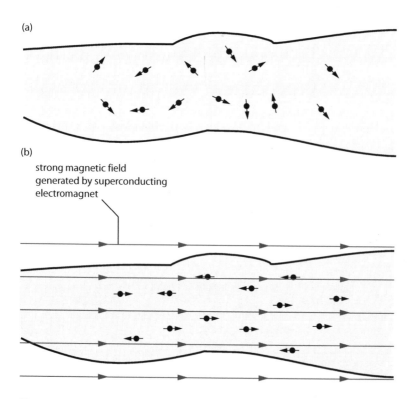

strong magnetic field
generated by superconducting
electromagnet

Figure 25.2. *Alignment of hydrogen nuclei in a MRI scan of a knee. Before the scan (a) there is no alignment. During the scan (b), the hydrogen nuclei align with the strong magnetic field generated by the superconducting electromagnet.*

range, perpendicular to the magnetic field. The energy is absorbed by some of the parallel protons, causing them to 'flip' their dipole to the opposite direction to the strong field, as shown in *Figure 25.3a*. These protons are now anti-parallel, so are in a higher energy state. The RF radiation must be close to the **Larmour frequency**; if so, the proton will 'resonate' and absorb energy; no other frequency will transfer energy effectively (resonant frequencies are discussed in *Chapter 5*).

After the electromagnetic pulse is switched off, the newly anti-parallel hydrogen nuclei revert to the parallel lower-energy state. They release the difference in energy as RF photons (see *Figure 25.3b*), which are detected by the scanner as tiny electromagnetic pulses. The RF-transmitting coil now becomes a highly sensitive passive sensor coupled to a computer, allowing a change in behaviour of just a very small proportion of hydrogen atoms to be detected and processed into an image. In effect the hydrogen atoms have been turned into mini radio transmitters, broadcasting where there is water, fat or other compounds containing hydrogen. As different tissues contain a different density of hydrogen atoms, anatomical structures can be revealed in the final image.

Producing the image

As energy must be conserved, the resonant Larmour frequency dictates the frequency of the emitted photons. The photons emitted have an energy (and therefore a frequency) that depends on the energy absorbed when the hydrogen dipole was flipped. This frequency is equal to the Larmour frequency which, as mentioned above, is in turn dependent on the applied field strength.

(a)

(b)

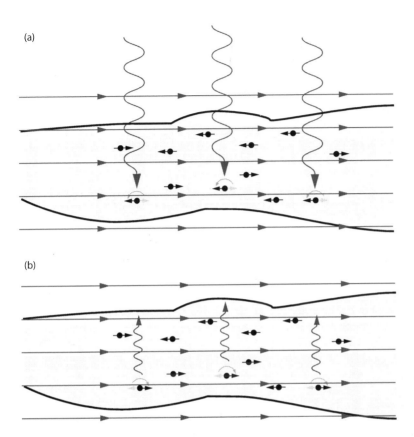

Figure 25.3. *RF radiation transmitted to the tissue (a) causes hydrogen nuclei to 'flip' into the anti-parallel (higher energy state). When the RF pulse is switched off (b) the hydrogen nuclei return to their initial state, releasing energy in the form of RF photons, which are detected by the scanner.*

The relationship between field strength and frequency is fundamental to the ability of MRI systems to produce an image. The exact position in three dimensions from which photons are released is found by applying additional fields during scanning. Electric currents are passed through additional coils, known as **gradient coils**. These fields make the magnetic field strength vary depending on the position within the patient. This means that the Larmour frequency and thus the frequency of emitted photons is dependent on their position, so their locations can be mathematically recovered from the acquired signal.

The RF pulse is switched on and off many times as the patient is successively scanned. For each scanning position, gradient fields are applied in two dimensions, producing a cross-sectional image built up from RF measurements made from every position within the 'slice'. A series of two-dimensional images can be combined, allowing high-resolution three-dimensional representations of the internal structure of the body to be obtained.

T1 and T2 relaxation

The amount of time taken for the hydrogen nuclei to relax and emit a photon can also reveal information about the tissue composition. Because the applied electromagnetic waves have a magnetic field component, which is perpendicular to the main field, they cause further alignment of the protons. There are now two magnetic fields perpendicular to one another, creating two vectors perpendicular to each other, which can be measured independently when the pulse is turned off. One is the restoration of **longitudinal magnetization (T1 relaxation)**, parallel to the main field, and the other is **transverse relaxation (T2 relaxation)**. Hydrogen atoms in different tissues return to their equilibrium states at different times, allowing differentiation between different tissue types. In a **T2-weighted scan**, for example, tissue with high water content appears brighter than fat-containing tissue, making this type of scan suitable for imaging injuries where oedema is present.

Contrast dye for MRI

Most MRI contrast agents work by shortening the T1 relaxation time of protons located nearby. The T1 shortening is stimulated by thermal vibration of strongly paramagnetic metal ions, which create oscillating electromagnetic fields at the correct resonant frequency (or energy) to cause the nuclei to rapidly flip back to their parallel state.

MRI contrast agents may be administered orally or by injection. Oral administration is well suited to scans of the GI tract, while intravascular administration is suitable for most other scans. The contrast substances used in MRI are **gadolinium chelates** which are very different from the iodine-derived contrast media used during CT scans or other X-ray type techniques. Gadolinium is useful because it has seven unpaired electrons which makes it strongly paramagnetic and results in a much stronger localized magnetic field. It is commonly used to help identify tumours and also in MRI angiography.

25.2 Safety considerations

MRI scanning rooms are restricted areas due to the high magnetic fields present. No ferrous metal objects are allowed in the room. The room is shielded from rogue electromagnetic radiation, particularly radio waves, which could interfere with the sensitive detection coils of the scanner. The room should include a quenching vent for coolant vapour release and also a **waveguide** (a copper tube that allows patient monitoring cable to pass from the scanner room to the observation/control room).

Exposure of equipment to magnetic fields

Projectile hazards are a potential danger to staff, patients and equipment within the scanner room. When ferromagnetic objects enter the scanner they will be attracted by the magnetic field and if loose they may be flung through the air. Non-ferrous metal objects in the scanner will not be attracted to the field; however, currents are induced in the objects when the fields are switched on and off. This produces a risk of burns from resistive heating; even limb-to-limb skin contact can create a burn, because tissue is an electrical conductor. Foam pads are placed between the limbs to prevent this. Because of the high magnetic field strength, pacemakers and internal cardioverters (DCIs) are generally contra-indicated for MRI scans. The strong field will also erase data on credit cards, ID cards, and anything else with magnetic encoding. Electronic devices including NIRS or pulse oximeter probes should also not be used unless they are labelled as MRI-safe.

Dedicated equipment for MRI scanners containing non-ferrous components should be available and clearly labelled as such. Titanium is non-ferromagnetic, making it ideal for implants and surgical

Table 25.1. *Four categories of medical device showing compatibility with MRI scanners.*

Category	Description
MR-compatible	The equipment can function within the MRI scanner
MR-safe	The equipment can enter the MRI scanner but may not function
MR-conditional	Advice needs to be sought as to whether the equipment may enter the scanner
MR-unsafe	Equipment must not enter MRI scanner

instruments for procedures carried out under MRI guidance. Aluminium can also enter an MRI scanner. *Table 25.1* describes the four categories describing the safe use of medical devices (including implanted devices) in MRI scanners.

Note that newer scanners have increased magnetic flux density (from around 1.5 T to around 3 T). This may mean that some equipment previously classified as MR-safe may now need re-classifying for the higher level of magnetic field.

Exposure of staff and patients to magnetic fields

Although MRI scanners create both a powerful magnetic field and emit electromagnetic radiation, they do not change the structure of the tissues they scan. This is because the electromagnetic waves are non-ionizing: that is, their energy is not great enough to change the structure of the molecules they interact with. Nevertheless, the abnormally high magnetic fields created by an MRI scanner can be harmful and there are guidelines for the maximum intermittent exposure and background exposure for staff and for patients. There are no known or expected harmful effects on humans using field strengths of up to 10 T. As opposed to steady fields, rapidly changing fields can cause hazardous effects. If the rate of change exceeds $20\,T\cdot s^{-1}$, the fields can induce eddy currents, which can cause micro-shock. This may be observed in patients during scanning because they often experience slight peripheral nerve stimulation.

Quenching

Quenching either occurs spontaneously due to a fault or by activation of the emergency magnet stop button. When this occurs the liquid cryogens that were cooling the magnet's coils boil off rapidly, and the resulting vapour then escapes very rapidly. The coils cease to be superconducting and become resistive. A quench

Definition
Quenching: occurs when the liquid cryogens that cool the magnet coils boil off rapidly.

will in general be accompanied by a loud bang, or a violent hissing sound as the cold gas escapes.

MRI scanners are fitted with quench pipes that lead vapours to the outside. In the event of these being blocked or some other failure, the cryogenic liquids and their vapours can deliver thermal burns to the skin or even frostbite. Inhalation of extremely cold vapours can damage the lungs and the rapidly released vapours can displace the majority of air present and, with the shortage of oxygen, asphyxiation can occur.

In some circumstances an emergency stop of the magnetic field is needed, such as if a patient becomes pinned against a magnet. It should be noted that stopping the magnetic field causes a considerable delay in scanning because it can take a few days for the coils to be cooled and the scanner to be brought back to working order.

The anaesthetized patient in the MRI scanner

The unit that holds the MRI scanner should ideally be specifically designed to allow easy access to the patient. The bore of the scanner is quite small and can feel claustrophobic to some patients and so sedation may be required. An MRI scanner is noisy due to the rapid on–off switching of the RF coils in the strong magnetic field, which causes significant mechanical movement. Some scanners cause up to 120 dB of noise so ear guards are usually worn. This also means that monitoring alarms will be difficult to hear so a clear view of the monitors is required. During scanning the patient is moved on a table in and out of the scanner very slowly, so access to the patient is severely limited.

Summary

- Superconductors have virtually no resistance to electric current and are used in MRI scanners to produce powerful magnetic fields.
- MRI utilizes the property of hydrogen nuclei that they spin and so have a small magnetic field, and align themselves with the scanner's magnetic field.
- Radiofrequency signals are emitted by hydrogen nuclei in response to a pulse of electromagnetic radiation in the radiofrequency range.
- The image is reconstructed from the detected radiofrequency signals.
- Different tissues have a different density of hydrogen nuclei, so MRI images produce good differentiation between soft tissues.
- The magnetic field strength inside an MRI scanner is very high, so ferromagnetic materials cannot be placed inside, or brought within close proximity to the scanner.
- Equipment used in the vicinity of an MRI scanner must be marked as MRI-safe or MRI-compatible.

Single best answer questions

For these questions, choose the single best answer.

1. Superconducting coils in MRI scanners:
   (a) can be metals, semiconductors or ceramics
   (b) can be cooled with liquid nitrogen
   (c) will allow currents to circulate indefinitely
   (d) are made from copper
   (e) can be switched on and off rapidly

2. Nuclear spin:
   (a) is a property shared by all atomic nuclei
   (b) is related to the strength of the applied magnetic field
   (c) creates a magnetic dipole in charged particles
   (d) can be transferred from one particle to another
   (e) causes precession of the nucleus in the absence of an applied field

3. Which one of the following could be safely placed in an MRI scanner?
   (a) A mobile phone.
   (b) A standard implantable pacemaker.
   (c) A titanium internal fixator.
   (d) A stainless steel wristwatch.
   (e) A pulse oximeter probe.

Multiple choice questions

For each of these questions, mark every answer either true or false.

1. Regarding magnetism, which of the following statements are true?
   (a) Magnetic fields are measured in coulombs.
   (b) There are no known side-effects to the magnetic fields generated in MRI scans.
   (c) Even very strong magnetic fields are not capable of lifting a drip stand off the floor.
   (d) All moving electric charges generate a magnetic field.
   (e) Superconductors allow strong magnetic fields to be generated.

2. The applied RF pulse:
   (a) causes photons to flip from the anti-parallel to the parallel state
   (b) is measured using a second coil
   (c) must be switched on and off to allow relaxation times to be recorded
   (d) is applied parallel to the strong field
   (e) is at a frequency related to the strong field

3. The gradient coils:
   (a) apply a magnetic field which varies from one part of the body to another
   (b) allow the density of hydrogen nuclei to be measured
   (c) speed up the relaxation time of the hydrogen nuclei
   (d) adjust the Larmour frequency of protons
   (e) allow the position of protons in three dimensions to be elicited

Chapter 26
Nuclear physics and radiation

Having read this chapter you will be able to:
- Define isotopes, radioactive decay and half-life.
- Appreciate the relative penetration abilities of alpha, beta and gamma rays.
- Describe what an X-ray is and how an X-ray image is taken.
- Understand the rudiments of tomographic imaging.
- Understand the science underlying PET scans.
- Appreciate how radiotherapy works.

26.1 Radioactivity

What is it that differentiates a radioactive material from other material? The answer is the stability of the atomic nucleus. Generally, larger heavier atomic nuclei such as uranium (atomic number 92) are more unstable than lighter nuclei and tend to make themselves more stable by emitting radiation, and reducing their atomic mass and/or their atomic number. This radiation can be in the form of a particle (either an **alpha** or **beta particle**) or as electromagnetic energy (a **gamma ray**).

Not all radioactive nuclei (**radionuclides**) are heavy. Unstable isotopes (*Section 1.1*) of low atomic number atoms exist, decaying to more stable isotopes, for example, carbon-14, a naturally occurring isotope of the more common and stable carbon-12. This isotope is present in small quantities in all living matter and has a **half-life** (the amount of time taken for half the nuclei to decay) of 5730 years. The relative amount of carbon-14 compared to carbon-12 is used for dating archeological samples of organic matter.

Most atoms have several naturally occurring isotopes in varying natural abundance. Those that decay are called radioactive (or parent) isotopes; those that are generated by decay are called radiogenic (or daughter) isotopes.

Hydrogen has three isotopes (see *Figure 26.1*). In its most common form it consists of a single proton with an orbiting electron, and no neutrons in the nucleus. The isotope **deuterium** (hydrogen-2) has one neutron, and hence twice the atomic mass. The other isotope, **tritium**, has two neutrons and a mass of 3. The charge of the nucleus is the same, and all isotopes have just one electron, and hence the same chemical properties. Deuterium is a stable isotope, but tritium is radioactive, with a half-life of 12.32 years.

Tritium decays to an isotope of helium by emitting an electron via a process known as beta decay:

$$^3_1\text{H} \rightarrow \, ^3_2\text{He}^+ + \beta^-$$

26.1

The daughter helium-3 nuclide is positively charged (as it lacks an electron) but is a stable isotope.

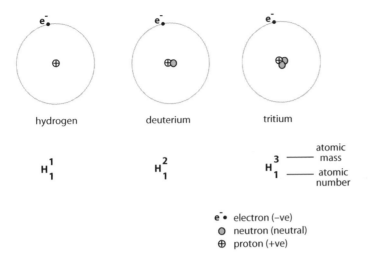

Figure 26.1. *The three isotopes of hydrogen differ by the number of neutrons in the nucleus.*

26.2 Radiation

In everyday use 'radiation' is usually associated with atomic radiation, but for physicists radiation is energy that travels as waves or high-speed particles. The most common forms of atomic radiation are alpha particles, beta particles and gamma rays. Alpha particles can be blocked by a single sheet of paper,

Definition
Radiation: energy that travels as waves or high-speed particles.

while beta particles require a sheet of aluminium several millimetres thick to stop them (see *Figure 26.2*). Gamma rays have by far the greatest penetration, requiring thick concrete or lead shielding to stop them.

Alpha particles

An alpha particle consists of two protons and two neutrons so is identical to a helium nucleus. Alpha particles have a positive charge and are emitted when radioisotopes undergo **alpha decay**.

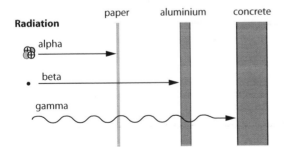

Figure 26.2. *Penetration of alpha particles, beta particles and gamma rays.*

Their penetration distance is short, with the outer layer of skin capable of stopping them. If alpha-emitting radionuclides are ingested, though, they can cause severe radiation poisoning.

Beta particles

Beta particle emission occurs when the ratio of neutrons to protons in the nucleus is too high; an excess neutron is transformed into a proton and an electron. The proton remains in the nucleus and the electron is emitted. The beta particle is essentially therefore a high-speed electron with the same negative charge. Beta particles can penetrate further than alpha particles and the speed of individual beta particles depends on how much energy they have. This energy can break chemical bonds and in the process form ions. Positively charged beta particles are also emitted by some forms of radioactive decay. These particles are high-speed **positrons**, the anti-matter counterparts of electrons.

Gamma rays

Gamma rays are the highest-energy electromagnetic waves and can pass through many kinds of materials including human tissue. Only very dense materials, such as concrete and lead, can act as a barrier. Gamma rays are very similar to X-rays, differing only in that they are more energetic and therefore more penetrating. X-rays are also distinct from gamma rays in that they are not produced in atomic nuclei. X-rays pose the same kind of hazard, however, and, like gamma rays, can pass through many materials.

26.3 Radioactive decay and half-life

Definition
Half-life: the time taken for half of the atoms in a radionuclide to decay.

When making popcorn the hard kernels are heated up and they eventually 'pop' to make the fluffy, edible popcorn. It is an irreversible act, as the popcorn will not turn back to kernel. It is not predictable on an individual level as to which kernel will pop first, but it is predictable how long it will take for half the popcorn present to pop (providing all the conditions are known).

This is equivalent to the decay of radioisotopes; predicting when an individual nuclide will decay is impossible. At the microscopic level, it is a seemingly random event. If a sample contains a large number of nuclides, however, it is possible to predict how many will remain. If we start with N_0 nuclides, the number N remaining after time t is given by

$$N = N_0 e^{-\lambda \tau}$$

26.2

where λ is the **decay constant**, a measure of an isotope's radioactivity.

Radioactive decay is an example of exponential decay (see *Chapter 27*). Clearly a sample of a radioisotope will become gradually less radioactive as the number of radionuclides decreases. The radioactivity will fall by a certain fraction after a fixed time has elapsed. The amount of time taken for half the nuclides to decay is known as the **half-life** of the radioisotope. If a further half-life elapses, the radioactivity will decrease by a half again and so on, never fully decaying away, instead reaching immeasurable levels after a very long time (see *Figure 26.3*). The half-life ($T_{1/2}$) is related to the decay constant by the following equation:

$$T_{1/2} = \frac{\ln 2}{\lambda}$$

26.3

Radionuclides with short half-lives present more immediate danger because they emit more radiation in a given time. Long half-life radionuclides pose other problems; for example, the half-life of some nuclear waste is many tens of thousands of years, causing problems with long-term storage.

Units

The becquerel (SI Unit, s^{-1}) is a unit used to measure radioactivity, and is the number of disintegrations occurring in one second. The becquerel has largely replaced the curie: 1 curie (Ci) = 3.7×10^{10} Bq.

26.4 Ionizing radiation

The ink on this page is observed by electromagnetic radiation being detected by the retina and computed by the brain. No cells are irrevocably altered in this process because the waves concerned are in the visible light spectrum and they carry relatively little energy.

Definition
Ionizing radiation: high-energy radiation which is capable of producing ions in the substance it is passing through.

It is a different matter for high-energy electromagnetic radiation. When a gamma ray, or X-ray photon, comes into contact with material including tissue, electrons can be knocked out of the outer shells of the atoms, creating ions, which cause further chemical reactions within the material. This is why gamma rays and X-rays are referred to as ionizing radiation. Alpha and beta particles are also classed as ionizing radiation, although the method of ionization is slightly different; because these particles carry an electric charge as well as kinetic energy, they can disrupt the electron structure of matter quite considerably as they pass through it.

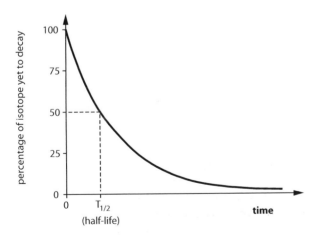

Figure 26.3. *Exponential decrease of a radioactive material: the half-life is plotted when 50% of the material has undergone radioactive decay.*

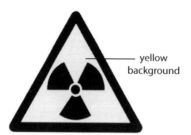
yellow background

Figure 26.4. *Universal warning sign for ionizing radiation.*

Biological effects

Ionizing radiation (*Figure 26.4*) is harmful to tissue because it can cause chemical changes within cells, causing a wide array of dysfunction and death. Radiation can also disrupt molecules in the DNA chain, causing harmful mutations including cancer. Hazards from ionizing radiation can arise from naturally occurring radioactive substances such as radon gas, which is a daughter nuclide of the decay of uranium-238 in rocks, and which can accumulate in caves and cellars. Radon contributes to the **background radiation**, as do cosmic rays, which are high energy gamma rays emitted by the sun.

The unit used to measure radiation doses is the gray ($1 \, \text{Gy} = 1 \, \text{J·kg}^{-1}$). One gray is the absorption of one joule of energy, in the form of ionizing radiation, per kilogram of tissue mass. Alternatively, the **dose equivalent** is sometimes quoted, which is measured in sieverts ($1 \, \text{Sv}$ is also equal to $1 \, \text{J·kg}^{-1}$). Sieverts weight different types of radiation for their damaging effect on biological tissue, so are more clinically relevant.

26.5 Radiotherapy

Radiotherapy (known as radiation therapy in the USA) describes the use of ionizing radiation to destroy malignant cells. As explained in the previous section, ionizing radiation damages DNA molecules in any exposed tissue. Radiotherapy uses high-energy X-rays, electron beams, or radioactive isotopes to attack malignant cells. These have been shown to be more susceptible to damage by radiation, because they do not possess the same mechanism for genetic repair as normal cells. In **external-beam radiotherapy**, several radiation beams are usually aimed from several angles to intersect at the target site, providing a much larger absorbed dose to the tumour than in the surrounding healthy tissue. The cells are killed outright or sufficiently damaged to prevent them from multiplying. Patients usually receive external-beam radiotherapy in daily treatment sessions over the course of several weeks. The number of treatment sessions depends on many factors, including the total radiation dose that will be given.

Radiotherapy can also be delivered systemically with radioisotopes ingested orally or injected intravenously. **Brachytherapy** is a type of radiotherapy where sealed radioactive sources ('seeds') are placed within, or in direct contact with cancerous tumours. The typical dose required to cure a solid epithelial tumour ranges from 60 to 80 Gy, while lymphomas are treated with 20–40 Gy.

26.6 X-rays: transmission, production and imaging

Imagine shooting wooden ducks at a fairground stall. Naturally, the larger the ducks are, the greater the chance of hitting them and, once hit, they will absorb the kinetic energy from the bullet more readily than any smaller ducks. If the nuclei of the atoms (that make up the molecules of the body) are analogous to the ducks then, when electrons are fired at them, the larger atoms will be hit more often and will absorb more energy.

> **Definition**
>
> **X-rays:** high-energy electromagnetic radiation capable of producing ionization in substances through which they pass; they have wavelengths between 5 and 10×10^{-9} m.

The interaction between the nucleus of an atom and the electromagnetic wave is referred to as attenuation. Attenuation of X-rays in solids takes place by several different mechanisms, some due to absorption, and others due to the scattering of the beam. Attenuation is the process by which radiation loses power as it travels through matter and interacts with it. Transmission is when an electromagnetic wave passes through an object unchanged.

Production of X-rays: Bremsstrahlung

In an X-ray tube, electrons are accelerated in a vacuum by an electric field and shot into a piece of metal called the target. X-rays are emitted as the electrons slow down (decelerate) in the metal. The technique used to do this is called Bremsstrahlung and this means 'braking radiation' in German (*bremsen:* to brake and *Strahlung:* radiation). X-rays are emitted by two processes: directly through conversion of kinetic energy to electromagnetic energy and indirectly through the creation of **characteristic X-rays**. This occurs when an incoming high-energy electron interacts with a

> **Definition**
>
> **Bremsstrahlung:** (German: 'braking radiation') refers to the electromagnetic radiation produced by deceleration of an electron; the radiation is in the X-ray region of the electromagnetic spectrum.

bound electron in an atom in the target and ejects it. After the electron has been ejected the atom is left with a vacant energy level. This vacancy is subsequently filled by an electron from a higher energy level, causing emission of an X-ray photon, whose energy (and frequency) is a characteristic of the target metal. Most elements emit X-rays when bombarded with electrons, but tungsten is one of the most suitable, as it emits a high intensity beam and can withstand high temperatures.

An X-ray tube is a large vacuum tube containing a tungsten filament cathode and an anode target (see *Figure 26.5*). A heated cathode causes electrons to 'boil off' in the vacuum, a process known as **thermionic emission**. The electrons are then accelerated to a high velocity by their attraction to the positively charged anode. The anode is angled so as to deflect the X-rays towards the target object. A by-product of this process is the generation of heat, so a means of cooling the tube is required. A thick lead shield surrounds the entire mechanism, which aims to stop leakage of radiation. There is a small window in the lead shield that allows the X-rays to escape. The narrow beam passes through a series of filters before exiting.

The traditional view of a radiograph (often referred to simply as an 'X-ray') is that of a film being examined on a light box. The principle is similar to an old-fashioned camera with film that reacts to light: X-rays are detected by a film that is sensitive to their wavelengths. It is then processed (developed) and an X-ray film is the result. X-ray films and plates are increasingly being replaced by receptors sensitive to X-rays that then produce a digital image that can be viewed on a monitor. Similar systems find application in airport baggage scanners.

The degree to which the X-rays are attenuated (blocked) whilst travelling through the body is dependent on both the density and thickness of the material. Thus bone, being relatively dense and thick, is shown as a light area on an X-ray film.

The operation of equipment delivering X-rays is stringently controlled and only adequately trained professionals may operate these machines. Protection such as lead aprons must be provided for staff required to be in the immediate vicinity of X-rays and extended protection is available including

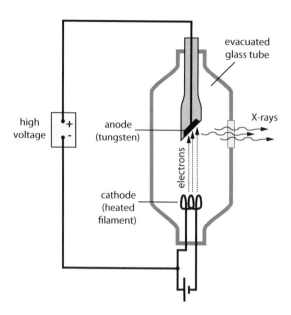

Figure 26.5. *An X-ray tube: electrons are accelerated against the tungsten and X-rays are produced.*

thyroid shields. These protective garments are heavy, though their weight has been reduced by the introduction of lower density lead composites.

26.7 Scintigraphy and SPECT scans

Definition
Scintigraphy: generation of an image from the detection of gamma rays emitted from an administered radioisotope; a scintillation camera obtains images.

When a gamma-emitting radioisotope (**radiopharmaceutical**) is injected, ingested or inhaled, the radioisotope decays, resulting in the emission of gamma rays. The gamma rays are detected by a gamma camera (also known as a scintillation camera or Anger camera) and processed to produce an image. The gamma camera can be used in planar imaging, or to acquire cross-sectional images using tomography, referred to as a **SPECT scan** (single photon emission computed tomography).

Functional brain imaging

A SPECT scan demonstrates the relative amount of radioisotope that has entered tissues and therefore relative blood flows. Usually, the gamma-emitting radioisotope used in functional brain imaging is ^{99m}Tc-HMPAO (hexamethylpropylene amine oxime). ^{99m}Tc is a radioisotope with a long half-life that emits gamma rays. Attaching it to HMPAO allows ^{99m}Tc to be taken up by brain tissue at a rate proportional to brain blood flow, allowing brain blood flow to be assessed with the scanner. A SPECT scan of the brain is used for diagnosis and patient monitoring in both neurology and psychiatry, including in assessment of neurological diseases (dementias), epilepsy, head trauma, neoplasms and cerebrovascular diseases.

Myocardial perfusion imaging (MPI)

Myocardial perfusion imaging is a form of functional cardiac imaging, used for the diagnosis of ischaemic heart disease. During exercise stress, diseased myocardium receives less blood flow than normal myocardial tissue. A radiopharmaceutical containing ^{99m}Tc is injected and then the heart rate is raised to induce myocardial stress, either by exercise or by administration of adenosine or dobutamine. Following the stress, SPECT imaging reveals the distribution of the radiopharmaceutical, and therefore the relative blood flow to the different regions of the myocardium.

26.8 Positron emission tomography

Positron emission tomography (PET) scans are similar to SPECT scans in that a radionuclide is injected and the result of the nuclear decay is measured. PET scans can assess the blood flow to areas of the brain and the uptake of labelled sugars by brain cells. They are increasingly used in conjunction with CT or MRI scans.

In PET scans the radionuclide decays and in the process emits a positron (a positron is a positively charged particle, and can be thought of as an electron's anti-particle). The positron interacts

Definition
Annihilation (positron-electron): occurs when an electron collides with a positron: this results in the production of two electromagnetic waves (gamma rays) travelling in opposite directions to each other.

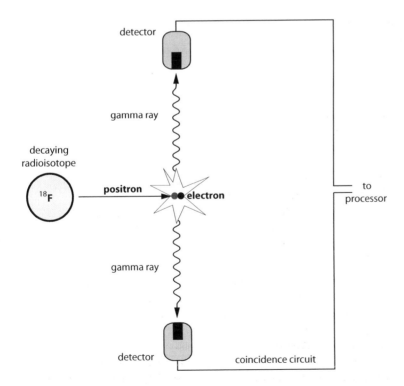

Figure 26.6. *Fundamentals of a positron emission tomography (PET) scanner.*

with an electron in the tissue, and **annihilation** of the electron and positron occurs, resulting in the production of two gamma rays travelling in opposite directions. As annihilation occurs very close to the point of decay, detecting the point of origin of these photons allows an image to be built up. They are detected by a series of receptors surrounding the patient. Detection of paired gamma rays simultaneously arriving at the different detectors confirms their origin. This type of detection system is known as a **coincidence circuit** (*Figure 26.6*).

Biologically active radiopharmaceuticals are used for PET. **Fludeoxyglucose**, an analogue of glucose that is labelled with fluorine-18 (half-life = 110 minutes), is common because the concentrations of radioisotope imaged give an indication of tissue metabolic activity, in terms of regional glucose uptake.

26.9 X-ray computed tomography

Definition
Tomography: the process of generating an image of a slice or cross-section through an object by the assimilation of multiple images.

Computed tomography (CT; see *Figure 26.7*), sometimes called computer-assisted tomography (CAT), has revolutionized medical imaging by generating detailed images of structures deep in the body that cannot be obtained using planar X-ray imaging systems. Tomography can refer to many imaging techniques whereby multiple views of a solid object are obtained from different angles, and the images are used to create a single image showing a cross-section or slice through the object. The computational power to process multiple images to form one clinically useful image has stretched the processing power of computers. Advances in computer processing have now largely caught up with the demands of tomography.

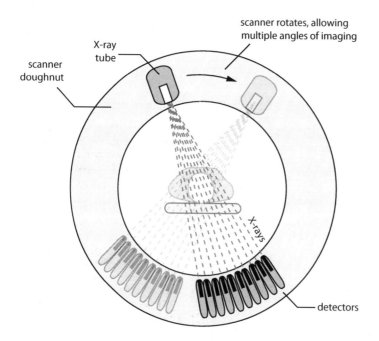

Figure 26.7. *An X-ray computed tomography scan.*

In a CT scanner, the patient is placed on a table, and a doughnut-shaped scanner moves so that the patient effectively passes through the ring. An X-ray tube and a detector opposite the tube both spin around the ring as the patient is scanned. A continuous 'spiral' scan is produced, taking no more than a few seconds to scan the body, minimizing the radiation dose. The spiral scan is a continuous series of views (called back projection scans) from which a 3-dimensional representation of the internal structure of the body may be constructed. Complex algorithms are needed to convert the back-projected views into cross-sectional images, which may be viewed on a screen. Like conventional planar X-ray images, lighter areas reveal denser tissue such as bones.

CT scans are suitable for imaging the brain, showing the extent and location of intracranial haemorrhages or other lesions in patients with head injuries. They are also suitable for detecting brain tumours, as well as malignant tumours in other parts of the body, such as the lungs.

Summary

- Radioactive decay involves the decay of an unstable nucleus of an element with the emission of radiation.
- Many elements have unstable radioisotopes, emitting alpha or beta particles or gamma rays.
- High-energy radiation can ionize the molecules it passes through, causing damage to tissue.
- X-rays are produced by a beam of electrons hitting a target through a process known as *Bremsstrahlung*.
- Radiotherapy works by ionizing atoms within the DNA chain, thus destroying the cancerous cells.
- X-rays and CT scans involve X-rays being passed through the body, whereas PET and SPECT scans involve the emission from a radioactive isotope within the body that has been injected, ingested or inhaled.

Single best answer questions

For these questions, choose the single best answer.

1. The best description of an isotope of an element is that:
   (a) it has more protons than neutrons
   (b) there is variation in the number of neutrons
   (c) electrons are all in the lowest energy levels
   (d) there is a paired increase in the number of protons and electrons
   (e) an isotope has an imbalance of charge as a result of changes to proton and electron numbers

2. Tomography is best described as:
   (a) multiple X-ray images computed to generate a 3D image
   (b) the process of generating an image using digital imagery rather than X-ray films
   (c) the process of radioactive decay unique to PET scans
   (d) the process of generating an image of a slice or cross-section through an object by the assimilation of multiple images
   (e) the augmentation of CT scans with advanced ultrasound techniques

3. An X-ray can be best defined as:
   (a) high-frequency, low-energy electromagnetic radiation capable of ionization
   (b) artificially generated beta particles capable of deep penetration of objects
   (c) low-frequency, high-energy electromagnetic radiation capable of ionization
   (d) the nucleus of a helium atom, two protons and two neutrons, travelling at speed
   (e) high-energy electromagnetic radiation capable of producing ionization

4. The radioactive decay central to a PET scan can be best described as:
   (a) electron–proton twin decay
   (b) characteristic energy particle decay
   (c) an emitted positron colliding with a nearby electron to produce a pair of electromagnetic gamma rays
   (d) an alpha particle decaying to form two beta particles travelling in opposite directions
   (e) an emission of electron pairs at high frequencies

Multiple choice questions

For each of these questions, mark every answer either true or false.

1. Which of the following statements concerning isotopes are true?
   (a) They have equal numbers of protons and neutrons.
   (b) Isotopes of an element have the same number of protons and electrons.
   (c) Isotopes vary: some are very unstable and others are extremely stable.
   (d) Radioisotope is a term used to refer to isotopes liable to undergo decay, emitting radiation.
   (e) On decay the type of radiation emitted is dependent on the isotope.

2. Which of the following statements concerning tomography are true?
   (a) It is a technique of imaging that can only be utilized when using X-rays.
   (b) An image of slices, or cross-sections, of the body can be generated.
   (c) Unlike standard X-rays, tomography tolerates patient movement well.
   (d) Restricted access to an intubated patient can be an issue during scans that incorporate tomography.
   (e) All cross-sectional imaging is tomography, including ultrasound.

3. Which of the following statements concerning the penetration of radiation are true?
   (a) Alpha waves have generally poor penetration of the skin.
   (b) Gamma waves need a highly dense medium to block them, such as lead or concrete.
   (c) Open wounds are less vulnerable to penetration by radiation than intact skin.
   (d) Gamma radiation with a higher energy has a poorer ability to penetrate compared with gamma radiation with a lower energy.
   (e) Gamma radiation has the greatest ability to pass through materials, and then alpha radiation, with beta radiation having the lowest ability to penetrate.

4. Which of the following statements concerning X-rays are true?
   (a) X-rays are fast-travelling electrons.
   (b) X-rays are generated by electrons bombarding a target such as tungsten.
   (c) To generate an X-ray the electrons in an atom have to drop down an energy level and in the process emit an electromagnetic wave.
   (d) Attenuation of X-rays is greatest when they pass through low-density materials.
   (e) X-rays are high-energy electromagnetic waves.

5. Which of the following statements concerning radiation are true?
   (a) Radiation therapy is viable as healthy tissue is generally resistant to the ionizing effect of radiation.
   (b) Scintigraphy is the image generated from the detection of gamma rays emitted from an administered radioisotope.
   (c) Annihilation (positron-electron) occurs when an electron collides with a positron: this result in the production of two electromagnetic waves.
   (d) The myocardial perfusion SPECT scan uses the radioisotope thallium-201.
   (e) Oxygen-16 is a typical radioisotope used in PET scans.

Chapter 27
Basic mathematical concepts

Having read this chapter you will be able to:
- Understand basic algebra, functions and graphs.
- Understand the concept of logarithms.
- Understand scientific notation.
- Appreciate integration and differentiation, including gradients and area under the curve.
- Understand the use of exponential functions including washout curves.

27.1 Basics

Fractions

$$\text{Fraction} = \frac{\text{numerator}}{\text{denominator}} = \frac{a}{b}$$

For example, $12.5\% = 0.125 = \dfrac{1}{8}$

Significant figures

Numbers may be rounded to a certain number of decimal places, or to a set number of significant figures. The number of significant figures refers to the total number of digits, regardless of whether they occur before or after the decimal point. For example:

2.4936 rounded to four significant figures is 2.494.

24.9357 rounded to four significant figures is 24.94

Algebra

Unknown variables in an equation are represented as either Arabic letters (e.g. x, y) or Greek letters (e.g. α, β). This allows mathematical laws containing variable quantities to be expressed.

Multiplication

For simple multiplication an 'x' is what we are used to, but beyond simple equations this can lead to confusion because x is commonly used in algebra. Instead, letters next to each other can signify multiplication: $a \times b = ab$.

Dots can also signify multiplication: $a \times b = a \cdot b$.

Variables and constants

Variable quantities (e.g. voltage V, current I, temperature T) and constants (e.g. speed of light c, gravitational constant, G) are written in *italics*.

Parentheses

The result of a calculation can be affected by the order in which it is executed. Multiplication and division take priority, but using parentheses (brackets) allows clarity, for example:

$$7 - 3 \times 4 + 12 = ?$$

Inserting parentheses:

$$(7 - 3) \times (4 + 12) = 4 \times 16 = 64$$

Using parentheses makes it clear that the calculations within the brackets should be carried out first.

Positive and negative numbers and multiplication

When a number is positive there is usually not a positive sign in front of it, but when a number is negative a minus sign precedes the number, i.e.

'minus one' is written as -1

$+2 \times +3 = +6$ is written as $2 \times 3 = 6$

When two negative numbers are multiplied together the result is a positive number but when a positive and a negative number are multiplied, the result is negative. For example:

$2 \times -3 = -6$

$-2 \times 3 = -6$

$-2 \times -3 = 6$

Recurring and irrational numbers

These are both kinds of never-ending decimal numbers. The fraction 1/3 expressed as a decimal is a recurring number equal to 0.33333333... etc. To simplify this, only the first recurring digit is needed and a dot is placed over the digit: $0.\dot{3}$

Irrational numbers are numbers that cannot be expressed as a simple fraction. They also have an infinite number of decimal places, e.g. the square root of 2 ($\sqrt{2} = 1.414213562373 \dots$ etc.) or pi ($\pi = 3.141592653589793$). These numbers are normally rounded to a practical number of decimal places e.g. $\sqrt{2} = \sim 1.414$.

27.2 Very large and very small numbers

Scientific notation

Scientific notation (or **exponential notation**) is used as a convenient way of writing numbers with very large or very small values. Any number can be written in the following form:

$$a \times 10^b$$

where a is the **coefficient** (usually in the range from 1 to 10) and b is the **exponent**, i.e. the power of 10. In this way, unnecessary zeros can be eliminated, for example:

$$4\ 750\ 000 = 4.75 \times 10^6$$

$$3.64 = 3.64 \times 10^0$$

$$0.000028 = 2.8 \times 10^{-5}$$

Note that for numbers smaller than 1, the exponent is negative. Note also that the coefficient is normally rounded to three, or at most, four significant figures. Since the scientific notation is based on multiples of 10 raised to a power, it is useful to consider some commonly encountered powers of 10:

$$10^6 = 10 \times 10 \times 10 \times 10 \times 10 \times 10 = 1\ 000\ 000\ (\text{million})$$

$$10^3 = 10 \times 10 \times 10 = 1000\ (\text{thousand})$$

$$10^1 = 10$$

$$10^0 = 1$$

$$10^{-1} = \frac{1}{10} = 0.1$$

$$10^{-2} = \frac{1}{10 \times 10} = 0.01$$

Logarithms

The two commonly used types of logarithms are so-called **common logarithms** (base 10 logarithms) and **natural logarithms** (base e logarithms, where e is the **Euler constant**, $e = 2.7818$). The logarithm of a number is the power that the base must be raised to, for example:

> **Definition**
>
> **Logarithm:** a mathematical function for transforming large or complex numbers; these transformations simplify the handling and multiplication of large numbers.

$$\text{If } \log_{10} \chi = n, \text{ then } 10^n = \chi$$

$$\text{If } \log_e \chi = n, \text{ then } e^n = \chi$$

The common logarithm is usually written simply as 'log', while the natural logarithm is usually written 'ln'. Some examples:

$$\log 100\ 000 = 5, \text{ because } 10^5 = 100\ 000$$

$$\log 236 = 2.373, \text{ because } 10^{2.373} = 236$$

$$\ln 7.839 = 2, \text{ because } e^2 = 7.839$$

Applications of logarithms

Before pocket calculators became available, multiplication and division of large numbers by hand was a difficult process. By converting numbers to logarithms and following the rules described below, calculations could be made relatively easily. The process requires having log tables or a slide-rule to hand (as used by NASA engineers and mission controllers during the Apollo era).

Table 27.1. *pH values for different hydrogen ion concentrations.*

pH	[H⁺] nmol litre⁻¹
3	1 000 000
6	1000
7	100
7.1	80
7.4	40
7.7	20
8	10
9	1

Logarithmic identities

The following are true for all logarithms

$$\log AB = \log A + \log B$$
$$\log\left(\frac{A}{B}\right) = \log A - \log B$$
$$\log A^b = b \log A$$

Logarithmic number scales

In science there are many variables that can have a very wide range of values. One example is the concentration of hydrogen ions in a solution. It is more convenient to represent this concentration by the pH scale. The pH scale is logarithmic, so what appear to be small numerical differences between two solutions can represent substantial differences in concentration. For example, a pH of 7.1 has twice the concentration of H⁺ ions as a pH of 7.4 (see *Table 27.1*). In general:

$$pH = -\log (\text{hydrogen ion concentration}) = -\log [H^+] \text{ (no units)}$$

27.3 Functions

A mathematical **function** is a generalized way of expressing the relationship between different variables. In its simplest form the function is shorthand for a mathematical expression whose value depends on the value of one or more variables. The following function finds the value of y in terms of x:

$$y = f(x)$$

where y is the dependent variable
          x is the independent variable

We say that 'y is a function of x.' For example: the area of a circle is a function of its radius r

$$A = f(r) = \pi r^2$$

A function can also depend on more than one independent variable, e.g. body mass index:

$$\text{BMI} = f(w, h) = w/h^2$$

where w is the patient's weight
          h is the patient's height

Linear functions

A function may be described as **linear** if it can be written in the following form:

$$y = mx + c$$

where m is the gradient of the graph of y against x
          c is the intercept on the y-axis

The gradient is constant for linear functions (see *Figure 27.1*), and is equal to the rate of change of y with respect to x, i.e.

$$m = \frac{\Delta y}{\Delta x}$$

Polynomial functions

A **polynomial function** is an expression of the following form:

$$y = a + bx + cx^2 + \dots$$

where a, b, c are the **coefficients** of the function

An example of a polynomial function is a **quadratic** function (or 2nd order polynomial), which has the form:

$$y = a + bx + cx^2$$

The order of the polynomial is equal to the highest-value **exponent** (power) of the variable (x) in the function. Thus a linear function is a 1st order polynomial (because the highest exponent of x is 1).

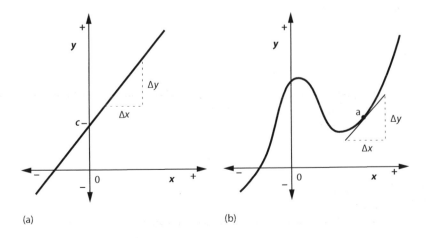

(a)   (b)

Figure 27.1. *(a) Linear and (b) non-linear functions.*

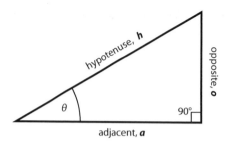

Figure 27.2. *A right-angled triangle.*

27.4 Trigonometry

Trigonometry, a branch of mathematics formalized by the ancient Greeks, is concerned with triangles and the relationship between their sides and angles. It is encountered in many areas of physics including mechanics, waves and simple harmonic motion. The sine function, for example, describes the behaviour of waves travelling through space.

Figure 27.2 shows a right-angled triangle with a marked angle θ. The longest side, known as the **hypotenuse**, is always opposite the 90° angle. The other two sides are labelled the **opposite** side (opposite the marked angle) and the **adjacent** side (adjacent to the marked angle).

The trigonometric functions (sine, cosine and tangent) are the ratios of different combinations of side lengths, as follows:

$$\sin\theta = \frac{\text{opposite}}{\text{hypotenuse}} = \frac{o}{h}$$

$$\cos\theta = \frac{\text{adjacent}}{\text{hypotenuse}} = \frac{a}{h}$$

$$\tan\theta = \frac{\text{opposite}}{\text{adjacent}} = \frac{o}{a}$$

These relationships are easily remembered by the meaningless but nevertheless useful mnemonic 'SOHCAHTOA' (Sine equals Opposite over Hypotenuse, Cosine equals Adjacent over Hypotenuse, Tangent equals Opposite over Adjacent).

Pythagoras' theorem

The Greek mathematician Pythagoras is credited with a fundamental rule of trigonometry, which states that 'the square on the hypotenuse is equal to the sum of the squares on the other two sides', i.e.

$$(\text{hypotenuse})^2 = (\text{adjacent})^2 + (\text{opposite})^2 , \text{ or}$$

$$h = \sqrt{(a^2 + o^2)}$$

Pi

The Greek letter π (pi) is the ratio between the circumference of a circle and its diameter, and is equal to 3.14159265359 (to 12 significant figures). Pi is an **irrational number** (meaning that it cannot be expressed as a fraction of two integers), and frequently appears in calculations, for example:

$$\text{area of a circle} = \pi r^2$$

$$\text{surface area of a sphere} = 4\pi r^2$$

$$\text{volume of a sphere} = \frac{4}{3}\pi r^3$$

$$\text{volume of a cylinder} = \pi r^2 h$$

where   *r* is the radius
          h is height (of the cylinder)

Radians

Radians, like degrees, are units for expressing angles. Scientists favour them over degrees because they greatly simplify calculations, especially those concerning circles and waves. One radian is the angle formed by a wedge with a circumference equal to the radius of the circle. The value of 1 radian is 57.3° (to three significant figures) but radians are often quoted in terms of π as:

$$\pi \text{ radians} = 180°, \ 2\pi \text{ radians} = 360°, \ ... \text{ etc}$$

At first radians seem less intuitive, because whole numbers of radians are rarely encountered. However, you will commonly come across them on graphs, especially those concerning waves, circular motion and phase relationships (*Figure 27.3*).

Note that in *Figure 27.3*, sine and cosine are out of phase by $\pi/2$ radians (90°), so the relationship between sine and cosine can be written as:

$$\cos(x) = \sin\left(x + \frac{\pi}{2}\right)$$

Trigonometric identities

The following equations are useful when simplifying complicated trigonometric functions where θ and ϕ are any two independent angles.

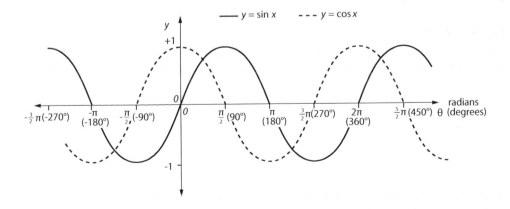

Figure 27.3. *Sine and cosine functions.*

$$(\sin\theta)^2 + (\cos\theta)^2 = 1$$

$$\tan\theta = \frac{\sin\theta}{\cos\theta}$$

$$\sin2\theta = 2\sin\theta\cos\theta$$

$$\cos2\theta = (\cos\theta)^2 - (\sin\theta)^2$$

$$\sin(\theta\pm\varphi) = \sin\theta\cos\varphi \pm \cos\theta\sin\varphi$$

$$\cos(\theta\pm\varphi) = \cos\theta\cos\varphi \pm \sin\theta\sin\varphi$$

27.5 Calculus

Mathematics is a key tool for physicists, but Isaac Newton found that the established mathematical toolbox of the time was inadequate for describing dynamic (changing) systems such as apples falling and the orbit of the moon around the earth. Out of Newton's need for more sophisticated ways of describing phenomena, calculus was born. Calculus was originally called the 'calculus of infinitesimals' and its inception resulted in a bitter argument between Newton and Gottfried Leibniz, a German philosopher and mathematician, who also claimed to be the father of calculus. Although Newton now gets most of the credit, it is Leibniz's notation that is still in use today.

Calculus can be highly complex, but put simply it can help find either the gradient of a line on a graph (differentiation) or the area under a line on a graph (integration). For graphs that involve straight lines calculus might not be needed but for non-linear graphs calculus is invaluable.

Rates of change: differentiation

Definition

Differentiation: a mathematical tool that allows the rate of change between one variable and other variables to be formulated.

For a curve on a graph **differentiation** can allow the gradient to be calculated, i.e. the rate of change of one variable relative to other variables. So for a simple graph plotting x against y the mathematical expression of the gradient is *approximately* equal to:

$$\text{gradient} \approx \frac{\Delta y}{\Delta x}$$

If the change Δx is made very small indeed Δy also becomes very small and the gradient may be found much more precisely. In calculus, we assume that the changes are **infinitesimally** small (as close to zero as possible). These changes are represented by dy and dx, so the gradient is *exactly* equal to:

$$\text{gradient} = \frac{dy}{dx}$$

An alternative notation for functions is sometimes used:

f'(x) represents the rate of change of **f(x)** or $\mathbf{f'(x)} = \dfrac{d}{dx}(f(x))$

Common differentials. Simple differentials may easily be differentiated. The general form for differentiating a polynomial is as follows:

$$\frac{d}{dx}(x^n + a) = nx^{n-1}$$

i.e. reduce the exponential (the power of *x*) by one and multiply *x* by the old exponential. If the power of *x* is already equal to 1, then the *x* disappears (because $x^0 = 1$). Constants become zero.
Some examples:

$$\frac{d}{dx}(x^2 + 3) = 2x$$

$$\frac{d}{dx}(2x^3 + 7x) = 6x^2 + 7$$

Differentials of trigonometric, exponential and reciprocal functions. There are special rules for these functions, e.g.

$$\frac{d}{dx}(\sin x) = \cos x$$

$$\frac{d}{dx}(\cos x) = -\sin x$$

$$\frac{d}{dx}(e^x) = e^x$$

$$\frac{d}{dx}(\ln x) = \frac{1}{x}$$

Area under a curve: integration

Integration allows the area under a curve to be calculated. Integration is described as the opposite of differentiation, so if you differentiate a function and then integrate the result, you end up with the original function.

A way of visualizing integration is to divide the area under the curve into a large number of very thin rectangles and then add the areas of the rectangles together. The width of each rectangle is dx and the height is the value of f(*x*) for that point. The integral of f(*x*) 'with respect to *x*' is written:

Definition

Integration: a mathematical tool that allows the area under a curve to be calculated; integration is the opposite to differentiation.

$$\text{Area under curve} = F(x) = \int f(x).dx$$

We can integrate a function to find the area under the curve enclosed between two points (x_1 and x_2) called the **limits** of the integration. The so-called **definite integral** is written:

$$\text{Area under curve between } x_1 \text{ and } x_2 = \int_{x1}^{x2} f(x).dx = F(x_2) - F(x_1)$$

The general form for integrating a polynomial is as follows:

$$\int (x^n + a)dx = \frac{1}{n+1}x^{n+1} + ax + c$$

Note that the constant becomes a coefficient of *x*, and an extra constant (the **constant of integration**) appears in the result. When integrating between limits, the constant of integration disappears (as shown by the equation for the definite integral above, the constant is effectively subtracted from itself).

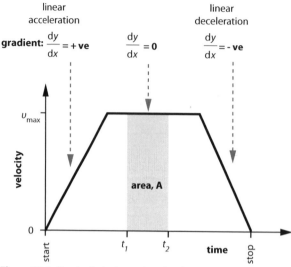

Figure 27.4. *Graph of velocity against time for a car. The area under the graph represents the distance travelled whilst the gradient represents the acceleration.*

Worked example

Velocity, acceleration and distance

Consider a car travelling along a straight road. The car accelerates from stationary to a maximum velocity v_{max}, maintains that velocity for a while, and then brakes (decelerates) until the car is stationary again. A graph of the velocity plotted against time is shown in *Figure 27.4*. The gradient of the graph gives the acceleration.

$$\text{acceleration (gradient)} = \frac{dv}{dt}$$

The area under the curve between two times (t_1 and t_2) gives the distance travelled by the car between these times. In the example shown:

$$\text{distance (area)} = \int_{t_1}^{t_2} v.dt$$

Clinical example

Respiratory flow and volume

Figure 27.5 shows a graph of flow rate against time for a cycle of ventilation. The volume change between two times is found by calculating the area under the curve between these times. In other words, volume is the integral of flow with respect to time. Put another way, flow is the differential of volume. It can be seen that the area under the inspired part of the graph is roughly equal to the area under the expired part, which means that the inspired and expired volumes are roughly equal.

The graph also shows the gradients (given by the time differentials of the flow curve). At the beginning of inspiration, the flow gradient is positive, meaning that the flow rate is increasing. The rate of change of flow rate then becomes negative as flow slows down and so on.

The area is the sum of these rectangles and this allows graphs that are non-linear (curved) to have the area calculated. The area under the graph shows the volume, so the area under the curve between t_{start} and t_{mid} gives the inspiratory volume and between t_{mid} and t_{end} the expiratory volume.

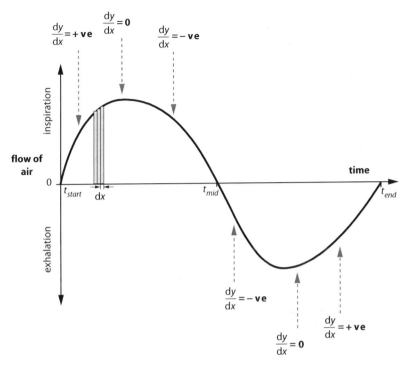

Figure 27.5. *Graph of flow against time for inspiration and expiration.*

27.6 Exponential growth

Exponential growth describes a function that increases by a multiple of that function's value, in other words:

$$x(t) = a \cdot b^{t/\tau}$$

where a is the initial value

          b is the **positive growth factor**

          t is time

          τ is the time constant (the time required for x to increase by a factor of b).

    Put very simply, the larger the quantity grows, the faster it grows. A few examples illustrate this point.

> **Definition**
>
> **Exponential growth:** the growth in a system where the amount being added to the system is proportional to the amount already present.

Coins on a chessboard

Imagine a chessboard has two coins placed on the first square and on the next square the number of coins are doubled (*Figure 27.6*). For the third square the coins are then double those on the second square, such that each square has twice as many coins as the previous square. The coins grow surprisingly rapidly in number: 2, 4, 8, 16, 32, 64, 128 and so on: very soon the squares are overflowing with coins. This is classed as an exponential rise and the number of coins x is related to the nth square thus:

$$x = 2^n$$

Exponential patterns are special because the growth rate depends on the current size of the variable. For the last (64th) square on the chessboard, the number of coins is equal to $2^{64} = 1.8 \times 10^{19}$. If all these coins are 2 mm high and are stacked on top of each other, they would reach over halfway to Alpha Centauri, the nearest star!

Compound interest on savings

If money is placed into a savings account, how is the interest calculated? There are two ways: either by **compound interest** or by **simple interest**. For annual compound interest, the new amount is based on the money in the account for the previous year. For simple interest it is solely based on the initial deposit.

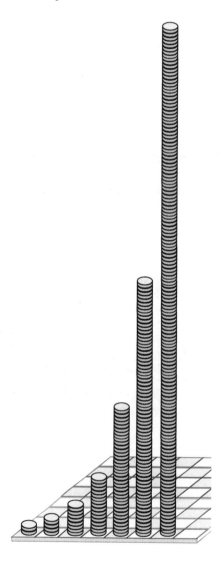

Figure 27.6. *Exponential growth illustrated by doubling the coins on successive squares of a chess board.*

Table 27.2. *Simple and compound interest.*

	Year 0	Year 1	Year 2	Year 3	Year 4	Year 5	Year 10
Simple interest	£100	£110	£120	£130	£140	£150	£200
Compound interest	£100	£110	£121	£133.10	£146.41	£161.05	£259.37

For the first year both compound and simple interest are the same: it does not matter which interest you are paid. If the interest is 10% then the account will grow by £10. For the second year it is a different matter:

- for simple interest, interest in the second year is again just paid on the starting deposit of £100.
- for compound interest, interest in the second year is paid on the starting deposit of £100 plus the interest from the first year – a total of £110. This growth in interest is exponential.

Looking at *Table 27.2*, in the first few years the difference is not astounding, but after ten years the gap between simple and compound interest is nearly £60.

Bacterial growth

Given a favourable environment bacteria will grow exponentially. A plate of bacteria is known to be growing at 10% per hour; how many bacteria would be present after 10 hours, given a starting number of 100 000? The answer is lying in *Table 27.2* because there is a direct analogy. If each £1 is taken to be 1000 bacteria, and instead of a year the time interval is an hour, then after 10 hours there will be nearly 260 000 bacteria present.

27.7 Exponential decay

A bath emptying provides a good illustration of the concept of exponential decay. The rate of flow out of the bath slows down as the water level in the bath drops. The rate at which it empties is dependent on the pressure exerted by the water above the plughole. The knock-on effect of the bath draining is that the pressure from the height of water also falls. The rate of change of volume in the bath (outflow) is dependent on the volume of water remaining in the bath as shown in the graph in *Figure 27.7*.

Definition

Exponential decay: occurs when a quantity decreases by the same proportion in each section of time; the rate of decay of a substance is proportional to the quantity of substance remaining.

In general, exponential decay may be represented by the following function:

$$x(t) = a \cdot e^{-t/\tau}$$

where a is the initial value

       $e = 2.7182$

       τ is the time constant (the time required for x to decrease by a factor of e)

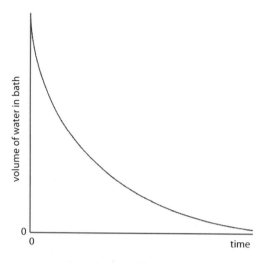

Figure 27.7. *The rate of flow of water from the bath is proportional to the volume of water remaining in the bath.*

Clinical example

Elimination of drugs

Exponential decay applies to the elimination of a drug with first order kinetics. The drug concentration decreases towards zero at a rate directly proportional to the plasma concentration such that:

$$C = C_0 e^{-k_e t}$$

where C is the plasma concentration

           C_0 is the initial plasma concentration

           k_e is the **elimination constant**

           t is time

The higher the elimination constant, the more rapidly the drug is metabolized. The **half-life** $t_{1/2}$ is sometimes quoted, being the amount of time needed for the concentration to fall by 50%, where:

$$t_{1/2} = \frac{\ln 2}{k_e}$$

Multiple choice questions

For each of these questions, mark every answer either true or false.

1. Multiplying two variables, A and B, can be written as:
   (a) $A \alpha B$
   (b) $A \times B$
   (c) $A \cdot B$
   (d) $A . B$
   (e) A/B

2. Brackets are required in equations because:
   (a) it is a traditional form of layout that is superfluous
   (b) it indicates which order to proceed with the calculations
   (c) it allows complex equations to be set out in a more straightforward way
   (d) it is only used in statistics
   (e) it is a format rarely used now and can be ignored

3. Examples of an exponential rise include:
   (a) bacteria in favourable conditions
   (b) compound interest
   (c) radioactive decay
   (d) a hysteresis loop
   (e) a washout curve

4. Which of the following statements regarding calculus are true?
   (a) Integration allows the area under a line on a graph to be calculated.
   (b) Integration allows the gradient of a line on a graph to be calculated.
   (c) Calculus includes integration and differentiation.
   (d) Calculus is a powerful tool when dealing with a dynamic system.
   (e) Differentiation is another term for exponential decay.

5. Which of the following statements regarding the gradient of a line on a graph are true?
   (a) A positive gradient represents a downward slope.
   (b) The higher the value of the gradient, the shallower the slope.
   (c) A horizontal line has a zero gradient.
   (d) Differentiation is a mathematical tool to calculate the gradient.
   (e) A sinusoidal wave only has a positive or zero gradient.

Chapter 28
Physical quantities and SI units

Having read this chapter you will be able to:
- Know the most important physical constants.
- Understand the importance of SI units.
- Know the difference between base SI units and derived units.
- Recall the standard prefixes used with SI units.
- Understand the quantities and notation used in respiratory physiology.

28.1 Physical constants

Table 28.1 lists some of the fundamental constants of physics. The values of these quantities are unchanging, and all are encountered in this book.

28.2 Fundamental and derived SI units

An age of rapid scientific discovery gave birth to a wealth of diverse units of measurement. The **International System of Units** known as **SI Units** (abbreviated from the French *Système international d'unités*) was devised with an aim to both simplify and unify the vast array of units that had developed. At the heart of the SI system are seven base quantities, shown in Table 28.2.

All other units can be expressed in terms of the base units. In addition to the base units, there are recognized combinations of the base units called **derived units**, and these are summarized in Table 28.3. Some derived units have been named after a prominent scientist associated with

Table 28.1. *Physical constants.*

Constant	Symbol	Value
Pi	π	3.1415927
Planck's constant	h	6.626×10^{-34} J·s
Speed of light	c	2.998×10^8 m·s^{-1}
Acceleration due to gravity	g	9.81 m·s^{-2}
Charge on an electron	e	1.602×10^{-19} C
Stefan–Boltzmann constant	σ	5.670×10^{-8} W·m^{-2}·K^{-4}
Avogadro's number	N_A	6.022×10^{23} mol^{-1}
Universal gas constant	R	8.314 J·mol^{-1}·K^{-1}

Table 28.2. *SI base units.*

Base quantity	Unit	Symbol
Length	metre	m
Mass	kilogram	kg
Time	second	s
Amount of substance	mole	mol
Thermodynamic temperature	kelvin	K
Electric current	ampere	A
Intensity of illumination	candela	cd

the quantity. An example is the unit for energy, the joule. It is named after the English scientist James Prescott Joule and can be expressed in base units as $kg \cdot m^2 \cdot s^{-2}$. Just to complicate matters, it is also referred to as the newton metre and is thus expressed as the multiplication of a base unit, the metre, and a derived unit, the newton. *Table 28.4* lists many commonly used units with special names.

Tips for choosing the correct units
- Check carefully that you are using a correct and appropriate unit.
- The base units on both sides of any equation should match. For example, if they are $m \cdot s^{-1}$ on one side then they must be $m \cdot s^{-1}$ on the other. This is a good way to check if an equation makes sense.
- SI units should be used where possible, but for historical reasons some measurements are recorded in other units. For example, blood pressure is quoted in millimetres of mercury (mmHg), not the SI unit (pascals), because until recently it was routinely measured using a mercury sphygmomanometer.

Table 28.3. *Commonly used derived quantities defined in terms of the seven base quantities.*

Derived quantity	Unit	Symbol
Area	square metre	m^2
Volume	cubic metre	m^3
Speed, velocity	metre per second	$m \cdot s^{-1}$
Acceleration	metre per second squared	$m \cdot s^{-2}$
Wave number	reciprocal metre	m^{-1}
Mass density	kilogram per cubic metre	$kg \cdot m^{-3}$
Current density	ampere per square metre	$A \cdot m^{-2}$
Magnetic field strength	ampere per metre	$A \cdot m^{-1}$

Table 28.4. *Derived units with special names.*

Derived quantity	Unit	Symbol	Alternative symbol	Base symbol
Frequency	hertz	Hz	–	s^{-1}
Force	newton	N	–	$kg \cdot m \cdot s^{-2}$
Pressure, stress	pascal	Pa	$N \cdot m^{-2}$	$m^{-1} \cdot kg \cdot s^{-2}$
Energy, work, quantity of heat	joule	J	$N \cdot m$	$m^2 \cdot kg \cdot s^{-2}$
Power, radiant flux	watt	W	$J \cdot s^{-1}$	$m^2 \cdot kg \cdot s^{-2}$
Electric charge, quantity of electricity	coulomb	C	–	$s \cdot A$
Electric potential difference, electromotive force	volt	V	$W \cdot A^{-1}$	$m^2 \cdot kg \cdot s^{-3} \cdot A^{-1}$
Capacitance	farad	F	$C \cdot V^{-1}$	$m^{-2} \cdot kg^{-1} \cdot s^4 \cdot A^2$
Electric resistance	ohm	Ω	$V \cdot A^{-1}$	$m^2 \cdot kg \cdot s^{-3} \cdot A^{-2}$
Electric conductance	siemen	S	$A \cdot V^{-1}$	$m^{-2} \cdot kg^{-1} \cdot s^3 \cdot A^2$
Magnetic flux	weber	Wb	$V \cdot s$	$m^2 \cdot kg \cdot s^{-2} \cdot A^{-1}$
Magnetic flux density	tesla	T	$Wb \cdot m^{-2}$	$kg \cdot s^{-2} \cdot A^{-1}$
Inductance	henry	H	$Wb \cdot A^{-1}$	$m^2 \cdot kg \cdot s^{-2} \cdot A^{-2}$
Celsius temperature	Celsius	°C	–	K
Activity (of a radionuclide)	becquerel	Bq	–	s^{-1}
Absorbed dose, specific energy (imparted), kerma	gray	Gy	$J \cdot kg^{-1}$	$m^2 \cdot s^{-2}$
Dose equivalent	sievert	Sv	$J \cdot kg^{-1}$	$m^2 \cdot s^{-2}$

28.3 Standard prefixes for SI units

An SI prefix is a name that precedes a basic unit of measurement to indicate a multiple of ten, or fraction of the unit. The standard prefixes (summarized in *Table 28.5*) are useful to reduce the number of zeros shown before or after a decimal point.

If used correctly, standard prefixes provide a convenient way of working with small or large quantities, for example:

$$0.0000000036 \text{ J (joules)} = 3.6 \times 10^{-9} \text{ J} = 3.6 \text{ nJ (nanojoules)}$$

$$43\,000\,000 \text{ Pa (pascals)} = 4.3 \times 10^7 = 43 \text{ MPa (megapascals)}$$

28.4 Respiratory and gas quantities

Quantities used for gas calculations should be treated with special care, because many different measurement systems are in use. For example, pressure is quoted in at least seven different types

Table 28.5. *Standard prefixes.*

Prefix	Symbol	Power
atto-	a	10^{-18}
femto-	f	10^{-15}
pico-	p	10^{-12}
nano-	n	10^{-9}
micro-	μ	10^{-6}
milli-	m	10^{-3}
kilo-	k	10^{3}
mega-	M	10^{6}
giga-	G	10^{9}
tera-	T	10^{12}
peta-	P	10^{15}
exa-	E	10^{18}

of units (see *Table 6.1*). As usual, during calculations, quantities should be converted into SI units where possible. *Table 28.6* shows the main variables used together with notes concerning their use.

Symbols used in respiratory physiology

Special notation is used in respiratory physiology, due to the great number of physiological quantities used. For example, the partial pressure of alveolar carbon dioxide is abbreviated to $P_A CO_2$.

Table 28.6. *The main quantities used in gas calculations.*

Quantity	Symbol	SI units	Derived units	In terms of base units	Notes
Pressure	P	Pa (pascal)	N·m^{-2}	m^{-1}·kg·s^{-2}	• often stated in kPa • 1 kPa = 1000 Pa
Temperature	T	–	–	K (kelvin)	• always use kelvin in calculations • to convert: [K] = [°C] + 273.15
Volume	V	–	–	m^3	• Litre (L) commonly used • 1 L = 0.001 m^3
Amount	n	–	–	mol (mole)	• mmol (millimole) is often used • 1 mmol = 0.001 mol
Mass	m	–	–	kg (kilogram)	• 1 kg = 1000 g
Partial pressure	P_{gas}	Pa (pascal)	N·m^{-2}	m^{-1}·kg·s^{-2}	• same for partial pressure in a gas or liquid • mmHg also widely used • to convert: 1 kPa = 7.5 mmHg

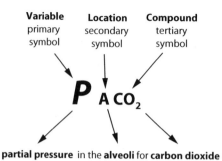

partial pressure in the **alveoli** for **carbon dioxide**

Figure 28.1. *Notation for physiological quantities used in respiratory physiology.*

The abbreviation consists of three parts: a primary symbol which identifies the variable, a secondary symbol identifying the location (alveoli), and a tertiary symbol identifying the compound (see *Figure 28.1*).

Table 28.7 summarizes the main primary, secondary and tertiary symbols used in respiratory physiology. Note that for the secondary symbols, upper case denotes a location pertaining to gases, while lower case denotes liquids. Other areas of medicine use similar notation, but few if any are as extensive as those listed here.

Table 28.7. *The main primary, secondary and tertiary symbols used in respiratory physiology.*

Variable: primary symbol (in italics)		Location: secondary symbol				Compound: tertiary symbol	
		Gas		**Liquid**			
C	Content (of gas in a blood)	*A*	Alveolar	*a*	Arterial	CO	Carbon monoxide
F	Fractional concentration	*B*	Barometric (atmospheric pressure)	*c*	Capillary	CO_2	Carbon dioxide
P	Pressure or partial pressure	*E*	Exhaled	*v*	Venous	O_2	Oxygen
Q	Volume (of blood)	*I*	Inhaled	\multicolumn{4}{l}{A dot above a symbol indicates a time derivative e.g. $\dot{V}$ is rate of change of volume (flow)}		
S	Saturation of haemoglobin with oxygen	*T*	Tidal	\multicolumn{4}{l}{A dash above indicates mixed or mean e.g. $\bar{v}$ is mixed venous}		
V	Volume (of a gas)	*ET*	End-tidal	\multicolumn{4}{l}{A ' after a symbol indicates end e.g. c' is end-capillary}		

Multiple choice questions

For each of these questions, mark every answer either true or false.

1. The following are SI base units, true or false?
   (a) Metres.
   (b) Inches.
   (c) Amperes.
   (d) Bar.
   (e) Second.

2. Regarding standard prefixes for units:
   (a) the prefix M, or Mega, signifies 1000
   (b) the prefix K signifies $\times 10^3$
   (c) nano is represented by the Greek letter μ
   (d) the prefix μ indicates $\times 10^{-6}$
   (e) micro and milli are interchangeable terms

3. Regarding the SI unit for pressure:
   (a) the SI unit for pressure is the pascal
   (b) the derived unit is $N \cdot m^{-2}$
   (c) in base units it can be expressed as $m^{-1} \cdot kg \cdot s^{-2}$
   (d) 1 bar is 100 kPa
   (e) 1 mmHg is approxiamtely equal to 1 kPa

4. Regarding the measurement of temperature:
   (a) Fahrenheit is a derived SI unit for temperature
   (b) kelvin is a base SI unit and measures temperature
   (c) Fahrenheit and kelvin are interchangeable units
   (d) Celsius is an SI derived quantity for temperature
   (e) the candela is an alternative SI unit for temperature

5. With regards to the use of SI units:
   (a) the base units on both sides of any equation should match
   (b) partial pressures are measured in different units to those of atmospheric pressure
   (c) $\dot{V}$ signifies the rate of change of volume
   (d) SI units is abbreviated from the French *Système international d'unités*
   (e) the joule measures: energy, work, quantity of heat

Chapter 29
Statistics

Having read this chapter you will be able to:

- Understand the basis of statistical concepts including measurement error and statistical uncertainty.
- Recall the basic aspects of study design and explain the outcome measures and the uncertainty in their definition.
- Explain the basis of meta-analysis and evidence-based medicine.
- Recall the types of data and their representation.
- Explain the normal distribution as an example of parametric distribution.
- Explain indices of central tendency and variability.
- Recall simple probability theory and the relationship to confidence values.
- Explain the null hypothesis and explain the choices for simple statistical tests for different types of data.
- Recall type I and type II errors.

29.1 Errors, uncertainty and averages

The purpose of statistics is to summarize and describe data while preserving information and reducing the volume of raw data. It is important to understand the basis of the main statistical tests available and the circumstances for their correct application. This enables results to be interpreted and a valid conclusion to be reached.

Uncertainty

The range in which the measurement lies.

Error

There is an error when there is a deviation of a measured result from the correct or accepted value of the quantity being measured. There are two basic types of errors: random and systematic.

Random errors. Random errors stray from the correct value in an arbitrary fashion. The distribution of multiple measurements with only random error contributions will be centred on the correct value. Examples include an inconsistent procedure followed by the operator, instruments with low resolution, and errors in recording the data.

Systematic errors. Measured results deviate by a fixed amount in one direction from the correct value. Examples include instruments that are wrongly calibrated or a signal loss in cables that has not been fully accounted for.

Mean, mode and median

How can a set of data be represented by a single number: a 'typical' value? There is more than one answer: the mean, mode or median.

Mean (or average). The mean is found by adding all the numbers together in a sample group and dividing by the sample size.

Mode. Mode is the most frequently occurring value in a frequency distribution. The data value, or a small data range, that occur the most often is the mode.

Median. If all the numbers in a sample are lined up from smallest to largest, the median is the middle number. Half the data will be greater than the median and half smaller.

29.2 Study design

The aim of a study should be clearly stated at the beginning. There could be a number of different designs that could look at the outcome of interest. The final choice of the study design will be made with resources (usually financial) taken into consideration as well as the views of the ethics committee; so, in the real world, a lot of studies have sub-optimal designs.

There are two main types of study design: **observational studies** (cross-sectional, case-control and cohort) and experimental studies (**randomized controlled trials**). The strength of a study depends upon its design, a relationship summarized in *Figure 29.1*.

Cross-sectional surveys

Cross-sectional surveys are also known as **descriptive studies** or **prevalence studies**. They look at data from a particular point in time and therefore represent a 'snapshot' of the population in question. The presence or absence of disease can be assessed to give the prevalence. These data can be compared with other data collected at the same time, such as sex, age, etc. These comparisons may then suggest a hypothesis that can be tested in another type of future study.

Case-control studies

This is a retrospective (look back in time) study. Subjects already have the disease or procedure. Controls are taken from the same population, from those that do not have the disease or procedure.

Case-control studies have the advantage that small numbers of subjects can be used. They are useful when it comes to rare conditions and they are much quicker (and usually cheaper) to perform than cohort studies. The disadvantages of case-control studies are that they are retrospective and the selection of cases and controls is difficult. Also, the overall incidence of the disease cannot be calculated from the data.

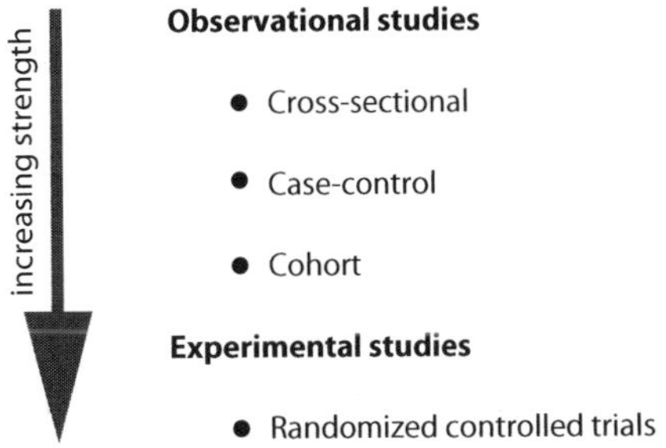

Observational studies

- Cross-sectional
- Case-control
- Cohort

Experimental studies

- Randomized controlled trials

increasing strength

Figure 29.1. *Study designs: a randomized controlled trial is the gold standard.*

Cohort studies

These studies are usually prospective (looking ahead in time). Often the subjects have been exposed to a drug or procedure and are then followed up. The characteristics of those who develop disease or cure, for example, can then be identified. Cohort studies allow the incidence of a disease to be calculated directly, and the effects of a rare exposure can be examined. The disadvantage is that large populations are studied over long periods of time, which is difficult and expensive. Furthermore, causal relationships can be difficult to identify and prove.

Randomized controlled trials (RCTs)

These are intervention studies and are experimental in their design. They are often prompted by the findings of observational studies. By randomizing, there is less chance of confounding variables. Usually there is an intervention group and a control (placebo) group. RCTs offer the best evidence of cause and effect, providing they are well designed.

29.3 Outcome measures and the uncertainty of their definition

Research in medicine is aimed at assessing the quality and effectiveness of health care, as measured by the attainment of a specified end result or outcome. Such measures help in continuous quality improvement programmes by providing data for researchers and feedback for practitioners. They help to improve evidence-based guidelines over time by identifying things that work well and things that don't.

Outcome measures can be simple biomedical measures such as body weight or head circumference, or they may be more complex such as the perception of improved health, satisfaction scores, pain/discomfort scores, treatment side-effects, or lowered morbidity or mortality. Economic outcomes are also increasingly used, such as cost of treatment or length of stay. Other outcome measures exist that are derived from study data. These are numerous and ever increasing in number, so only the commonly encountered are described below.

Risk and numbers needed to treat (NNT)

Risk is a measure of the probability or the chance of something happening. Risk factors are associated with an increased chance of developing a given disease. Number needed to treat (NNT) is a measure of the number of patients who would need to undergo an intervention to prevent one bad outcome from occurring. It is a way of measuring the effectiveness of an intervention.

Standardized mortality ratio (SMR)

The SMR is the ratio of observed deaths to expected deaths. The expected deaths are calculated relative to a typical area with equivalent age and gender mix. Examining the death rates for different ages and genders in the larger population does this.

Hospital standardized mortality ratios (HSMRs)

This is the ratio of in-hospital observed deaths to the expected deaths × 100. It is now used as a screening tool for hospital care in many countries. However, their interpretation can be complicated by a differing hospital case mix such as all elective admissions, or admissions consisting of multiple care episodes, such as with trauma patients.

29.4 The basis of meta-analysis and evidence-based medicine (EBM)

Systematic review is the formalized process of combining information after an exhaustive search for studies concerning the same health condition. One of the statistical tools to present the findings from this systematic review is called **meta-analysis.**

Meta-analysis is a method of combining results from a number of independent studies to give one overall estimate of effect. More simply put, it can be thought of as an overview of the available evidence. Meta-analysis reduces lots of data down to a manageable chunk, while reducing time and costs by hopefully preventing the need for a new study. It also reduces the effect of any errors in one particular study and allows greater power to detect effects of interest. One disadvantage is that the results may contain some inherent bias.

Evidenced-based medicine (EBM) emerged as a phenomenon in the 1990s and was a response to 'anecdote-based medicine' mixed with personal opinions. By using systematic reviews available on databases produced by the Cochrane Collaboration, EBM categorizes different types of clinical evidence and ranks them according to the strength of their freedom from the various biases that are commonly found in medical research.

In the UK, the NHS (www.evidence.nhs.uk) uses a ranking system for evidence labelled A, B, C, and D.

- Level A: consistent randomized control clinical trial, cohort study or none (see note below), clinical decision rule validated in different populations.
- Level B: consistent retrospective cohort, exploratory cohort, ecological study, outcomes research, case-control studies; or extrapolations from level A studies.
- Level C: case-series studies or extrapolations from level B studies.
- Level D: expert opinion without explicit critical appraisal, or based on physiology or bench research or first principles.

The Oxford-based **Centre for Evidence Based Medicine** (www.CEBM.net) similarly uses a ranking system from 1 (best evidence) to 5 (least evidence), which relates to the NHS system as follows.

- Level A: consistent level 1 studies.
- Level B: consistent level 2 *or* 3 studies *or* extrapolations from level 1 studies.
- Level C: level 4 studies *or* extrapolations from level 2 or 3 studies.
- Level D: level 5 evidence *or* troublingly inconsistent *or* inconclusive studies of any level.

29.5 Types of data and their representation

It is important to correctly identify the data type in order to ensure that the correct statistical test is used. There are two basic types of data, but note that different books have used different names for the same two basic types.

Quantitative or numerical data

These can be further subdivided into:
- continuous data: there is no limitation on the value the data can take, such as length in metres
- discrete data: the values can only be whole numbers, such as days of annual leave

All these data are arithmetically related in a conventional manner, for example, a 120 kg individual is three times heavier than a 40 kg person.

Qualitative or categorical data

These types of data can be further subdivided as follows.

- **Nominal data** consist of discrete items which belong to different categories that are otherwise unrelated. A common example would be sex (male or female) or ABO blood type. The data are mutually exclusive and unordered.
- **Ordinal data** are assigned a numbered value to which there is an inherent order but no mathematical relationship. The data are mutually exclusive and ordered. A commonly cited example is visual analogue pain score such as Wong–Baker pain faces. A child is invited to pick a face with corresponding number (0–5) and description that most closely resembles the pain they are experiencing. However, if a novel local anaesthetic agent was tested and found to reduce a child's average pain score from a 4 (hurts a lot) to a 2 (hurts a little), it would be incorrect to conclude that there was an average of 50% reduction in pain in the trial group. The correct inference is that there was an average reduction of two points on the Wong–Baker pain faces scale.
- **Dichotomous data** are in binary format; that is, they can only be one or the other, such 'yes or no' or 'dead or alive'.

Tables

Data can easily be stored, retrieved and manipulated statistically when in a tabulated format. Usually this will be as some kind of spreadsheet or database program and from this raw state, further kinds of representation can be made.

Graphics

A graphic is a visual representation of numerical data. An example is a graph such as a histogram or scattergram, which shows the relationship between two sets of data. Other examples of graphics include a pie chart, which is an intuitive representation of relative proportions or a bar chart. *Figure 29.2* shows some examples of graphical representations of data.

Graphical representation provides an opportunity to present a large amount of statistical data in a simple way. A commonly used device is the **box and whisker plot**, shown in *Figure 29.3*, which shows the range and median as well as the upper and lower quartiles (the values which 25% of the data are greater than or less than, respectively).

It is often not obvious which style of graph/table to use until the distribution of the raw data is categorized into either a **unimodal, bimodal** or **multimodal** distribution (*Figure 29.4*).

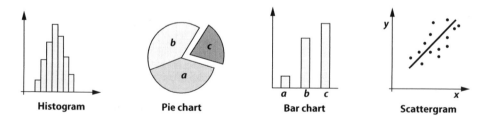

| Histogram | Pie chart | Bar chart | Scattergram |

Figure 29.2. *Various graphical forms of presenting data.*

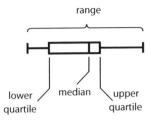

lower
quartile

median

upper
quartile

Figure 29.3. *Box and whisker plot.*

Additionally, the distribution can be symmetrical or be skewed (either positive: right tail, or negative: left tail), as shown in *Figure 29.5*.

29.6 Parametric and non-parametric distributions

When data conform to the standard rules of statistical probability, the distribution is called **parametric**. In the medical world, many distributions will not conform to the standard probability and these are described as **non-parametric** distributions.

Broadly speaking, parametric tests make more assumptions than non-parametric tests. Parametric tests can produce more accurate and precise results if their assumptions hold true for the data. Conversely, parametric methods can be very inaccurate if their underlying assumptions are false.

The normal distribution: a parametric distribution

Most continuous data are represented by a normal or Gaussian distribution producing the familiar 'bell-shaped' curve. This is an example of unimodal distribution. It conforms to the assumptions underlying a distribution based on probability and is therefore an example of a parametric distribution.

Statistically the normal distribution is described by two parameters: the mean (μ) and the variance (σ^2). The variance is a measure of the spread of the data and is used in statistical tests to determine the likelihood of results coming from different populations as well as providing an indication as to the confidence we can have in our results. Variance is more commonly expressed as the standard deviation: the square root of the variance.

The standard deviation is used because it has the advantage of being in the same units as the data. *Figure 29.6* shows a well-known example of normally distributed data, the Wechsler IQ score of a large population of subjects. From this figure we can see that 68% of the data lie within +/− 1 standard deviation of the mean, 95% within +/− 2 standard deviations and 99.7% within +/− 3 standard deviations. It is easy to deduce that the larger the figure for the standard deviation, the

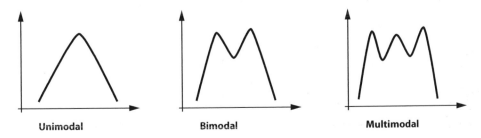

Figure 29.4. *Unimodal, bimodal and multimodal distributions.*

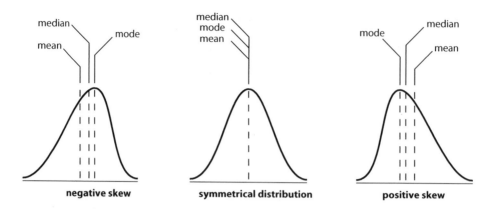

Figure 29.5. *Distribution of data, including positively and negatively skewed data.*

greater the spread of the data. A number that is frequently encountered is a standard deviation multiplied by ± 1.96 because this represents the range that will contain 95% of our data; data from outside this range have a less than 5% chance ($p < 0.05$) of having come from our intended sample population.

Non-normally distributed data

So far we have discussed normally distributed or parametric data. However, quite often in medical research we come across data that are not normally distributed so our statistical tests mentioned so far could not be applied. The first challenge is to spot that you are dealing with non-normal data. Clues can be obtained by simply looking at the data and seeing a non-bell-shaped distribution curve. Another trick is to calculate the standard deviation and then see if data 2 standard deviations either side of your mean (which should contain 95.4%) of your values, actually contain feasible measurements. Formal tests include the Kolmogorov–Smirnov 'goodness-of-fit' test.

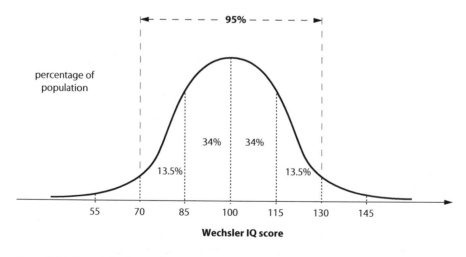

Figure 29.6. *Normal distribution of IQ scores.*

Table 29.1. *Parametric tests and their non-parametric equivalents.*

Parametric test	Non-parametric equivalent
Two sample *t*-test	Mann–Whitney *U* test
Paired *t*-test	Wilcoxon rank-sum test
ANOVA	Kruskal–Wallis test
Pearson's correlation coefficient	Spearman's rank correlation coefficient

When faced with a non-normal distribution, it is possible to attempt to transform the data into a normal distribution. Whilst this sounds like a bit of a mathematical fudge, it is in fact entirely valid. Mathematical transformation may be achievable by taking the square root, taking reciprocals or producing logarithmic versions of the data. If these data then fit, a parametric test can be used.

When stuck with non-parametric data there are, fortunately, a variety of tests available. Although non-parametric tests are not considered to have as good 'statistical power' as parametric tests, they are still valid. Parametric tests and their non-parametric equivalents are summarized in *Table 29.1*.

29.7 Indices of central tendency and variability

Probability theory and confidence intervals

When conducting a study, the aim is to draw conclusions about the characteristics of the general population from your sample study population. Any difference that does occur may be due to one or more of the following factors:

- chance sampling variation
- bias(es) in the study
- confounding factors
- true difference

The effect of the first three factors must be assessed before concluding that any difference is a true one.

Hypothesis tests and **p** *values*

When conducting a study, data from two groups are often compared. Any difference between these groups of data may be due to chance variability. In order to check if the populations are truly different, a hypothesis (significance) test can be performed.

> **Definition**
>
> **Null hypothesis:** this states that there is no difference between the two groups in the study.

The first step is to state the null hypothesis. This essentially states that the two sample groups are in fact from the same population and so the intervention will have no effect. In formulating the null hypothesis it is usually paired with an alternative hypothesis that will be accepted if the null hypothesis is shown to be false.

A useful non-medical demonstration of null hypothesis testing is in the application of the 'innocent until proven guilty' model of criminal justice. If a man is tried for a crime our default position (null hypothesis) is that he is innocent. We test the null hypothesis by hearing the evidence (experimentation) and based on what we hear, either accept the null hypothesis (innocence) or reject it in favour of the alternative hypothesis (guilt).

Table 29.2. *Type I and II errors in the 'innocent until proven guilty' model of criminal justice.*

	Null hypothesis is true: accused did not commit the crime	Null hypothesis is false: accused committed the crime
Accept null hypothesis: not guilty	Right decision	Wrong decision: type II error
Reject null hypothesis: guilty	Wrong decision: type I error	Right decision

Type I and type II errors

In a courtroom drama a type I error is produced when the null hypothesis is *incorrectly* rejected and the alternative hypothesis is accepted, i.e. the innocent man is found guilty. This has obvious and disastrous ramifications; the accused goes to prison for a crime he did not commit. The aim is to make the chance of a type I error occurring as small as possible; in law this is termed 'proof beyond reasonable doubt' but in science this can be quantified as 'the degree of confidence'. A confidence level is normally set at 5% or $p < 0.05$; in other words, there is a less than 5% possibility that this result could have occurred by chance alone. A type I error represents a 'false positive' result.

A type II error is produced when there is a failure to reject the null hypothesis but in fact it should have been rejected. In the legal example this would equate to failing to find the accused guilty of a crime he actually committed. By keeping the chance of a type I error small this necessarily makes the probability of a type II error quite large. In effect, letting guilty men go free is more palatable than incarcerating the innocent. A type II error represents a 'false negative' result (see *Table 29.2*).

Type I and II errors are covered in greater depth in the context of power calculations later in this chapter.

Confidence intervals

> **Definition**
>
> **Confidence interval:** a range of values so defined that there is a specified probability that the value of the parameter lies within it.

Ideally a hypothesis would be tested against the total relevant population, but this is usually impractical. Instead a sample of manageable size is chosen from the relevant population on which to test the hypothesis. What guarantee is there that the results obtained from our experiment are representative of the true mean of our population? The confidence interval calculation uses standard deviation (spread) of the sample and the sample size to calculate the probability that our obtained mean is representative of the total population. A 95% confidence interval tells you that there is a 95% chance that the true value lies within the stated limits (or a 5% chance of lying outside these limits).

Sensitivity and specificity of a test

A perfect test would have a sensitivity of 100% and specificity of 100%. However, in practice there is usually a trade off between the two and increasing the sensitivity is often only possible at the expense of a reduction in specificity. A good example of a highly sensitive but extremely non-specific test is D-dimer measurement to detect a thromboembolic event.

- A D-dimer test is extremely sensitive, i.e. a negative result virtually excludes a thromboembolic event.
- A positive D-dimer is caused by such a multitude of physiological circumstances that it is impossible to attribute a positive result with any certainty to a thromboembolic event, i.e. it is very non-specific.

Power calculations

As discussed earlier, a type I error (also called α) is the probability that a difference has been detected where in fact none exists.

- This equates to a false positive result and in natural sciences is usually quoted for the figure of 0.05. A type II error (or β) is the probability of failing to detect a difference when in fact one does exist: a false negative.
- β is usually set at 0.2 and the power of a study is defined as (1- β) that in this case would be 0.8. As demonstrated by *Figure 29.7*, the levels at which type I and type II errors are set in finite samples are related; decreasing the probability of one occurring increases the probability of the other, and vice versa. The only way to decrease the probability of both is to increase the sample size, which may not be practical. As such, this leaves us having to accept a trade-off, which in medical research is usually set as a 4 to 1 weighting in favour of making a type II error (0.2) versus a type I error (0.05).

The ethics of clinical trials is an immensely complex subject and certainly beyond the scope of this book. A core principle, however, is that any experimentation done on humans or animals must be for genuinely useful research and, as such, any study must be optimally designed to detect a difference and correctly reject the null hypothesis if this is the case. It is possible to precisely calculate the power of a study retrospectively. So when appraising a piece of research, if the null hypothesis is accepted but the study is found to be underpowered, it cannot be concluded with any degree of certainty that a difference does not in fact exist.

Essentially, a power calculation gives the sample size required to detect the minimum difference that it is deemed to be clinically significant. After all, there would no point in detecting a clinically insignificant difference, whatever the level of statistical significance. In order to perform a power calculation you need to know:

- the difference to be detected
- the desired α and β values – these will depend on the type and aims of the study

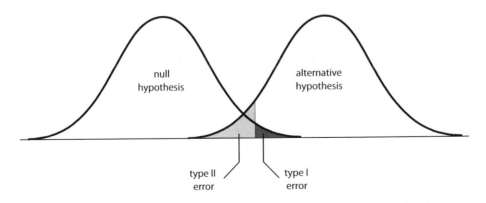

Figure 29.7. *Type I and type II error levels.*

- an estimate of the standard deviation of the samples (this estimate is derived from the literature, pilot studies and common sense and is the reason why it is only possible to retrospectively perform a precise power calculation)

29.8 Common statistical tests

The following examples are illustrations of statistical tests commonly seen in clinical papers. Working through these examples will aid understanding of the tests that have been outlined in this chapter.

Worked example

A new asthma inhaler (two-tailed Student's t-test)
Take the example of testing a new asthma inhaler. The formulation is designed to improve the patient's peak flow. The trial design is very simple: the sample population is 200 patients with asthma currently on standard treatment. The groups (two groups of 100 patients each) are matched as far as possible and then randomized so as to receive either our drug (the **trial group**) or placebo (the **control group**). The peak expiratory flow rate is measured before and after a treatment period of 2 weeks. The primary end point is defined as an improvement in peak expiratory flow after 2 weeks (*Figure 29.8*).

Scenario I
The treatment is a roaring success.
- Trial group – mean improvement in PEFR = 100 (SD 20).
- Control group – mean improvement in PEFR = 2 (SD 20).

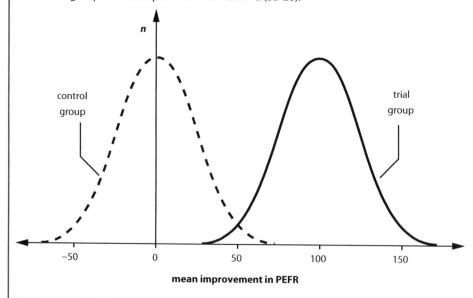

Figure 29.8. *The trial was a success: there was a significant difference between the two groups.*

Observation alone allows you to conclude that these mean values are taken from two very different groups; clearly we must reject the null hypothesis that our new treatment has no effect on the peak flow rate in asthmatic patients and accept the alternative. However, there is a need to apply a statistical test even though it might be obvious what the result will be. In this case, the correct test would be a **two-tailed Student's *t*-test** because our data are **normally distributed**. This unsurprisingly delivers a result of $p < 0.0001$ which is extremely statistically significant.

Scenario II
Let's say that the treatment is not such a roaring success (*Figure 29.9*) and the results obtained are:
- Trial group – mean improvement 10 (SD 20).
- Control group – mean improvement 5 (SD 30 – slightly greater spread of results than the trial group).

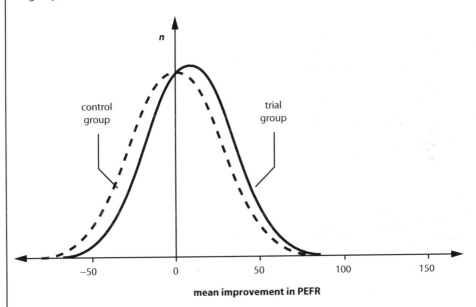

Figure 29.9. *The trial did not show a significant difference between the two groups.*

Now it can be seen that there is a much smaller difference between the groups and a greater spread of data in the control group. The *p* value is 0.16, meaning that there is almost a one in five chance that this result could occur by chance alone; a far less convincing result for a new inhaler.

Statistical significance and clinical significance
This example also raises the important distinction between **statistical significance** and **clinical significance**. If we use the same increase in mean value (five points of PEFR) in the second part of the example, but radically increase the number of trial participants to 2000 in total, then the *t*-test gives us a highly significant result of $p > 0.001$.

Why is this? By increasing our sample size by a factor of ten the sensitivity is increased to detect even small differences between populations. However, just because statistical significance has been achieved and the new treatment is demonstrated to make a difference to patients' peak flows, it doesn't mean that the difference is large enough to warrant manufacture and sale.

An extra five points on a PEFR probably does not relate to any significant improvement in symptom control for these patients. When this is considered in the context of side-effects, hassle of taking another drug and idiosyncratic reactions, an improvement of 5 peak flow points is probably not sufficiently *clinically significant* to warrant mass production.

Worked example

Shark repellent (Chi-squared test)

For this experiment we have invented a shark repellent spray that we feel reduces the chance of a swimmer being attacked in the sea. Our problem is that the incidence of shark attack on humans is exceptionally low (about 1 in 1.3 billion) so we will have to use an animal model to detect a difference. For this we visit Seal Island which has a population of 20 000 seals, many of which are regularly eaten by sharks. We diligently set about randomizing our seals into two groups, treatment and placebo, and then spraying them accordingly.

Scenario I (large population)

Having allowed for confounding factors (like marking and identifying 20 000 seals) we then set about observing what happens for the duration of the experiment. The seals have only two outcomes: 'attacked' or 'not attacked'. After the period of the experiment is over we construct a contingency table to analyse our results.

$n = 20\,000$	Attacked	Not attacked
Placebo	680	9320
Test spray	600	9400

The most well-known statistical method for testing categorical variables is probably the **chi-squared test**.

Plugging these data into the chi-squared formula gives us a *p* value of 0.02, so we can conclude that it is highly likely that our result did not occur by chance and our shark repellent spray makes a real difference. In this example, we have used extremely large numbers (20 000) to tease out a relatively small effect (7.3% vs. 6.4% of seals being eaten). In cases where the incidence of an event occurring is relatively low, large numbers are required to detect a small effect.

Scenario II (small population)

The test has smaller numbers, with just 100 seals. A contingency table can be constructed as follows:

$n = 100$	Attacked	Not attacked
Placebo	4	46
Test spray	2	48

Re-doing our chi-squared calculation gives a *p* value of 0.4 – not statistically significant in spite of a larger percentage difference (8% vs. 4% of seals being eaten). This helps demonstrate the importance of sample size in powering studies.

Worked example

Ear length, height and age (Pearson's correlation coefficient)

In 1996 the BMJ published a study where Japanese investigators measured 400 patients' ear length, height and age. They first corrected ear length for height (as initial correlation analysis showed that ear length positively correlated with height) and then plotted these values against each patient's age to obtain the following scatter plot (*Figure 29.10*).

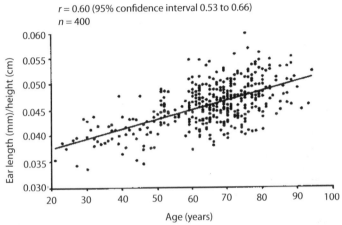

Figure 29.10. *Graph of ear length against age (reproduced from: Asai, et al., Br. Med. J. 1996; 312: 582).*

As the line of best-fit shows, there is clearly a positive correlation that is quantified by **Pearson's r statistic**, given here as 0.6. Interpreting Pearson's *r* statistic is traditionally:

  $r = 0$–0.2 very low and probably meaningless
  $r = 0.2$–0.4 a low correlation that might warrant further investigation
  $r = 0.4$–0.6 a reasonable correlation
  $r = 0.6$–0.8 a high correlation
  $r = 0.8$–1.0 a very high correlation

Whilst correlation tells us about the strength of association between the variables (ear length increasing with age in the above example), it is worth noting that it does not give any clue as to the aetiology of the relationship.

Worked example

Size Zero trial (power calculation)

In the sample calculation a new medication called Size Zero is being trialled. The clinical application of Size Zero is as a 'miracle' weight loss drug that increases the speed at which patients lose weight. It is known that, on average, it takes patients on the current weight loss programme 100 days to reduce their BMI by 5 points. It is decided that for Size Zero to be a useful medication, it must decrease the time for patients to drop their BMI by 5 points to 90 days or less.

Sample size calculation
   Mean of placebo group = 100 days *from previously collected data*
   Minimal clinically significant mean of test group = 90 days

Standard deviation of both groups = 20 *from previously collected data*

$\alpha = 0.05$

$\beta = 0.2$

In order to achieve the desired power a minimum total of 98 participants (49 in each arm of the study) will be needed. Once again, to demonstrate the effect of sample size we perform the same power calculation, but this time we decide we are happy to detect a clinical effect of only two days, so our minimum clinically significant mean in the test group becomes 98 days. Now, in order to be assured of not committing a type II error, our sample size must be 2474. This is why studies that are attempting to tease out minor changes or are investigating conditions or outcomes with a small incidence need massive numbers!

Worked example

NG tubes and delirium (sensitivity and specificity)

There is an evaluation of the presence of delirium in an ITU patient at night handover as a predictor for them pulling out their nasogastric tube. There are 100 patients in the test.

n=100	Pulled NGT out	Did not pull NGT out
Delirious at handover	30 (true positive)	20 (false positive)
Not delirious at handover	5 (false negative)	45 (true negative)

The sensitivity of the test = true positives/(true positives + false negatives)
= 0.86

The specificity of the test = true negatives/(true negatives + false positives)
= 0.69

From this it can be deduced that the criteria are quite sensitive (orientated patients rarely pull out their NGTs), but only moderately specific (just because the patients are delirious doesn't necessarily mean they are going to pull their NGT – they may sleep all night).

We can also calculate the positive predictive value (PPV) and negative predictive value (NPV) of our test.

PPV = if you are delirious, what chance is there you will pull out your NGT?
= true positive/ (true positive + false positive)
= 60%

NPV = if you are not delirious, what is the chance you will leave your NGT in?
= true negative / (true negative + false negative)
= 90%

It can be concluded that it is unlikely that staff will be spending the night replacing the nasogastric tubes of patients still in command of their faculties. However, the patients whose NGTs are replaced are more than likely going to need a dose or two of Haloperidol to guarantee a happy, smiling ITU nurse by 8 am the following morning.

Answers to self-assessment questions

Chapter 1

Single best answer questions
1. a
2. b
3. c
4. d
5. c

Multiple choice questions
1. c and e
2. d and e
3. a, c, d and e
4. b, c and e
5. b and c

Chapter 2

Single best answer questions
1. d
2. b
3. c
4. c
5. b
6. c
7. c
8. a

Multiple choice questions
1. d and e
2. b and d
3. a and e
4. c and e
5. a, c and e
6. e only

Chapter 3

Single best answer questions
1. c
2. d
3. e

Multiple choice questions
1. a, c and d
2. a, b and e
3. b and d

Chapter 4

Single best answer questions
1. c
2. c
3. d
4. d
5. b

Multiple choice questions
1. a, c and d
2. a and d
3. b and e
4. a and c
5. c only

Chapter 5

Single best answer questions
1. a
2. b
3. c
4. b
5. a

Multiple choice questions
1. a and d
2. a and c
3. a and e
4. b and c
5. a, c and d

Chapter 6

Single best answer questions
1. b
2. c
3. e
4. b

Multiple choice questions
1. a and c
2. a and b
3. a, c and d
4. c and d

Chapter 7

Single best answer questions
1. c
2. d

Multiple choice questions
1. b and c
2. e only
3. b and c
4. b and d
5. a, c and e

Chapter 8

Single best answer questions
1. d
2. a
3. b

Multiple choice questions
1. d and e
2. b and e
3. b, c and d

Chapter 9

Single best answer question
1. b

Multiple choice questions
1. b only
2. c only
3. a only
4. d only

Chapter 10

Single best answer questions
1. d
2. c
3. a
4. c
5. b

Multiple choice questions
1. a and c
2. a and d
3. b and d
4. a and c
5. a, b and c

Chapter 11

Single best answer questions
1. d
2. e

Multiple choice questions
1. a and b
2. a, d and e

Chapter 12

Single best answer questions
1. b
2. d
3. d

Multiple choice questions
1. a and c
2. c and d
3. a, c, d and e

Chapter 13

Single best answer questions
1. d
2. e
3. b

Multiple choice questions
1. c only
2. a, b and c
3. b, c and e
4. b, c and d

Chapter 14

Single best answer questions
1. b
2. a
3. e

Multiple choice questions
1. d and e
2. a and d
3. a, b, c, d and e
4. b and e
5. a, b, c and e

Chapter 15

Single best answer questions
1. d
2. b

Multiple choice questions
1. b and e
2. a, c and e

Chapter 16

Single best answer questions
1. c
2. d
3. c

Multiple choice questions
1. a and c
2. b and e
3. c and e

Chapter 17

Single best answer questions
1. d
2. a

Multiple choice questions
1. b and e
2. a, b and d

Chapter 18

Single best answer questions
1. d
2. e
3. d

Multiple choice questions
1. c and e
2. a, b and d
3. a and e

Chapter 19

Single best answer questions
1. e
2. c
3. a

Multiple choice questions
1. b, c and d
2. a and c
3. c and d

Chapter 20

Single best answer questions
1. d
2. c
3. b

Multiple choice questions
1. d and e
2. c and e
3. a and d

Chapter 21

Single best answer questions
1. b
2. c
3. e

Multiple choice questions
1. c, d and e
2. a, b, c and e
3. b only

Chapter 22

Single best answer questions
1. e
2. b
3. e

Multiple choice questions
1. c, d and e
2. a, d and e
3. c and e

Chapter 23

Single best answer questions
1. b
2. d
3. c

Multiple choice questions
1. a and c
2. b and e
3. a, b and e

Chapter 24

Single best answer questions
1. a
2. d
3. c
4. b
5. e

Multiple choice questions
1. c and d
2. c and d
3. d and e
4. d and e
5. a and e

Chapter 25

Single best answer questions
1. c
2. c
3. c

Multiple choice questions
1. b, d and e
2. c and e
3. a, d and e

Chapter 26

Single best answer questions
1. b
2. d
3. e
4. c

Multiple choice questions
1. b, c, d and e
2. b, d and e
3. a and b
4. b, c and e
5. b, c and d

Chapter 27

Multiple choice questions
1. b, c and d
2. b and c
3. a and b
4. a, c and d
5. c and d

Chapter 28

Multiple choice questions
1. a, c and e
2. b and d
3. a, b, c and d
4. b and d
5. a, c, d and e

Index

pulmonary (*continued*)
   fibrosis, 25
   surfactant, 15–17
   valve, 287
pulse oximeter, 194
pulsed laser, 294
pump, 22
Pythagoras' theorem, 322

quenching, MRI, 303

radians, 325
radiant flux, 58
radiation of heat, 34–36
radio waves, 50
radiopharmaceutical, 312
Raman spectroscopy, 148
random errors, 338
randomized controlled trials (RCTs), 340
Raoult's law, 135
rayl (unit), 284
RCD, 246
rechargeable battery, 143
Recklinghausen, 75
recurring numbers, 318
red blood cell
   osmosis, 130
reflective blanket, 37
refraction, 187
refractive index, 187
Regnault's hygrometer, 84
residual current device (RCD), 246
resistance, electrical, 219
resistors
   in parallel, 226
   in series, 225
resolution
   axial, 285
   depth, 285
   of displays, 275
   far-field, 286
   lateral, 285
   near-field, 286
   temporal, 285
resonance, 54
resonant frequency, 54
respiratory physiology, notation, 335–336
return plate, diathermy, 250
Reynolds number, 96–97, 104
rise time, 141
root mean square (voltage), 234
rotameter, 102
rotating-vane respiratory flowmeter, 103–104
rubber (absorbing volatiles), 128
Rutherford's model of the atom, 1

safety critical systems, 212
Sanz electrode, 145
saturated vapour pressure, 81, 113, 150

scalar, 9
scattergram, 342
scavenging, 179
Schimmelbusch mask, 150
Schrader socket, 159, 164, 166
scientific notation, 318
scintigraphy, 312
scuba diving tanks, 119
security of data, 211
Seebeck effect, 40
semi-permeable membrane, 125, 131, 135
semiconductor, 222
sensitivity drift, 214
sensitivity, statistics, 346–347, 352
Severinghaus electrode, 145
sevoflurane, 134, 154, 173
servicing of equipment, 210
shivering, 31
shock, micro-, 246
SI units, 332–334
side-stream, 138
signal
   artifact, 272
   conditioning, 271
   to noise ratio, 272
significant figures, 317
simple harmonic motion, 53–54
sine wave, 53, 56
single photon emission computed tomography
   (SPECT), 312–313
sinusoidal, 53
siphon effect, 71–72
Snell's law, 186
soda lime, 151, 171–173
soft limits, 213
software, 275
solenoid, 231
solubility, 125, 131
solute, 125, 131, 135
solvent, 125, 131
Spaulding classifications, 214–215
SPECT, 312–313
specific heat capacity, 4–5, 30–31
specificity, statistics, 346–347, 352
speed, 9
sphygmomanometer, 74
spirometry, 106
spirometer, Benedict-Roth, 106–107
splitting ration, 151
spontaneous breaths, 182
spring constant, 11–12, 54
standard temperature and pressure (STP), 109
Stefan constant, 34
Stefan–Boltzmann law, 34
standardized
   equipment, 210
   mortality ratio (SMR), 340
static electricity, 248
sterilization of equipment, 216